The prevention of mental illness in primary care

The prevention of mental illness in primary care

Edited by Tony Kendrick, André Tylee and Paul Freeling

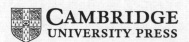

CAMBRIDGE
UNIVERSITY PRESS

Published by the Press Syndicate of the University of Cambridge
The Pitt Building, Trumpington Street, Cambridge CB2 1RP
40 West 20th Street, New York, NY 10011–4211, USA
10 Stamford Road, Oakleigh, Melbourne 3166, Australia

© Cambridge University Press 1996

First published 1996

Printed in Great Britain at the University Press, Cambridge

A catalogue record for this book is available from the British Library

Library of Congress cataloguing in publication data

The prevention of mental illness in primary care / edited by Tony
    Kendrick, André Tylee, and Paul Freeling.
        p.   cm.
    Includes index.
    ISBN 0 521 47057 9 (hc)
    1. mental illness – Prevention.   2. Mental illness – Diagnosis.
3. Primary care (Medicine)   I. Kendrick, Tony.   II. Tylee, André.
III. Freeling, Paul.
    [DNLM: 1. Mental Disorders – prevention & control.   2. Mental
Disorders – diagnosis.   3. Primary Health Care.   4. Primary
Prevention.   WM 140 P9446 1996]
    RC454.4P69 1996
    616.89 – dc20   95-38679 CIP
    DNLM/DLC
    for Library of Congress

ISBN 0 521 47057 9 hardback
ISBN 0 521 57648 2 paperback

To our wives,
Sharon, Sue and Shirley,
with love and thanks for all your support
during the preparation of this book

Contents

Foreword

David Goldberg, Director of R&D, Institute of Psychiatry, London

Primary care, once seen as a venue where established cases of illness received treatment, is now being seen as a setting where health-promoting advice can be made available so that illnesses can be prevented, and where illnesses may be caught in an early stage and prevented from developing into those disorders familiar to psychiatrists. These two activities – primary and secondary prevention – are an additional function for primary care, and the potential for each has barely been explored.

Primary prevention is, of course, the business of many others besides the primary care team: teachers, politicians, community leaders, members of housing departments and housing associations, as well as many engaged in voluntary organisations; all have important parts to play in the prevention of ill-health. The extent of harm done to children who have suffered physical and sexual abuse in children has only really been appreciated in the past 10 years or so, with fairly convincing accounts of the frequency of such occurrences in the early life of those who later develop anxiety or depression. However, apart from activities of social workers in carrying out work with abused children, society has still not thought through the problems involved in preventing these abuses.

The possibilities of systematic education being given to schoolchildren in child-rearing and parenthood have not really been explored in this country. Similarly, little systematic information is made available to the general public on the harm done to children by divorce. Relatively little has been done in primary care with this sort of health-promoting information, and the authors of this book have therefore confined themselves to high-risk groups.

Tirril Harris gives a comprehensive account of research done by George Brown's group over the past 20 years which will be unfamiliar to general practitioners and other members of the primary care team, and which focuses on problems of prevention. She herself has carried out innovative and well-researched work on the contribution to be made by befrienders in preventing repeated episodes of depression. Deborah Sharp gives a thoughtful account of the research done on mothers with puerperal depression, once more with special emphasis on the preventive work which can be done both by the general practitioner and by specalised nurses and health visitors in preventing this disorder. Colin Murray Parkes has written a jewel of a chapter, condensing a life-time's experience of bereavement into a format most useful to the working general practitioner.

Where secondary prevention is concerned, primary care offers many exciting possibilities for intervention. Information about safe limits of alcohol intake have allowed many people to control their drinking, by giving them some standard by which to judge their present behaviour. Many illnesses can be caught in an early stage, and the descent into chronic invalidism prevented. Chronic fatigue states and chronic somatisation are both good examples of this. Simon Wessely has shown that people with chronic fatigue states seen in primary care are more responsive to interventions than are people who are referred to psychiatrists, typically after months or years of symptom experience. The teaching package for primary care physicians on the management of somatised forms of psychological distress produced by Linda Gask and myself is also predicated on the notion that, if these disorders are properly managed in their early stages, many cases of chronic somatisation can be prevented. Similar arguments apply to the early stages of eating disorders, described in this volume by Frances Raphael.

André Tylee provides a useful account of research into the prevention of depression, which is especially useful since general practitionerss are likely to see the majority of such cases. Tom Burns contributes an ingenious chapter on the management of psychotic patients who are seen in primary care but who refuse to see a psychiatrist.

The last section of the book deals with relapse prevention and dealing with disability: both aspects of tertiary prevention. Here, there are also exciting developments to keep abreast of. Eugene Paykel summarises what is known about the longer-term drug management of depression, while Jan Scott describes recent progress in cognitive behaviour therapy. Two later chapters deal with the shared care of psychotic patients between mental health teams and primary care.

This is an exciting and comprehensive book, which starts with an admirable general overview by the editors of prevention from the primary care perspective.

Preface

It is now recognised that between 25% and 30% of patients presenting in primary care are suffering from psychological problems, which while they are not severe enough to require specialist referral, nevertheless make considerable demands on the primary health care team. In addition, the recent shift to care in the community for sufferers of severe long-term mental illness has added to the tasks of the primary care system.

These tasks include:

Primary prevention: the identification and modification of known risk factors for the development of illness.

Secondary prevention: the early identification of problems, and interventions to prevent their progression.

Tertiary prevention: preventing the development of complications for patients with established conditions, and of recurrence in patients with relapsing conditions.

The prevention of mental illness in primary care is therefore an important topic which has not been well addressed in the past.

This book is intended as a handbook for general practitioners, other members of the primary health care team, mental health professionals working in primary care, and academics and educationalists.

The contributors have reviewed the current state of research in the prevention of mental illness and emphasised what practical measures primary health care teams, and mental health professionals working in primary care, can take to practise prevention.

Editors:

Dr Tony Kendrick BSc MRCGP
General Practitioner and Senior Lecturer in General Practice and Primary Care, St George's Hospital Medical School

Dr André Tylee MD FRCGP
General Practitioner, Senior Lecturer in General Practice and Primary Care, St George's Hospital Medical School, and Senior Mental Health Education Fellow, Royal College of General Practitioners

Professor Paul Freeling OBE FRCGP
Emeritus Professor of General Practice, St George's Hospital Medical School

Acknowledgement
Many thanks to Jill Rolfe for all her help in preparing the manuscript.

Contributors

Tom Burns *MD FRCPsych*
Professor of Community Psychiatry, St George's Hospital
Medical School, Cranmer Terrace, London SW17 0RE, UK

Roslyn Corney *MSc PhD*
Professor of Psychology, University of Greenwich, Southwood
Site, Avery Hill Road, Eltham, London SE9 2HB, UK

Jenny Curran *MRCPsych*
Lecturer, Division of Psychiatry of Disability, St George's
Hospital Medical School, Cranmer Terrace, London SW17 0RE, UK

Paul Freeling *OBE*
Emeritus Professor in General Practice, St George's Hospital
Medical School, 59 Spencer Park, Wandsworth, London SW18 2SX

Hamid Ghodse *MD PhD DPM FRCP FRCPsych*
Professor of Psychiatry of Addictive Behaviour, St George's
Hospital Medical School, Cranmer Terrace, London SW17 0RE, UK

Tirril Harris *MA*
Research Scientist, Department of Social Policy & Social Science,
Royal Holloway & Bedford New College, 11 Bedford Square,
London WC1B 3RA, UK

Peter Hill *MD FRCPsych*
Professor of Child & Adolescent Psychiatry, St George's Hospital
Medical School, Cranmer Terrace, London SW17 0RE, UK

Sheila Hollins *MRCPsych*
Professor of Psychiatry of Disability, St George's Hospital Medical
School, Cranmer Terrace, London SW17 0RE, UK

Tony Kendrick *BSc MRCGP*
Senior Lecturer in General Practice and Primary Care, Division of
General Practice, St George's Hospital Medical School, Cranmer
Terrace, London SW17 0RE, UK

Helen Kennerley *PhD*
Clinical Psychologist, Warneford Hospital, Headington,
Oxford OX3 7JX, UK

Elizabeth Kuipers *BSc MSc PhD FBPsS*
Reader in Clinical Psychology, Institute of Psychiatry, De
Crespigny Park, London SE5 8AF, UK

Colin Murray Parkes *MD FRCPsych*
Honorary Consultant Psychiatrist, St Christopher's Hospice,
Sydenham and St Joseph's Hospice, Hackney, London E8 4SA, UK

Sangeeta Patel *MRCGP*
General Practitioner and Lecturer in General Practice, St George's
Hospital Medical School, Cranmer Terrace, London SW17 ORE, UK

Eugene Paykel *MD FRCP FRCPsych*
Professor of Psychiatry, University of Cambridge, Addenbrooke's
Hospital, Cambridge CB2 2QQ, UK

Frances Raphael *MRCPsych*
Lecturer in Mental Health, Department of Mental Health Sciences,
St George's Hospital Medical School, Cranmer Terrace, London
SW17 ORE, UK

Jan Scott *MD MRCPsych*
Professor, University Department of Psychiatry, Royal Victoria
Infirmary, Newcastle upon Tyne NE1 4LP, UK

Philip Seager *MD FRCPsych*
Professor of Psychiatry, 9 Blacka Moor Road, Dore, Sheffield
S17 3GH, UK

Deborah Sharp *MA MRCGP PhD*
Professor of Primary Health Care, Department of Epidemiology
and Public Health Medicine, University of Bristol, Canynge Hall,
Whiteladies Road, Bristol BS8 2PR, UK

Quentin Spender *MRCPsych*
Lecturer in Child Psychiatry, St George's Hospital Medical School,
Cranmer Terrace, London SW17 ORE, UK

Geraldine Strathdee *MRCPsych*
Consultant Psychiatrist in Rehabilitation & Community Care, The
Maudsley Hospital, Denmark Hill, London SE5 8AZ, UK

Jeremy Turk *BSc MRCPsych*
Senior Lecturer, Division of Child & Adolescent Psychiatry, St
George's Hospital Medical School, Cranmer Terrace, London
SW17 ORE, UK

André Tylee *MD, FRCGP*
Senior Lecturer in General Practice and Primary Care, Division of
General Practice, St George's Hospital Medical School, Cranmer
Terrace, London SW17 ORE, UK

Hugh Williams *MRCPsych*
Clinical Lecturer, Division of Psychiatry of Addictive Behaviour,
St George's Hospital Medical School, Cranmer Terrace, London
SW17 ORE, UK

[1] Introduction

Paul Freeling and Tony Kendrick

Background

In a well-developed primary care system such as that in the United Kingdom, health professionals assume long-term continuing responsibility for a registered population of patients, usually of whole families, in community based facilities rather than hospitals, and working in primary health care teams including general medical practitioners, nurses, and other professionals.

Among western industrialised nations those countries with better developed primary care systems in general enjoy lower costs of care, higher patient satisfaction with health services, better health levels, and lower use of medication (Starfield, 1994). These benefits derive partly from the 'gatekeeper' role whereby primary care physicians refer only a proportion of their patients to specialists in the secondary care services, and partly from the long-term continuity of care offered by primary care professionals which encourages the development of therapeutic relationships (Freeling & Harris, 1984). In the UK, Ireland, the Netherlands, Denmark, Portugal, and Canada, patient care is largely supervised by general practitioners, and in the United States the government's policy is to increase the number of generalists as a way of increasing the population's access to medical care (Rivo, Henderson & Jackson, 1995).

Changes in health services in the United Kingdom

Through the second half of the 1980s it became increasingly obvious that a radical revision of the focus and organisation of health services was needed in the UK. The costs of the National Health Service were spiralling upwards. Current practice in health care was not always subjected to rigorous scientific evaluation and often did not utilise current scientific research findings. Since the inception of the NHS, hospitals and other secondary care services had received funds directly from central government and there were few incentives for them to respond to the needs and preferences of their local populations.

These concerns culminated in the NHS reforms which intro-duced the internal market through the purchaser–provider split (Department of Health, 1989). The reforms aimed to introduce more accountability in the provision of secondary care services. Purchasers were expected to shape the provision of health care taking into account the needs of the local population and the available evidence for the effectiveness of services offered by providers. General practice fundholders were given budgets to purchase secondary care services directly for their patients, and other general practitioners participated in the commissioning of services through advising District Health Authority purchasers. This introduced an element of *managed care* with incentives for primary care physicians to purchase the least costly but effective services for their registered population of patients, in a way similar to physicians working in the health maintenance organisations in the US (Sabin, 1994).

As primary care was gaining more influence over the provision of services in the UK, bodies responsible for health policy at all levels were increasingly aware of the need for greater emphasis on the promotion of health, the prevention of illness, and the limi-tation of handicap to parallel the advances continuing to be made in 'high tech' medicine. This led to the Health of the Nation preven-tive initiative (Department of Health, 1992), roughly coinciding with the 'New Contract' for general practitioners which included payments for health promotion (Department of Health, 1990a).

At the same time, long-standing changes in the nature of mental health care provision were also reaching culmination. The number of long-stay beds maintained by the NHS for the care of the long-term mentally ill was being radically reduced with whole institu-tions being closed as patients were resettled in the community (Department of Health, 1990b). This shift to community care was also taking place in other European countries and in the US. In parallel with this shift was what Strathdee and Williams (1984) termed 'the silent growth of a new service' with specialist psy-chiatrists and other members of community mental health teams moving their bases out of hospitals and increasingly spending time working in general practice settings. The New Contract also introduced discretionary reimbursement towards the costs of directly employing practice counsellors and psychologists. In 1992 we surveyed a representative sample of 1542 practices in England and Wales and found the following professionals to be working on site: practice nurses (in 97% of practices), health visitors (in 83%), community psychiatric nurses (34%), counsellors (17%), clinical psychologists (12%), psychiatrists (9%), psychiatric social workers (6%), and psychotherapists (3%) (Kendrick et al., 1993).

Working together to prevent mental illness

The white paper *The Health of the Nation* included three targets for improvements in mental health by the year 2000: to reduce the suicide rate by 15%; to reduce the suicide rate of severely mentally ill people by 33%; and to improve significantly the health and social functioning of mentally ill people (Department of Health, 1992).

The government's main strategy has been to target specialist mental health services at the severely mentally ill, in particular those with psychosis, who have the highest risk of suicide. *The Health of the Nation Mental Illness Key Area Handbook* (Department of Health, 1994) recommended that primary health care teams, whilst helping secondary care teams identify and monitor the long-term and severely mentally ill, should take responsibility themselves for the care of other less severe psychiatric disorders. However, it is the less severe disorders which form the bulk of mental illness and between them constitute a major public health problem, incurring enormous economic costs in terms of time off work, social security payments, consultations and drug costs (Croft-Jeffreys & Wilkinson, 1989), to say nothing of the misery endured by millions of people in the UK at any one time. In recognition of this public health problem, which specialist services could not possibly cope with alone, the government handbook also included a section on *Mental Health Promotion* including educational and preventive strategies to which primary health care teams were asked to contribute.

The result of all these changes therefore has been not only increased implementation of preventive approaches to medical care but also a new insistence on basing such endeavours in the community. General practitioners, like other members of the primary health care team, have become more involved in prevention themselves and have begun to use their new purchasing powers to bring more consultants and other health care professionals into their practices to help them (Kendrick, 1994). Managed care is usually *shared care*, and the US experience suggests that purchasing power can effectively shape the provision of secondary and community mental health care (Schreter, Sharfstein & Schreter, 1994).

Aims of this book

A focus on preventive approaches to health care requires an understanding of psychological and social aspects as well as of biological and technical ones: it requires, of course, familiarity with the preventive perspective. This book aims to foster knowledge and understanding of the preventive perspective and attempts to apply the preventive model to the care of the mentally ill in primary care. Such application will usually require a multidisciplinary approach bringing together health care professionals from a range of backgrounds who have explored together areas of mutual interest, have developed a fuller awareness of each other's existing skills and concerns, and who have the capacity to acquire collectively further appropriate knowledge and skills. The aims therefore are to illustrate the available preventive strategies in mental health and to give specific practical advice which should help primary health care teams either to develop services themselves where appropriate, or to decide what to purchase from secondary care teams, or both. We have asked authors to provide references to the available research evidence to justify the adoption of particular strategies wherever possible. The practical suggestions are highlighted in boxes to make them readily appreciable.

A preventive approach

A preventive approach assumes that each individual has the capacity for a particular, personally optimal, course of development, and that health care is directed to maintaining that course or returning that person to his or her natural trajectory of development. A preventive approach assumes that adverse change in the individual's natural development follows an interaction between that individual (the host), an agent, and the environment. It is this interaction which causes pathogenesis and initiates an adverse alteration to the individual's developmental trajectory. The host can be described in both somatic and psychological terms and the environment in both physical and social ones. The term 'agent' may subsume a number of different factors. Most of the conditions which cause major public health problems today are multifactorial in origin and this seems especially true of those affecting mental health. Once pathogenesis has occurred, there is often a period during which the individual is either asymptomatic or uncomplaining. This is followed by a symptomatic period. The symptomatic period may result in death (a cessation of the developmental

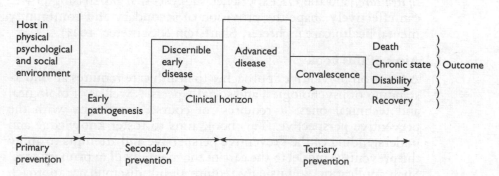

Fig. 1.1 *A model of 'unhealth'.* (Modified from Leavell & Clark, 1965.)

course); complete cure (a return to the individual's normal course of development); or something in between which leaves some degree of impairment, disability, or handicap (a deviation from the individual's original course of development) (see Fig. 1.1).

Primary prevention

Primary prevention interventions aim to prevent pathogenesis and include health education, the promotion of healthy behaviours, and specific protection such as immunisation.

Secondary prevention

Early diagnosis and prompt, appropriate treatment comprise secondary prevention. The hope is to shorten the severity and duration of acute disorder and to limit any subsequent impairment.

Tertiary prevention

Once impairment has occurred, attempts will be made to limit consequent disability (adverse effects on performance) and subsequent handicap (adverse outcome in terms of social role and social function). This is one aspect of tertiary prevention: another is to set out to remove or reduce recurrence or relapse.

A preventive approach requires knowledge of the stages which comprise the developmental trajectory, of the factors which may affect it, of the effects likely to be produced by those factors, and of the nature and outcomes (desired and undesirable) of available interventions. The reader should be able to select any aspect of mental illness and apply to it the preventive approach outlined so far. Doing so may reveal difficulties, strengths and weaknesses. Some of these will stem from the fact that our knowledge of the aetiology, pathogenesis, and natural history of many mental illnesses is far from complete.

Weaknesses

An apparent weakness of the preventive model as applied to mental illness lies in the area of primary prevention because many of the predisposing factors in the physical and social environment such as poor housing or unemployment seem beyond the control of professionals working in primary care. It has been demonstrated that the prevalence in a population of above-threshold scores on the Chronic General Health Questionnaire (CGHQ – a measure of psychological distress (Goodchild & Duncan-Jones, 1985)) is highly correlated with mean CGHQ scores in that population (Anderson, Huppert & Rose, 1993). This implies that the number of psychiatric cases is strongly associated with the general characteristics of the population in which they arise. This finding is not limited to psychological disorders (Rose & Day, 1990). Anderson and colleagues argue that their findings indicate that 'The mental health of society is integral and reflects its social economic and political structure. At this point psychiatric epidemiology and prevention merge into social policy – they cannot exist apart.' Interventions are most likely to be effective if they affect the whole of a population rather than the 'high risk tail' (Anderson, Huppert & Rose, 1993).

Nevertheless, individual doctors still have the responsibility of seeking to help their individual patients, and the preventive model allows us to turn to consideration of what characteristics of the host lead to susceptibility. Many of these in turn may be beyond the control of primary health care teams. The model leaves us then to consider the wisdom of identifying high risk groups on which secondary preventive endeavours can be focused.

Attempts at early identification of deviation from the expected developmental trajectory can be conducted opportunistically, by taking advantage of an individual's self-initiated contacts with primary care: this is *case-finding* or opportunistic screening. Alternatively, primary care can be completely pro-active and call individuals to attend for testing. This is *screening*.

Screening

Screening is 'the presumptive identification of unrecognised disease or defect by the application of tests, examinations, or other procedures which can be applied rapidly' (Commission on Chronic Illness, 1957). Screening tests attempt to distinguish in a population between a group of people who probably have a condition and the remainder who probably do not. Screening needs to be followed by an attempt to confirm the positive probability, i.e. to make a diagnosis. In the case of mental health, the screening instrument will nearly always be a questionnaire. There are a number of well-validated questionnaires in use, often self-complete in form, and widely employed for the purposes of research. Diagnostic instruments may be a 'free-form' clinical interview or a validated questionnaire. To a degree which does not seem common in other specialist disciplines, psychiatric conditions are specified against international criteria. Only when categorical labels mean the same thing to all who use them can workers discuss their subject with meaning. There seems to be considerable evidence that many general practitioners do not share with their psychiatric colleagues a common categorical language. In part this may be the result of different judgements as to 'caseness'.

When is a case?

When preventive activity was focused mainly on acute infectious disease, it was relatively easy to decide when to make a diagnosis. The diagnosis could be considered as having a bimodal distribution in the population with a specific, easily defined cut-off which separated those with the disease from those without it. Today, prevention is concerned also with chronic disease, and most of the parameters measured are distributed continuously or unimodally so that an arbitrary determination of the level to use as a cut-off point is necessary in order to indicate when pathogenesis has taken place, although the condition is presymptomatic and without pathognomonic physical signs. Only in relatively few chronic somatic disorders is there a clearly defined phase when pathogenesis has been initiated but serious disease not yet begun: an example of such a clearly signposted condition is carcinoma of the cervix.

Arbitrary cut-offs

The arbitrary nature of cut-offs in screening for chronic disease affects the effectiveness and efficiency of secondary prevention. The problem is similar to the 'band-width fidelity' dilemma described in testing for competence (Katz & Snow, 1980): to decrease the number of patients with false negative findings, it is necessary to set a cut-off point which includes many false positives who have to undergo the anxiety, discomfort, and cost of an unnecessary diagnostic procedure. This dilemma can lead to doctors and patients both being reluctant to continue their involvement. Where mental illness is concerned, matters may be further complicated by the stigmatising nature of the conditions involved. The nature and magnitude of the problem is such as to make any general practitioner think twice before risking attaching incorrect labels to patients even temporarily.

The matter of caseness does not bear only on the problems of producing false positives. The need to categorise carries with it a need to make sure that the categorisation is valid. Caseness has been defined as the subject displaying 'a collection of symptoms which a psychiatrist would recognise as a characteristic and abnormal mental state for which intervention would be appropriate if it were available' (Copeland, 1990). However, not all patients have neat constellations of symptoms which conform to case definitions, especially if those definitions reflect experience with different populations of patients. General practitioners will often make decisions to treat, which while not supported by descriptions in diagnostic schedules, seem justified by the severity of disturbance of family or function. Nevertheless, general practitioners need to be aware when a particular treatment has been demonstrated to be effective in one category of disorder but not in another (Paykel et al., 1988) rather than being anarchic in their selection of therapy.

An avoidable burden?

Whatever the level of caseness chosen, there is no doubt that psychiatric disorder in the community represents an important burden of ill-health in the population and results in a highly significant consumption of health service resources (Croft-Jeffreys & Wilkinson, 1989). Some of this consumption may be avoidable and much of the burden is reducible. It has been shown that about a third of people consulting their general practitioner with a new inception of illness have some form of psychological disorder (Bridges & Goldberg, 1985) but patients with mental disorders (Group V in the International Classification of Diseases (ICD-9) (World Health Organisation, 1978)) comprised only 6.8% of all patients attending practices in the Third National Morbidity Study in General Practice in 1981–82 (Royal College of General Practitioners, 1986). It has been estimated (Mann, 1992) that the rate of general practitioner consultation in 1981 for ICD-9 Mental Disorders was 22 980/100 000, that outpatient attendance was 2532/100 000, day hospital attendance was 4943/100 000 and psychiatric admissions were 397/100 000. One-fifth of patients prescribed antidepressants by general practitioners had no vestige of depressive illness when subjected to extensive and validated research diagnostic interviews (Sireling et al., 1985) whilst half of those patients with major depressive illness went unacknowledged (Freeling et al., 1985). This is important because it has been demonstrated that a majority of patients with major depression will respond rapidly to inexpensive drug treatment (Paykel et al., 1988). The fate of these unacknowledged depressives is likely to include prolonged emotional ill-health and may contribute to non-psychiatric outpatient referral and its variability.

Three bands

When considering the provision of mental health care in primary care, it can be useful to work to the concept that there are three 'bands' of psychological or psychiatric disorder which can be distinguished within the community as remaining within the care of general practitioners and the primary health care team: ill-defined emotional malaise; defined disorder not requiring psychiatric referral; and the long-term mentally ill. A better understanding of the nature of these three bands and of the boundaries between them will help to improve diagnostic accuracy and treatment. The construct helps emphasise that over and above the problems of diagnosing and managing acute psychological disorder are those of managing in the community patients with long-term mental illness who are entitled not only to receive help in maintaining stability (tertiary preventive care) but, also, of being assured that they are not deprived of the general benefits of primary and preventive care of physical disorder, with consequent later costs to the NHS.

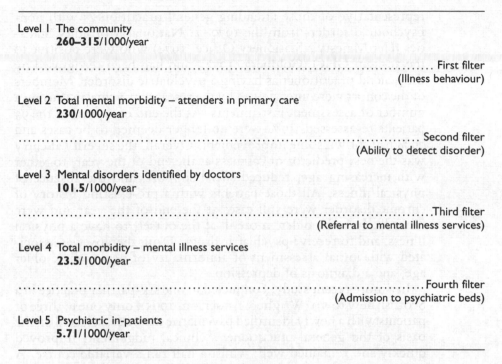

Level 1 The community
260–315/1000/year

.... First filter
(Illness behaviour)

Level 2 Total mental morbidity – attenders in primary care
230/1000/year

.... Second filter
(Ability to detect disorder)

Level 3 Mental disorders identified by doctors
101.5/1000/year

....Third filter
(Referral to mental illness services)

Level 4 Total morbidity – mental illness services
23.5/1000/year

....Fourth filter
(Admission to psychiatric beds)

Level 5 Psychiatric in-patients
5.71/1000/year

Fig. 1.2 *Mental illness: levels and filters.* (After Goldberg & Huxley, 1980.)

Five levels

When considering the contribution of primary care to the provision of mental health overall, a most useful model is that devised by Goldberg and Huxley (1980) which incorporates five levels separated by four filters (Fig. 1.2).

Particular virtues of the model are that it emphasises that individuals in the community exercise a choice between consulting and not consulting a general practitioner, and that general practitioners control the proportion of their work apparently due to psychological disorder by their ability or willingness to detect such conditions.

To further the prevention of mental illness in primary care it is necessary to describe the natural history of psychiatric illness among patients attending general practice with a view to identifying those characteristics associated with poor prognosis and hence the need for medical intervention.

The natural history of psychiatric disorder

Mann and his colleagues (1981) set out to establish the 12-month outcome of patients with neurotic illness in two general practices in Warwickshire. Their cohort of 100 patients was designed to be representative of those attending general practitioners with non-psychotic disorders from the 1970–71 National Morbidity Statistics (Her Majesty's Stationery Office, 1974) who were positive to the 30-item GHQ (Goldberg, 1972), and had been recognised by the general practitioner as having a psychiatric disorder. Members of the cohort were interviewed by the research psychiatrists using a number of assessment instruments. At the end of a year, of the 93 patients re-assessed, 49% were no longer deemed to be cases and 79% had shown some improvement. Overall, the severity at entry was the best predictor of caseness at the end of the year, together with increasing age, reduced social support, and the absence of physical illness. All those patients with a pre-existing history of chronic disorder were still cases at the end of the year and were more likely to be older, more ill at the outset, to have a physical illness, and to receive psychiatric drugs. Drug therapy was associated with initial assessment of abnormality of personality, older age, and a diagnosis of depression.

In a more recent study, conducted in one six-partner practice in a Scottish new town (Wright & Anderson, 1995), only one in three of patients with a newly identified psychiatric disorder, selected on the basis of the general practitioner's clinical judgement, improved quickly and remained well, whilst a half ran a variable course. A strong association was found between high neuroticism (N) scores on the Eysenck personality questionnaire and poor outcome. Within the preventive model this would be described as a characteristic of the host but unfortunately probably not one susceptible to primary prevention.

Probably about half of all psychiatric morbidity seen in general practice is mild and transient. The crucial difficulty for the general practitioner is to distinguish between the mild disorder requiring minimal intervention and potentially severe but early psychiatric disorder that requires professional input and consequent expense. It may be that Mann and his colleagues, and Wright & Anderson have taken a step towards a classification system which is outcome based and which could, therefore, lead to agreed targeting of secondary prevention. Age, personality, past psychiatric history and the presence of physical illness should be taken into account.

The tasks of a general practitioner

There is now a statutory requirement for general practitioners to have undergone vocational training before they can practise in any country in the European Union. Vocational training in the UK has been directed towards a job description widely endorsed in Europe (Leuwenhorst Working Party, 1974). Key tasks in this definition include accepting a responsibility for giving 'care to individuals, irrespective of age, sex and illness'; including and integrating 'physical, psychological, and social factors in his considerations about health and illness' and knowing 'how and when to intervene through treatment, prevention and education'. It has long been clear that, to meet such responsibilities, general practitioners needed to gain high skills in interviewing as well as a comprehensive understanding of normality and the nature of deviations from it.

Behaviour in interviews

The behaviours which seem likely to lead to successful elicitation of the patient's experience and elucidation of the patient's problem, along with the conduct of a discussion leading to a change in the patient's understanding, have been recognised and agreed for some time (Fletcher & Freeling, 1988). These behaviours prove desirable not only for interviews with patients complaining of somatic symptoms but also for those complaining of psychological problems. Many are consonant with the practice of non-directive counselling.

Factors established as associated with accuracy in detecting mental disorder (Goldberg & Huxley, 1980) include behaviours at the outset of the interview such as establishing eye contact, clarifying the present complaint, directing questioning to areas such as the home and family, using open-ended questions initially, allowing the patient to set the agenda, before clarifying particular details with closed questions. Other factors include making frequent empathic responses, being sensitive to both verbal and non-verbal cues, not reading the medical records whilst taking a history, being able to control over-discursiveness, and asking fewer questions about the past history. Despite all these good auguries, however, many general practitioners seem unable to produce these behaviours when confronted with, for instance, depressed patients, whilst others seem to obtain the co-operation of the patient even though not all their evinced behaviours would be found in a list of 'desirable' ones (Goldberg et al., 1993).

The benefits of good interview behaviours extend beyond the making of diagnoses since it has been demonstrated that doctors who are good detectors are also better at giving information and advice: they give more information and specific instructions; they negotiate management with the patient and check the patient's understanding; and they explain both the purposes and possible side-effects of treatment (Millar & Goldberg, 1991).

It appears then, that some doctors compared to others have a reduced ability to involve themselves with psychologically ill patients. This may manifest itself as bias affecting the threshold for case identification (Marks, Goldberg & Hillier, 1979).

Counselling

Bias probably affects general practitioners' willingness to counsel their patients with emotional difficulties. This may be one explanation of the recent but not uniformly distributed increase in the number of counsellors employed in primary care. Unfortunately there has been, as yet, little systematic assessment of the outcomes achieved by these workers. This may be because the experience and training of such counsellors varies enormously and has yet to be extensively described (Sibbald *et al.*, 1993). There has, however, been reported a properly controlled study of the efficacy in primary care patients suffering from major depressive disorder of a relatively brief problem-solving treatment. The treatment was given by a psychiatrist experienced in the field and by two trained general practitioners. Their outcomes were as good as those produced by drug treatment with 150 mg of amitriptyline per day and were twice as effective as placebo tablets (Mynors-Wallis *et al.*, 1995). It may be worth noting that, in this study, about one-third of the patients referred by their general practitioner were excluded, 'mostly because they did not meet the research criteria for major depression'. This is concordant with the finding pointed out above that problems with caseness, in depressive illness at least, are not confined to general practitioners failing to make diagnoses in depression of a severity likely to benefit from treatment but are found also in a tendency to make diagnoses when there is little or no evidence for psychiatric disorder by the yardstick of validated research diagnostic instruments.

Variability among general practitioners

Given the breadth of their responsibilities and the large numbers of doctors involved, it is hardly surprising that general practitioners vary in their ability and willingness to diagnose and manage psychiatric illness. There is currently a widespread endeavour to improve their knowledge, upgrade their skills, and foster appropriate attitudes in the UK, as part of the Royal College of Psychiatrists' and Royal College of General Practitioners' joint 'Defeat Depression Campaign' (Priest, 1991). The Royal College of General Practitioners has appointed André Tylee as Senior Mental Health Education Fellow. He has recruited a network of Regional Mental Health Fellows who, in turn, are providing educational materials and support to Postgraduate Centre General Practitioner Tutors and other key educators at District Health Authority level so that they may offer education to their local practitioners. This 'top–down' approach is being balanced by attempts to identify and take into account the particular personal educational needs of practitioners in a learner-driven approach to continuing medical education.

It is possible, however, that driving for improved accuracy in diagnosis may not be the complete answer and can even afford some disadvantages. A major reason for making a diagnosis is that doing so predicates the appropriate treatment. If the treatment is unrelated to the diagnosis, the working clinician may prefer to apply the treatment and justify it with a diagnosis later (Howie, 1972; Marinker, 1973). If a counselling approach, an empathic carer and social support are all that is necessary for the group of patients who suffer from ill-defined psychological disorder, then this term is in itself sufficient as a diagnosis. To take the diagnosis further may be to medicalise unhappiness or social deprivation (Illich, 1975).

The future shape of mental health services in the UK

Given the multiplicity of changes in the structure and financing of the NHS, and taking into account the shift in the care of the mentally ill to the community, it seems likely that there will need to be changes in the balance between primary care and specialist mental health services if the most effective and efficient care is to be received by our patients with mental health problems. Studies have shown that the impact of holding psychiatric clinics in general practice includes a reduction in the number of admissions to psychiatric hospital (Tyrer, Seivewright & Woolerton, 1984), mainly by achieving a reduction in the number of non-psychotic patients admitted (Williams & Balestrieri, 1989). Moving the bases of community mental health teams into general practices in Manchester was associated with an increase in the specialist team's caseload, both of patients with minor disorders and of the long-term mentally ill. The primary care-based community teams met more of the needs of the practices' long-term mentally ill patients, although at increased cost (Goldberg et al., 1992). However, there is a risk that, rather than strengthening the primary health care team's own management of their patients, community mental health teams might simply replace them and take on an increased caseload inappropriately. Although some general practitioners may welcome a reduction in demands on their time, transferring more patients to long-term supervision by mental health teams may 'de-skill' general practitioners and make them less effective when, inevitably, patients do need to call on them. Warner et al. (1993) found no evidence that the Manchester experiment led to de-skilling in terms of general practitioners' abilities to detect and treat less severe emotional disorders but their study was very short-term and did not examine skills likely to be useful with the long-term mentally ill, such as the assessment of more severe symptoms and the review of long-term drug treatments. The corollary is that the specialist team may find it has less time to offer to the most difficult and disturbed patients who need most help, often at very short notice.

The tasks of primary care

If changes in the balance of care are necessary, they would best be achieved if the tasks of the primary care system within the NHS as a whole are borne in mind. These tasks can be cast within the framework of the preventive model which forms the matrix for this book.

Primary prevention might include offering sympathetic support or systematic counselling to people at increased risk of mental illness such as the unemployed, the bereaved, new mothers, single-parent families, the isolated elderly and the disabled. The decision as to whether to limit the intervention to sympathetic support or to proceed to more formal counselling interventions would no doubt rest upon judgements of the effectiveness of the person's coping strategies and these in turn may be hinted at by the person's help-seeking behaviours. Many general practitioners have some picture of these from previous contacts with their patients. One wonders how many record such knowledge so that changes can be recognised by colleagues.

General practitioners and their primary care colleagues have the opportunity to practise *secondary prevention* in a non-stigmatising environment. Their skills in identification need to be fostered and this is more likely to occur where it is clear that there is also rapid and easy access to specialist support. Such support may permit the use of screening or case-finding for depression, eating disorders, or abuse of a range of substances. An understanding of illness behaviour and the possible meaning of variations in its habitual manifestations will be of great value and this too may develop in the environment of close co-operation and support between primary care and specialist services.

The provision of continuing care and support for those with chronic illness and persisting impairment, disability or handicap is essential if care is to be effective and humane. It seems likely that such *tertiary prevention* will be best achieved through joint management plans formulated between specialist workers and primary health care team members who know and trust each other. Finally, if patients are to benefit fully from their carers applying a preventive approach, then it will be important to provide easy access to those people with conditions known to relapse or recur (also tertiary prevention). These conditions might be arbitrarily subdivided into those in whom a repeat manifestation of illness is a failure to keep up monitoring contacts and those in whom the manifestation is a change in help-seeking behaviour.

The chapters in this book outline current knowledge which needs to be applied to achieve these tasks. The aim is to give specific practical ideas for members of primary health care teams to follow, together with their specialist colleagues where appropriate, in order to improve the mental well-being of our patients.

References

Anderson, J., Huppert, F. & Rose, G. (1993). Normality, deviance and minor psychiatric morbidity in the community: a population-based approach to General Health Questionnaire data in the Health and Lifestyle Survey. *Psychological Medicine*, **23**, 478–85.

Bridges, K. & Goldberg, D. (1985). Somatic presentations of DSM-III psychiatric disorders in primary care. *Journal of Psychosomatic Research*, **29**, 563–9.

Commission on Chronic Illness. (1957). *Chronic Illness in the United States. Volume 1. Prevention of Chronic Illness.* p. 45. Cambridge, Mass: Harvard University Press.

Copeland, J.R.M. (1990). Suitable instruments for detecting dementia in community samples. *Age and Ageing*, **19**, 81–3.

Croft-Jeffreys, C. & Wilkinson, G. (1989). Estimated costs of neurotic disorder in UK general practice 1985. *Psychological Medicine*, **19**, 549–58.

Department of Health. (1989). *Working for Patients*. London: HMSO.

Department of Health. (1990b). *Terms and Conditions of Service for General Medical Practitioners in the National Health Service.* London: HMSO.

Department of Health. (1990b). *Caring for People: Community Care in the Next Decade and Beyond.* London: HMSO.

Department of Health. (1992). *The Health of the Nation: A Strategy for Health in England.* London: HMSO.

Department of Health. (1994). *The Health of the Nation Key Area Handbook: Mental Illness* (2nd edition), London: HMSO.

Fletcher, C. & Freeling, P. (1988). *Talking and Listening to Patients: A Modern Approach.* London: Nuffield Provincial Hospitals Trust.

Freeling, P. & Harris, C. (1984). *The Doctor–Patient Relationship.* (3rd edition). London: Churchill Livingstone.

Freeling, P., Rao, B.M., Paykel, E.S., Sireling, L.I. & Burton, R.H. (1985). Unrecognized depression in general practice. *British Medical Journal*, **290**, 1880–3.

Goldberg, D.P. (1972). *Detecting Psychiatric Illness by Questionnaire. Maudsley Monograph No.21.* London: Oxford University Press.

Goldberg, D. & Huxley, P. (1980). *Mental Illness in the Community: The Pathway to Psychiatric Care.* London and New York: Tavistock Publications.

Goldberg, D. & Jackson, G. (1992). Interface between primary care and specialist mental health care. *British Journal of General Practice*, **42**, 267–8.

Goldberg, D.P., Tantam, D., Gater, R. *et al.* (1992). *The Interface between Primary Care and Specialist Mental Health Services in the Community*. Manchester: Mental Illness Research Unit.

Goldberg, D.P., Jenkins, L., Millar, T. & Faragher, E.B. (1993). The ability of trainee general practitioners to identify distress among their patients. *Psychological Medicine*, **23**, 185–93.

Goodchild, M.E. & Duncan-Jones, P. (1985). Chronicity and the General Health Questionnaire. *British Journal of Psychiatry*, **146**, 56–61.

Her Majesty's Stationery Office. (1974). Morbidity Statistics for General Practice, Second National Study 1970–71. *Studies on Medical Population Subjects No.26*, London: HMSO.

Howie, J.G.R. (1972). Diagnosis – the Achilles heel. *Journal of the Royal College of General Practitioners*, **22**, 310–15.

Illich, I. (1975). *Medical Nemesis. The Expropriation of Health*. London: Calder & Boyars.

Katz, F.M. & Snow R. (1980). Assessing Health Workers' Performance. *A Manual for Training and Supervision*, p.27. Geneva: World Health Organisation.

Kendrick, T., Sibbald, B., Addington-Hall, J., Brenneman, D. & Freeling, P. (1993). Distribution of mental health professionals working on-site within English and Welsh general practices. *British Medical Journal*, **307**, 544–6.

Kendrick, T. (1994). Fundholding and commissioning general practitioners. *Psychiatric Bulletin*, **18**, 196–9.

Leavell, H.R. & Clark E.G. (1965). *Preventive Medicine for the Doctor in his Community*. New York: McGraw-Hill.

Leuwenhorst Working Party. (1974). The General Practitioner in Europe. *Journal of the Royal College of General Practitioners*, **27**, 117.

Mann, A. (1992). Depression and anxiety in primary care: the epidemiological evidence. In *The Prevention of Depression and Anxiety; the Role of the Primary Care Team*. Jenkins, R., Newton, J. and Young, R. eds. pp. 1–10, London: HMSO.

Mann, A.H., Jenkins, R. & Belsey E. (1981). The twelve-month outcome of patients with neurotic illness in general practice. *Psychological Medicine*, **11**, 535–50.

Marinker, M. (1973). The doctor's role in prescribing. In *The Medical Use of Psychotropic Drugs*. suppl. 2, **23**. London: Royal College of General Practitioners.

Marks, J., Goldberg, D.P. & Hillier, V.F. (1979). Determinants of the ability of general practitioners to detect psychiatric illness. *Psychological Medicine*, **9**, 337–53.

Millar, T. & Goldberg, D. (1991). Link between the ability to detect and manage emotional disorders; a study of general practitioner trainees. *British Journal of General Practice*, **41**, 357–9.

Mynors-Wallis, L.M., Gath, D.H., Lloyd-Thomas, A.R. & Tomlinson, D. (1995). Randomised controlled trial comparing problem solving treatment with amitriptyline and placebo for major depression in primary care. *British Medical Journal*, **310**, 441–5.

Nuffield Provincial Hospitals Trust Working Party (1980). *Talking with Patients; A Teaching Approach*. p.40. London: Nuffield Provincial Hospitals Trust.

Paykel, E.S., Hollyman, J.A., Freeling, P. & Sedgwick P. (1988). Predictors of therapeutic benefit from amitriptyline in mild depression: a general practice placebo-controlled trial. *Journal of Affective Disorders*, **14**, 83–95.

Priest, R.G. (1991). A new initiative on depression (editorial). *British Journal of General Practice*, **41**, 487.

Rivo, M.L., Henderson, T.M. & Jackson, D.M. (1995). State legislative strategies to improve the supply and distribution of generalist physicians. *American Journal of Public Health*, **85**, 405–7.

Rose, G. & Day, S. (1990). The population predicts the number of deviant individuals. *British Medical Journal*, **301**, 1031–4.

Royal College of General Practitioners. (1985). *Education and Training for General Practice. Policy statement 3*. London: RCGP.

Royal College of General Practitioners, Office of Population Censuses and Surveys, Department of Health and Social Security (1986). *Morbidity Statistics from General Practice. Third National Study 1981–1982*. London: HMSO.

Sabin, J.E. (1994). A credo for ethical managed care in mental health practice. *Hospital and Community Psychiatry*, **45**, 859–60.

Schreter, R.K., Sharfstein, S.S. & Schreter, C.A. (eds) (1994). *Allies and Adversaries: The Impact of Managed Care on Mental Health Services*. Washington DC, American Psychiatric Press.

Sibbald, B., Addington-Hall., J. Brenneman, D. & Freeling, P. (1993). Counsellors in English and Welsh general practices: their nature and distribution. *British Medical Journal*, **306**, 29–33.

Sireling, L.I., Paykel, E.S., Freeling, P., Rao, B.M. & Patel, S.P. (1985). Depression in general practice: case thresholds and diagnosis. *British Journal of Psychiatry*, **147**, 113–19.

Starfield, B. (1994). Is primary care essential? *Lancet*, **344**, 1129–33.

Strathdee, G. & Williams, P. (1984). A survey of psychiatrists in primary care: the silent growth of a new service. *Journal of the Royal College of General Practitioners*, **34**, 615–18.

Tyrer, P., Seivewright, N. & Woolerton, S. (1984). General practice psychiatric clinics: impact on psychiatric services. *British Journal of Psychiatry*, **145**, 15–19.

Warner, R.W., Gater, R., Jackson M.G. & Goldberg, D.P. (1993). Effects of a community mental health service on the practice and attitudes of general practitioners. *British Journal of General Practice*, **43**, 507–11.

Williams, P. & Balestrieri, M. (1989). Psychiatric clinics in general practice: do they reduce admissions? *British Journal of Psychiatry*, **154**, 67–71.

World Health Organisation. (1978). *Mental Disorders: Glossary and Guide to their Classification in Accordance with the Ninth Revision of the International Classification of Diseases*. Geneva: WHO.

Wright, A.F. & Anderson, A.J.B. (1995). Newly identified Psychiatric illness in one general practice: 12 month outcome and the influence of patients' personality. *British Journal of General Practice*, **45**, 83–7.

Part one

At-risk groups

[2] Primary prevention of childhood mental health problems

Quentin Spender and Peter Hill

Introduction

Child mental health can be defined as: 'The optimal achievement of the child's developmental potential, intellectually, emotionally and behaviourally'. A variety of circumstances may inhibit or impair a child's optimal development. Identifying these risk factors at a sufficiently early stage to stop them affecting childhood mental health constitutes primary prevention. In relation to child mental health, primary prevention has been defined as: 'The actual recognition of potential developmental and other problems and intervention to prevent the emergence of these problems as disabling disorders' (Berlin, 1990). Before looking at risk factors, we will briefly identify some of the commoner child mental health problems.

The scope of childhood psychiatric disorder

Childhood mental health problems are conventionally divided into two broad groups: disorders of conduct or externalising problems, and disorders of emotion or internalising problems. Children whose behaviour concerns adults around them are often regarded as having a conduct disorder. Hyperactivity is usually put in the same group, probably because of its strong association with behavioural difficulties. Children with separation anxiety excessive for their age, phobias, obsessive–compulsive disorder, anorexia nervosa, depression, or somatic presentations of psychological disturbance are said to have an emotional disorder.

In addition to the two major groupings there are disorders affecting the social control of sphincters (enuresis and encopresis), and those affecting motor impulses such as tic disorders and Tourette's syndrome. There are problems associated with the sleep and feeding of young children and the rarer disorders of social and linguistic development, including the pervasive developmental disorders such as autism. Organic psychoses and schizophrenia are rare in childhood but become increasingly recognised in adolescence. The same is true for substance misuse and dependency.

The classification of psychiatric disorders in childhood has limitations when applied to individual children. One reason is comorbidity: the co-existence of several recognised conditions in one child. This may reflect a common aetiology. For instance, a child who is emotionally disturbed because of losses in his family or other disruptions to care may express this in a variety of ways, including:

- withdrawal
- evident misery
- recurrence of behaviours such as enuresis or temper tantrums which the child had grown out of (regression)
- disobedience
- aggressive behaviour.

A particular child may manifest several of these at the same time, so fitting into both the conduct-disordered and the emotional-disordered group.

Alternatively, a condition such as hyperkinetic disorder can render the child more vulnerable to another, such as conduct disorder. This also applies to conditions such as general learning disability or dyslexia which are sometimes classified with psychiatric disorder and which certainly predispose affected children to further psychological difficulties.

As with diagnoses in other branches of medicine, careful categorisation can be used as a guide to both treatment and prognosis.

Disturbance tends to follow different patterns in boys and girls. Both epidemiological studies and referral patterns show that boys outnumber girls until mid-adolescence, when mental health disorders start to be as frequent in girls, and then more frequent as the adult pattern develops – which is of course that women outnumber men. Boys tend to present with externalising disorders, and girls are more likely to have internalising symptoms. This may be due to a combination of gender-specific differences in temperament and sex-role expectations. It is possible that internalising disorders in girls are as frequent as externalising disorders in boys, but less well detected until puberty. This is consistent with the findings of a study of the prevalence of psychiatric disorder in children aged 7 to 12 attending general practice, which showed that girls outnumber boys by 3 : 2; most affected children presented with somatic symptoms concealing emotional disorder (Garralda & Bailey, 1986).

Risk factors for the development of child mental health problems

Primary prevention consists of the identification and modification of known risk factors. These can conveniently be divided into those intrinsic to the child, qualities of parenting, and other factors in the environment (Pearce, 1993). There is some overlap between these categories. Multiple risk factors have a multiplicative effect – increasing the total risk by more than merely adding to each other. In other words, a risk factor which trebles the chance of a psychiatric disorder developing can interact with another risk factor which also trebles the risk so that the combination of the two increases the risk to nine times, not six times, the base rate. It is not surprising that children with identified mental health problems often have several different risk factors operating. It is also important to consider protective factors.

Risk factors in the child

Many of the risk factors in Box 2.1 cannot be prevented, but they can often be modified by providing as much support to the child and parents as possible, as soon as possible after the risk factor has been recognised. Sometimes this is primary prevention of the psychological and social sequelae, and sometimes these are already well established before it is possible to offer help.

The route from risk factor to psychiatric disorder varies. Low intelligence can lead to difficulties in finding ways of coping with practical and emotional stresses. This may result in poor socialisation, or the retention of immature strategies which yield short-term gains at the expense of longer-term benefit. An example would be the child who irritates another in the classroom as a means of gaining attention rather than seeking approval through trying to do the work set. Difficult temperament is likely to elicit impatient, punitive parenting, and can lead to a scapegoated child – the one child in the sibship who is blamed for everything. Language disorder or communication difficulty may lead to frustration in child, or parent, or both which can be expressed as behavioural or emotional symptoms. Chronic illness can lead to resentment, which can also be expressed in a variety of ways. Low self-esteem breeds a number of maladaptive behaviours. This may serve to try to minimise failure by avoiding educational or personal challenges (as in the above example), or by conforming to the labels given by adults (as in the child who has to be naughty because that's how he is always described).

Parents of a child with a *difficult temperament* may be helped enormously by professional recognition of this as a constitutional problem rather than as the consequence of inadequate parenting. About 10% of small children can be categorised as difficult according to the characteristics listed in Box 2.1. It is immediately apparent that such a child will be hard to live with and unrewarding to parent. Given that most parents believe that their child's personality is the product of their parenting, they will blame themselves and become demoralised. This will diminish their ability to persist

Risk factors in the child	Examples and comments
Low IQ	severe learning difficulties treble the risk of psychiatric disorder
Difficult temperament	resistance to imposed change or novelty slow to adapt to new situations marked tendency to whinge and grizzle high intensity emotional responses unpredictable biological rhythmicity, e.g. • *tiredness* • *hunger* • *elimination* doubles the risk of psychiatric disorder
Specific developmental delay	language disorder specific reading, spelling or writing disorder (dyslexia) clumsiness
Communication difficulty	hearing loss autistic symptoms
Physical illness	affecting the CNS • e.g. *epilepsy (especially frontal or temporal lobe focus)* chronic illness
Low self-esteem	may be a consequence of any of the above, or of inadequate encouragement from adults
Male gender	except for depression in adolescence

Box 2.1 *Risk factors in the child.*

with appropriate child-rearing because they see no gains and believe they are doing something wrong. They therefore change tactics and thus expose their child to just the sort of inconsistency he resents. They are typically exposed to a welter of advice which implicitly (or explicitly) undermines their confidence in themselves and their ability to parent. Eventually they may take against the child and become critical or punitive in an attempt to impose their will. The child reacts to harsh handling and his sense of parental rejection with anger, and his attempts to improve the situation or alleviate his unhappiness usually make matters worse.

Professional labelling of the child as 'difficult' in his own right by virtue of nature rather than personal motive can be very helpful, providing the child is not then seen as the source of all family ills. We have often heard parents saying 'If our second child had been born first, we wouldn't have had a second.' These parents can see that it is not their fault, because the first child was easy. If the difficult child comes first, parents inevitably feel they are doing something wrong (and the child's awkward nature makes it hard for them to be the good parents they wish to be). The most helpful initial intervention for the general practitioner or health visitor in these circumstances may be to sympathise with how difficult the child is and explain that this is a problem which some children are born with, rather than immediately giving advice on handling which may reinforce the sense of blame. In general terms the parents should be advised to be patient, trust their own judgement and not to look to immediate change in their child as to judge whether they are doing the right thing. The prognosis for change in the temperament of a toddler or young child is good, given reasonably consistent and positive handling. The parents can be reassured that the difficult behaviour can be temporary so long as they keep their nerve and their faith in their own child and themselves. They should look for change over a period of months, or even years, rather than days.

Low self-esteem is a problem for children who have lost faith in themselves and anticipate failure or rejection. In such circumstances children can go to enormous lengths to avoid further humiliation. It has been argued that most social behaviour in humans is motivated by a need to generate and maintain an adequate sense of self-worth. Children with poor self-esteem may make comments which reveal this ('I'm a rubbish child'), or their poor sense of their own worth may be revealed in drawings or writings at school. They may behave oddly. Although the concept of attention-seeking behaviour has been overused to the point of meaninglessness, children with poor self-esteem will carry out odd actions, particularly in the company of other children, in order to win their acclaim. In school, there is often an obvious unwillingness to try new activities in case of failure, and a fear of praise in case it means the children have to live up to a new standard of achievement they expect will be unattainable. Such children may destroy their own work or become obstructive in the face of encouragement. Other children with low self-esteem appear unsociable, bad-tempered or devious, resisting attempts to draw them into activities that carry a risk of failure. They lack the self-confidence to practise generosity, to postpone gratification, to contain their anger, or to risk placing another person in a more powerful position than themselves.

Adequate self-esteem can be promoted by frequent use of appropriate praise. It is better to focus this on achievements rather than attributes because this encourages further endeavour. This is very difficult for some parents, particularly if they themselves have a poor sense of self-worth. Indeed, the commonest reason for a child's low self-esteem is having parents who have poor self-esteem. Parents may have difficulty giving praise if they have had no experience of being praised themselves. A wise professional knows how to find opportunities to congratulate a parent on the handling of a difficult child.

Risk factors such as *specific learning difficulties* in language, reading, spelling or writing increase the likelihood of failure, and expose the child to misplaced criticism which attributes their difficulties to laziness or not trying hard enough. It therefore becomes important to recognise the problem for what it is – an inborn, constitutional disability – as early as possible and ensure that remedial steps are taken by a speech and language therapist or an educational psychologist accordingly. Nothing is gained and much placed in jeopardy by a policy of wait and watch.

Almost any *chronic illness* or condition increases the risk of psychiatric disorder through a number of pathways. Associated pain or disability can cause frustration or misery. Some medication is behaviourally toxic, including many anticonvulsants, and salbutamol syrup. Opportunities for social activities may be curtailed. The well-intentioned restrictions of parents or medical advisers can compound this. The sick role provides opportunities for secondary gain which become evident to the child and may be exploited. The needs of well siblings in this context should not be ignored – they should in general be as involved as possible, and should not have to feel they must become ill to receive as much love or special attention.

The locus of the illness may be in the brain, the organ of the mind, and affect emotions or behaviours directly. It is increasingly recognised that some rare inherited conditions which affect brain development can also have a direct influence on behaviour: Williams' syndrome, fragile-X and Turner's syndrome, for instance.

Factors associated with parenting

It is commonly assumed by parents that psychiatric disorder in their children is a result of deficiencies or mistakes in parenting. This is sometimes true, as in the case of children who have been abused, but is often an unwarranted assumption. The strongest association with poor quality parenting is in conduct disorder. Even when behavioural abnormalities in the child can clearly be traced to his experiences within the family; the role of the child needs to be taken into account: some children bring out the worst in their parents. Also environmental factors (see below) may make adequate parenting impossible. It may be more helpful to think in terms of parenting lack rather than parenting deficiency, in order to eschew an attitude which always blames parents.

Parenting can conveniently be divided into the *good*, the *bad* and the *ugly*. No parents are perfect; it is sufficient to be *good enough*. Ten qualities of competent parenting are shown in Box 2.2. It is not necessary to do all of these, all of the time, to be a 'good-enough' parent!

Primary prevention should include fostering these parental attitudes and skills. In principle, this could be done by providing parenting classes in secondary school. In practice, it is not at all clear whether parentcraft training can teach those children who have

---

Competent parents:

Are there when needed

Protect their children from harm

Love their children
- *provide affection*
- *provide emotional support*
- *provide comfort*
- *provide food and shelter*
- *provide information*

Use their authority so that they are in charge of their children (rather than vice versa)

Respect their children's immature status and judge it accurately

Keep adult business (sex, marital conflict, etc.) away from their children

Set reasonable limits of tolerance on their children's behaviour

Establish a moderate amount of justifiable household rules

Have their own lives and do not live through their children

Maintain their own self-esteem and personal development

Box 2.2 *Aspects of good-enough parenting.*

experienced poor parenting to be better parents. Teaching all
children, before they leave school, the principles of good-enough
parenting is unlikely to lead to significant benefit in those who
most need it, because they are least likely to be able to apply
theoretical principles, to get beyond their own experience of being
parented when they were children themselves, and to see how
individual children's needs differ. They are unlikely to see how
bringing up a child is relevant to them until they actually have
children of their own. Similarly, antenatal classes do not benefit
those who need tuition in parenting most, since they are the least
likely to attend. Competence at parenting is an aspect of general
social competence and those who deal with life reactively rather
than with foresight and planning will be unlikely to make the
effort and arrangements to attend classes in parenting. The
'inverse care law' applies.

However, it is helpful for professionals to have ideas about what
good-enough parenting is, based on empirical findings in scientific
child development research. Baumrind's work on parenting styles
in families of pre-school children has shown that children of parents
who are authoritative do better than children whose parents are
either too permissive or too authoritarian (Baumrind, 1967). The
most competent and mature children had parents who were authoritative, i.e. firm about setting limits, but prepared to justify these if
necessary; who were loving, but encouraged autonomy; and who
were understanding, but demanded a good deal of their children.
Children who were unhappy or socially withdrawn were found to
have parents who were authoritarian. In other words, these parents
were controlling in a punitive way; did not justify their imperatives
or encourage their children to express themselves; and were not
affectionate. Children who were dependent or immature had permissive parents who were disorganized in running their homes;
mothers who used withdrawal of love and ridicule as methods of
control, rather than power or reason; and fathers who were lax in
discipline, and tended to baby their children rather than encouraging their independence. Some of these results could be interpreted
as the effects of the child on the parent – as with the temperament-
ally difficult child – but it is generally agreed that an authoritative
parenting style, of the sort described by Baumrind, is best for
children.

Most parenting skills are probably learnt either from the experience of being a child, or from opportunities within the extended
family to practise looking after younger children. Sadly, the
ubiquity of the nuclear family, and the social isolation it entails, has
meant that many adolescents grow up with no opportunities to
look after young children at all. If their experience of being parented
lacked the above features, then they are likely to develop a parenting style with the same lacks. Reasons for *'bad' parenting* are shown

in Box 2.3. Not all are the fault of the parents and the term 'bad' merely describes the situation as a brief mnemonic term.

As with so many other risk factors in child psychiatry, these are mostly very difficult to prevent, but can sometimes be modified according to common-sense principles. It is an item of faith or common sense that this should be attempted: there is a lack of hard

Forms of 'bad' parenting	Examples and comments
Parental mental ill health	(postnatal) depression psychotic illness agoraphobia
Parental conflict or divorce	it is very difficult to keep the child's interests separate from the antagonistic feelings between the parents
Death or loss	of mother of other family members
Repeated separations of child from parents	admission to hospital accommodation or reception into local authority care
Lack of interpersonal skills	poor (grand) parental example no experience or tuition
Failure to adapt to child's developmental needs	development delay or other handicap; any child's needs will change with age
Coercive or harsh disciplinary style	due to: • *ignorance* • *lack of alternatives* • *experience of similar coercions in childhood*
Paternal criminality, alcoholism, or psychopathy	parental example financial problems family discord or separations

Box 2.3 *Parenting lack that can be described as 'bad'.*

evidence. The effects of postnatal depression on the infant are well established (Murray, 1992), though we know of no studies show- ing that treatment of the depression alleviates the effects on children – but it is intuitively obvious that it should. Similarly, older children of mentally ill parents are known to suffer parenting lack in various ways, but it is not clear to what extent this is remediable by psychiatric treatment for the parents, or even additional parenting (e.g. from the extended family).

Repeated, lengthy separations from parents should be prevented if possible. Some separations are essential, for instance starting nursery or primary school. The child is more likely to experience them as a step on the path to independence than a sad loss if, first, he has a secure emotional attachment to a parent, and, secondly, he has a gradual introduction to what it is like to be separated. For instance, a child is more likely to cope with nursery school if he has been to a child-minder or play-group before, and more likely to cope with primary school if he has spent at least one night away from home. Provision of such brief separations is likely to be easier and have a more satisfactory outcome if the child has a secure emotional attachment.

Admission to hospital used to be an unpleasant experience of separation. Most children no longer find it so. Nearly all wards admitting children now have facilities for mothers to stay if they wish. Children who are admitted electively are usually given the opportunity to look around the ward beforehand, so that it does not seem so frightening. Parents should be encouraged to talk about the forthcoming admission if the child brings the topic up and not rely on dismissive reassurance. It is, of course, more important for a parent to accompany the child if he is young, has not been to the hospital before, or is being admitted as an emergency.

Formal *parent training* can be used to remedy parental lack of skills, and help parents find alternatives to coercive styles of child behaviour management, but is generally vulnerable to the inverse care law (see above). It can be based on a combination of behavioural techniques and attention to the parents' emotional needs (Webster-Stratton, 1991). This seems to be more effective if it is targeted at parents of children with antisocial behaviour, such as aggression. It seems particularly effective when carried out in groups, as the parents then feel able to profit from each other's successes and mistakes, and feel less criticised by professionals. But it can be very time-consuming and costly – and so not readily applicable to primary care. Parent training therapy, combined with some school-based input, has also been used as part of a primary prevention programme in schools (Hawkins, von Cleve & Cata- lano, 1991). Small gains seem to have been achieved at great cost – but the long-term follow-up results may show savings in pro- fessional input needed during adolescence.

Parental mental disorder can prove a pernicious influence on childhood mental health. Chronic anxiety, depression, substance abuse and personality disorder in parents are more of a risk for psychiatric disorder in their children than acute psychosis. Prompt treatment is, of course, indicated. Some voluntary organisations such as Newpin (UK) are specifically interested in the impact of mentally disordered parents upon their children. Others, such as Alcoholics Anonymous and some of the substance abuse support agencies, run special programmes for older children of affected parents.

The third form of parenting of relevance to child mental health problems is *ugly* parenting, or abuse (see Box 2.4).

Forms of 'ugly' parenting	Possible explanations (usually several)
Physical abuse	very difficult child indeed parental depression hatred of what the child represents parents' own childhood experience of violence

Neglect	poverty
	lack of support from nuclear
	   or extended family:
	   • *emotional*
	   • *practical*

Sexual abuse	family boundaries not established
	   or kept
	child's needs seen as less important
	   than parental gratification
	a child who is in need of affection
	parent was sexually abused as a child
	no sexual satisfaction in marriage

Emotional abuse	negative feelings towards what the child represents parental depression parental personality disorder

Box 2.4 *Parenting lack that can be described as 'ugly'.*

Primary prevention of physical abuse and neglect

A recent review (MacMillan *et al.*, 1994*a*) suggests that at-risk families can be successfully targeted. If teenage parents, single parents and families living in poverty are identified before delivery of the first child, long-term home visiting by professionals has been shown to reduce the number of injuries and hospital visits, and reports of physical abuse or neglect. Although the majority of the studies have been done in North America, this has major implications for the organisation of primary care in Great Britain. It suggests that health visitors, if informed by community midwives of families thought to be at risk, can play an important preventive role by forming a supportive relationship with mothers, and visiting more frequently than they would otherwise have time for over the first two years.

Primary prevention of sexual abuse

Educational programmes for pre-school children have been shown to increase awareness of sexual abuse and prevention skills (MacMillan *et al.*, 1994*b*), though it is not clear whether the number of episodes of sexual abuse is actually decreased. These programmes have not been able to target children at risk, mainly because the risk factors listed in Box 2.4 are not specific enough. Another option would be to prevent adults from becoming perpetrators. For instance, some boys who have been abused go on to become perpetrators, and it is possible that appropriate treatment may prevent this, which could be regarded as an example of primary prevention (of victim psychopathology).

Primary prevention of emotional abuse

Emotional or psychological abuse is a frequent concomitant of other forms of abuse, but does occur on its own (Claussen & Crittenden, 1994). It is also associated with child mental health problems of various sorts. It can be defined as one or more of the following (Skuse & Bentovim, 1994):

- rejection (chronic denigration)
- social isolation
- terrorising by threatened abandonment
- chronic deprivation of attention
- corruption by exposure to deviant child-care practices
- 'adultifying' – making persistent age-inappropriate demands upon the child.

It is unclear whether emotional abuse can be prevented either by specific child abuse prevention programmes such as home visitation, or by more general preventive programmes directed towards disordered parenting. Important examples of these are *befriending schemes for mothers* (Cox, 1993). These include Homestart and Newpin. They both share the use of befrienders as the main source of support for mothers under such stress that they have lost control of their lives. The befrienders have been through the scheme themselves, and therefore have overcome similar problems. Professional support is provided both organisationally, and in the form of supervision, often in groups. There are usually also playgroups, and discussion groups for the mothers. Preliminary evaluation suggests that a high proportion of mothers entering Newpin can sustain their involvement, despite their very troubled childhoods and high level of psychiatric morbidity. Improvements in the mothers' psychiatric state occurred only after six months' involvement in the programme, so that encouragement to persist is important. Changes in the relationship between parent and child were more difficult to substantiate, perhaps because the follow-up was too short. Overall, these programmes appear to offer an opportunity to break the cycle of abuse in mothers who would not readily be able to engage with professional help.

A third component of risk affecting children with mental health problems are *environmental risk factors*. They often occur in combination. Box 2.5 shows a list of such factors (Quinton, 1988; Pearce, 1993).

Many of these factors require political will to alleviate them, but from the standpoint of primary care the first task is to recognise them and not trivialise their significance. A social factor is more likely to enhance the impact of other adversities than to cause psychiatric disorder on its own. For instance, there are strong associations between conduct disorder and socio-economic factors. But such factors are commonly associated with other child or parental risk factors that predispose to conduct disorder, so that it is difficult to judge the relative importance of the multiple factors. However, in extreme circumstances of poverty, temporary housing, criminal neighbourhoods or racial abuse, good-enough parenting may be impossible.

Bullying, as another example, is common, and not all victims develop psychiatric disorders. In epidemiological terms it is a risk factor, not a cause in its own right. Yet it should not be trivialised, nor dismissed as a necessary part of growing up. The temptation for doctors is to shrug it off because it is beyond their control; but what they can do is identify it as a problem of relevance to mental health, and encourage the parents to take it up with the school. If the school takes it sufficiently seriously, it can then be dealt with by a whole school approach. A policy combining openness about the issue, parental involvement, and teachers' readiness to condemn specific episodes promptly but non-punitively, has been shown to reduce the prevalence of this source of so much childhood misery

Environmental risk factors	Examples and comments
Poverty	often underestimated as a source of psychiatric morbidity
Social deprivation	lack of social support overcrowding homelessness or temporary housing living in the upper floors of high-rise accommodation
Socio-cultural influences	migration may sever family and social supports racial discrimination may be an added stress
Bullying	affects about 10% of primary school pupils
Peer group pressure	law-breaking may be socially acceptable to a deviant peer group
Environmental toxins	lead possibly dioxins have only a slight effect

Box 2.5 *Risk factors in the environment.*

(Olweus, 1993). Such a whole-school programme may at times involve the school nurse.

On a more positive note, Box 2.6 shows *protective factors* for the child. These factors need to be fostered.

Secure emotional attachment arises from the phase of normal clinging to one or both parents evident between about six months of age and associated for a year or two with separation anxiety – which is normal. Thereafter, anxiety about separation should subside, though resurface when the child is tired, frightened, in pain or ill. Securely attached children seem able to form an internal mental representation of their attachment figure (usually their mother) which is sufficiently kind and nurturing for them to tolerate increasingly long separations from her without undue fretting. This is a gradual process which takes place over several years from

---

Factors protecting a child against psychological disorder

Adaptable temperament

Positive self-image

Having a special skill or high IQ

Secure emotional attachment

Attitude and actions of adults
- *affection*
- *adults building you up rather than putting you down*
- *enough supervision*
- *authoritative discipline*

Box 2.6 *Protective factors for the child.*

the initial proximity-seeking that appears in the first year of life up to about the age of four. It is promoted by affectionate, tolerant firmness on the part of the mother, who encourages her child to tolerate brief separations of a few hours in settings where he is safe and to which she returns predictably. A secure attachment enhances exploratory behaviour, anxiety management, self-esteem, and peer group relationships.

Insecurely attached children continue to cling, cannot tolerate even brief separations, are difficult to settle to sleep and are reliant upon their mothers to relieve their anxieties and unhappiness. They lack the resourcefulness and confidence to manage their own emotional upsets. Insecurity is more likely if the mother uses threats of abandonment as a punishment or is an anxious, uncertain parent who is generally inconsistent, so that the child does not know what to expect. Not that all insecurity is the result of parental handling. Other incidents can undermine a child's confidence that his mother will return from a brief separation and that there will continue to be someone to care for him.

They include:

- illness or injury to a parent
- threats overheard by the child during a marital argument
- an unpleasant experience of separation
- a traumatic experience
- a death in the family.

The temperament of the child comes into play too, so that anxious or difficult children are more likely to elicit inconsistent or unconfident handling by their parents. An evidently clingy 4-year-old

needs help to tolerate brief separations which become inevitable at
school entry. The parents should be encouraged to arrange brief
separations of gradually increasing duration in supportive surroundings (playgroup, the homes of relatives or friends) even in the
face of protest from the child. Similar issues usually arise at
bedtime, since sleep is a separation from parents, and the parents
will need structured advice to manage the problem (see Chapter 9).

Parents are occasionally concerned that a mother who returns to
work when her child is young might be failing to meet his needs
appropriately. The position is a little complicated. Various studies
have shown that the young children of working mothers are not at
risk for mental health problems so long as their care during the day
is adequate, and there are arrangements for their mother to take
time off to care for them when ill. Indeed, the possession of a job
can enhance mother's self-esteem and protect against depression.
The decision about whether to return to work or not cannot be
taken in isolation from decisions about substitute child-care. Fears
that the child of a working mother will have an insecure attachment
are groundless; it is the quality of the interactions and relationship
between mother and child which counts, not the amount of time
spent with the mother. A mother who is affectionate, child-
centred, firm and reliable (see authoritative parenting above) will
promote good-quality interactions and relationships.

Early intervention programmes in the United States (e.g. Head-
start) have shown that it is possible for attempts at counteracting
environmental privations to have long-term effects. For instance, a
trial of well-staffed nursery education for disadvantaged children
aged three and four years resulted in a rise in IQ after one year of
27 points, followed by a fall to the same levels as controls
(Schweinhart & Weikart, 1988). Follow-up at age 15 years showed
a more positive attitude to school, better grades and less need for
special education. Follow-up at age 19 years showed higher liter-
acy, less mental retardation, less unemployment, higher earnings,
and less pregnancies among the girls.

Also, impoverished Mexican–American children were enrolled
at the age of one year in a study of a two-year educational programme in parenting (Johnson, 1988). The results at the end of the
programme showed, on videotaped interactions, that mothers
were more affectionate, used more praise, used less criticism, were
less rigidly controlling, and were more encouraging of their child's
verbalisations. Follow-up when the children were aged four to
seven years old showed that the treated boys did better than
controls on parental reports of destructive behaviour, overactivity
and negative attention seeking. Follow-up at ages eight to eleven
years, using a teacher's rating, showed less restlessness, im-
pulsivity, disruption and fights, and greater independence. It was
calculated that, if secondary services such as child psychiatry had

been available (which they were not), referrals would have been fewer among the treated group.

It is difficult to see the practical implications of some of these studies for primary care in the UK, particularly as they were initiated in the USA at a time of enthusiasm for large research grants. The difficulty lies partly in the boundary between politics and health. It is clear that nursery education is of benefit to children who would otherwise receive less attention by staying at home; and that there is a greater financial benefit than cost – by a ratio of 3 : 1 for the two-year nursery programme (Schweinhart & Weikart, 1988). But it is not within the power of primary care health workers to provide this – beyond taking advantage of playgroups and nurseries which offer a higher quality of stimulation than is available in the family home. Some caution is advisable here. For a number of years children with language delays were very commonly placed in day nurseries because it was felt that these provided more language stimulation than the children's homes. Systematic study showed this not to be true (Tizard et al., 1972). The implication is that careful evaluation of the home environment is required before a decision is made.

The special case of suicide

The reduction of suicide is one of the targets in the Health of the Nation programme. Suicide is exceptional before puberty but the rate rises with age subsequently to a high level in young adult life. Half of all suicides in a New York study of 170 adolescent suicides (aged 19 and under) had had previous contact with a mental health professional, and most had some psychiatric symptoms at the time of death, according to psychological autopsies (Shaffer & Piacentini, 1994). This included not only depression, but also anxiety, conduct disorder, drug and alcohol abuse – the latter being a particularly important factor in males. Depressive disorder was present in a third of the girls and a sixth of the boys, but was found in 50% of a different series of 67 adolescent suicides in Pittsburgh (Brent et al., 1993). There are three main patterns of symptoms and signs which typify adolescents who eventually kill themselves (Shaffer & Piacentini, 1994). One has an irritable, impulsive, volatile nature and a tendency to self-referential interpretations of the actions of others, reacting with unjustified sensitivity to perceived criticism. A second group consists mainly of girls who have a depressive disorder identical to the familiar adult picture but usually associated with social withdrawal and concealed from casual enquiry. Thirdly, there is a group of adolescents who are perfectionists, who find it hard to adjust to new circumstances, and become extremely anxious about forthcoming events.

The most effective endeavour at primary prevention has been the substitution of natural gas, with a carbon monoxide content of 2%, for gas with a carbon monoxide content of 40% in Great Britain between 1957 and 1970. During this period, the total suicide rate in Great Britain declined by 26%. School-based intervention programmes do not alter attitudes to suicide, and have not been shown to reduce suicides (Shaffer *et al.*, 1988). It is possible that more effective community psychiatric services for teenagers may prevent suicide, but this has yet to be proven. As there is strong evidence of some suicides having an imitative element, Shaffer *et al.* (1988) recommend de-glamourising suicide. Imitation is less likely if suicide is portrayed as a deviant act by someone with a mental disturbance than an understandable, tragic, heroic or romantic response to stresses emanating from uncaring adults or institutions.

So-called successful suicides are in general quite different from most teenagers who take overdoses – who are usually communicating distress, or some other message (Kingsbury, 1993). However, there is an overlap, and a small proportion of teenagers who take an overdose die by mistake. In a few, the overdose was indeed an inadequate suicidal attempt, or the teenager recovers from the overdose but goes on to kill themselves at a later date. Follow-up studies show attempted adolescent suicides subsequently completing suicide in 1 to 11% (Shaffer *et al.*, 1988), a 17-fold increased risk (Brent *et al.*, 1993). What this means is that all teenagers who take an overdose should be assessed for suicidal intent, as should all teenagers who express ideas or fears of killing themselves. Transient suicidal ideas occur in perhaps 10% of all teenagers (Hill, 1994), though good data are lacking. Definite plans or recurring thoughts are dangerous but may not be mentioned spontaneously and should be specifically asked for.

The most specific predictors of suicide are a previous overdose in males, and the presence of depression in either sex (Shaffer & Piacentini, 1994). It seems possible for general practitioners to reduce the incidence of suicide due to depression in adults (Rutz, von Knorring & Walinder, 1989), but this may be less easy in adolescents, who may not bring their depressive symptoms to the general practitioner. If they do, it would seem logical to press for psychiatric referral, but such referral may be resisted by the teenager or the parents – whose reasons and fears will then need examination.

Conclusions

Knowledge of risk factors is insufficient for the achievement of primary prevention. Resources and opportunities are also required. One example for which this is possible is the value of increased involvement by health visitors in potentially preventing episodes of physical abuse. The difficulty is to be clear which families are sufficiently at risk to justify the extra expense (Skuse & Bentovim, 1994). It seems possible that health visitors will eventually prove potent agents in the primary prevention of child mental health problems. Other examples include the role of the school nurse in increasing awareness of bullying; and the role of the general practitioner in fostering good-enough parenting, arranging for parents of difficult children to receive enough support, and making referrals of teenagers thought to be at risk of suicide.

References

Baumrind, D. (1967). Child care practices anteceding three patterns of preschool behavior. *Genetic Psychology Monographs,* **75**, 43–88.

Berlin, I.N. (1990). The role of the community mental health center in prevention of infant, child and adolescent disorders: retrospect and prospect. *Community Mental Health Journal,* **26**, 89–106.

Brent, D.A., Perper, J.A., Moritz, G., Allman, C., Friend, A., Roth, C., Schweers, J., Balach, L. & Baugher, M. (1993). Psychiatric risk factors for adolescent suicide: a case-control study. *Journal of the American Academy of Child and Adolescent Psychiatry,* **32**, 520–9.

Claussen, A.H. & Crittenden, P.M. (1994). Physical and psychological maltreatment: relations among types of maltreatment. *Child Abuse and Neglect,* **15**, 5–18.

Cox, A.D. (1993). Befriending young mothers. *British Journal of Psychiatry,* **163**, 6–18.

Garralda, M.E. & Bailey, D. (1986). Children with psychiatric disorders in primary care. *Journal of Child Psychology and Psychiatry,* **27**, 611–24.

Hawkins, J.D., von Cleve, E. & Catalano, R.F. (1991) Reducing early childhood aggression: results of a primary prevention programme. *Journal of the American Academy of Child and Adolescent Psychiatry,* **30**, 208–17.

Hill, P. (1994). *Adolescent Psychiatry.* Edinburgh: Churchill Livingstone.

Johnson, D.L. (1988). Primary prevention of behaviour problems in young children: the Houston parent–child development center. In *Fourteen Ounces of Prevention: a Casebook for Practitioners.* Price, R.H., Cowen, E.L., Lorion, R.P. and Ramos-McKay, J., eds. Washington, DC: American Psychological Association.

Kingsbury, S. (1993). Parasuicide in adolescence: a message in a bottle. *ACPP. Review and Newsletter,* **15**, 253–9.

MacMillan, H.L., MacMillan, J.H., Offord, D.R., Griffith, L. & MacMillan, A. (1994*a*). Primary prevention of child physical abuse and neglect: a critical review. *Journal of Child Psychology and Psychiatry*, **35**, 835–56.

MacMillan, H.L., MacMillan, J.H., Offord, D.R., Griffith, L. & MacMillan, A. (1994b). Primary prevention of child sexual abuse: a critical review. *Journal of Child Psychology and Psychiatry*, **35**, 857–76.

Murray, L. (1992). The impact of postnatal depression on infant development. *Journal of Child Psychology and Psychiatry*, **33**, 543–61.

Olweus, D. (1993). *Bullying at School*. Oxford: Blackwell.

Pearce, J. (1993). Child health surveillance for psychiatric disorder: practical guidelines. *Archives of Disease in Childhood*, **69**, 394–8.

Quinton, D. (1988). Urbanism and child mental health. *Journal of Child Psychology and Psychiatry*, **29**, 11–20.

Rutz, W., von Knorring, L. & Walinder, J. (1989). Frequency of suicide on Gotland after systematic postgraduate education of general practitioners. *Acta Psychiatrica Scandinavica*, **80**, 151–4.

Schweinhart, L.J. & Weikart, D.P. (1988). The High/Scope Perry Preschool Program. In *Fourteen Ounces of Prevention: a Casebook for Practitioners*. Price, R.H., Cowen, E.L., Lorion, R.P. and Ramos-McKay, J., eds. Washington DC: American Psychological Association.

Shaffer, D. & Piacentini, J. (1994). Suicide and attempted suicide. In: *Child and Adolescent Psychiatry: Modern Approaches*, Rutter, M., Taylor, E. and Hersov, L. eds., 3rd edn. pp. 407–424. Oxford: Blackwell Scientific Publications.

Shaffer, D., Garland, A., Gould, A., Fisher, P. & Trautman, P. (1988). Preventing teenage suicide: a critical review. *Journal of the American Academy of Child and Adolescent Psychiatry*, **27**, 675–87.

Skuse, D. & Bentovim, A. (1994). Physical and emotional maltreatment. In *Child and Adolescent Psychiatry: Modern Approaches*, Rutter, M., Taylor, E. and Hersov, L., eds. 3rd edn. pp. 209–229. Oxford: Blackwell Scientific Publications.

Tizard, B., Cooperman, O., Joseph, A. & Tizard, J. (1972). Environmental effects on language development: a study of young children in long stay residential nurseries. *Child Development*, **43**, 337–58.

Webster-Stratton, C. (1991) Strategies for helping families with conduct-disordered children. *Journal of Child Psychology and Psychiatry*, **32**, 1047–62.

[3] Primary prevention: assessing the relevance of life events and difficulties among primary care attenders

Tirril Harris

Introduction

While the notion of stress-related disease dates back to classical times, it is only in the last two decades that research into the role of life events has been systematic enough to inform general medical practice. Alongside these improvements in the study of environmental stressors, there has been increasing sophistication in the understanding of the impact of psychosocial factors in general upon health and illness. In parallel, work in neuropsychopharmacology has thrown up wide-ranging hypotheses, which have allowed the elaboration of integrated biopsychosocial models with compelling implications for preventive interventions.

In a brief chapter of this kind, it is clearly impossible to do justice to all these developments, and the focus of this contribution has had to be restricted accordingly. The theme selected highlights the personal meaning of adverse life events and ways in which this might be explored by a person's doctor and other health care professionals. This theme will be developed by describing in some detail the work of one particular research tradition.

Life events, difficulties and meaning

The studies to be discussed here were undertaken during the last 25 years in London, by the Royal Holloway and Bedford College Medical Research Council research team, both in general population and in psychiatric patient samples. Their original purpose was to investigate the psychosocial aetiology of mental disturbance, although the study of the course of illness and recovery also became possible later. Early work in the late 1960s focused on depressive disorder, and since the bulk of incidence of mental disorder found in primary care consists of depression (anxiety without depression is mostly chronic, and psychosis is relatively rare), it is easiest to begin by describing this.

The research (among women in Camberwell, London) was

designed to explore the impact upon depressive onset of, on the one hand, recent stressful experience and, on the other, background psychosocial factors such as socio-economic status, employment, education and supportive social networks, using the LEDS (Life Events and Difficulties Schedule), (Brown & Harris; 1978).

The assessment of meaning in life stress

At that time most life events research had used a checklist questionnaire approach to data collection (see, for example, the classic Social Readjustment Rating Scale, Holmes & Rahe, 1967) with the respondents ticking a list of predefined experiences (such as housemove or birth of a child) if they had occurred in a defined period. But this approach fails to deal with the *meaning* of events for individuals. A planned first pregnancy in a secure marital and financial situation has a totally different meaning from an unplanned pregnancy for a single parent where there are already three children, in cramped housing and short of money, but both would get the same score on the checklist system. The LEDS' chief merit is its attempt to capture these variations in 'context' without specifically taking account of the actual emotional appraisal of the individual concerned (Box 3.1).

A depressed person's account of the meaning of events will itself be coloured by the depression. Therefore it is necessary to obtain a *contextual* method of rating, based on knowledge of a wide range of circumstances surrounding each event. A judgement is made by the investigator about the likely meaning of each event for the person concerned, on the basis of what most people would feel in such a situation given his biography, prior plans and current circumstances, but ignoring what he himself reports as his actual reaction to the event.

The checklist procedure has a number of other disadvantages, involving measurement bias and imprecision, particularly as far as the relative timing of life stress and onset of disorder are concerned. These are minimised by the nature of the LEDS, which is a semi-structured face-to-face interview, with a set of previously developed rules embodied in training manuals. These ensure high rates of inter-rater reliability (Tennant *et al.*, 1979).

Provoking agents and vulnerability factors: an early model of depression

Severe life events and depression

The Camberwell study involved both psychiatric patients from the Maudsley Hospital and a random sample of the surrounding general population, among whom 17% had been depressed at some point during the 12 months before interview. For a number of

---

A. Severe events
1. Humiliating rejections/separations
2. Major revelations, e.g. *R* learns son is a paedophile
3. Death of someone close
4. Entrapment events, e.g. is told nothing more can be done for own crippling arthritis

B. Non-severe but unpleasant events
1. Separations without humiliating elements e.g. husband posted abroad for one year when respondent is working and in good health
3. Surprising news/minor revelations e.g. *R* hears daughter-in-law has left son but will not deny *R* access to grandchildren
4. *R* involved in helping with death/illness of someone less close
5. *R* is told he/she has ulcer but that various medications may help

C. Events neutral or positive in the long term
1. House move to preferred area
2. Job change actively sought by respondent
3. Upon marriage daughter leaves home to live in same town
4. Child starts school – settles in well

D. Reassessment-forcing experiences
(non-severe events, or even 'incidents', which bring home the meaning of a severe ongoing difficulty)

1. Returns to bad housing after holiday staying in relatives' comfortable cottage
2. Learns of widowed friend's remarriage while herself in undermining marital relationship

Legend: R means respondent

Box 3.1 *Typical examples of life events.*

practical reasons only women were included in the community sample. However later work with men suggests that the findings concerning meaning can be generalised across the sexes. The type of events which proved to be most important in the aetiology of depression involved those which are *severe* in terms of *long-term* contextual threat and unpleasantness. Box 3.1 illustrates the contrast between severe and other unpleasant events. (For a precise definition see Brown & Harris, 1978.)

Only *major* difficulties (i.e. severe and ongoing) appear to be of

critical importance for depression. These provoking agents constitute only a small minority of all events and ongoing difficulties
recorded by the LEDS instrument and largely involve experiences
of loss (including losses of cherished ideas as well as losses of person
or object). Interpersonal crises, such as discovering a partner's
infidelity, children's stealing or estrangements from former good
friends or family of origin, were frequent, but depression was also
linked with more material stressors such as threats of eviction or
unemployment. It was noteworthy that events such as house
moves, which were not rated severe (because although involving a
certain amount of hassle were no more than mildly unpleasant),
were not associated with depression. Nor were events which were
severe in the short but not the long term, such as finding a breast
lump and learning from biopsy within two weeks that it was
benign. Although extremely distressing during the first few days,
such events were, by definition, largely resolved by the end of 14
days. As will emerge later, this finding has implications in terms of
possible intervention within a few days of a potentially severe event
occurring.

Major difficulties and the timing of depression

Especially interesting was the exploration of the puzzle as to why
major difficulties, which by definition had to have been going on
for at least two years, could come to provoke depression at one
particular point in time. It seemed that some 'reassessment-forcing
experience' (a minor event or even a positive incident) might have
caused the women to reappraise situations they had been avoiding
facing for some time (See Section D. in Box 3.1).

Thus one woman with a cold and unsupportive partner
became depressed when her younger sister announced her
engagement to a successful warm young man, as if only now by
comparison could she see her own situation clearly.

Another became depressed shortly after a routine operation
with no complications – a dilatation and curettage ('D and C')
which seemed to have really helped her menorrhagia, an
experience common among many non-depressed women in the
sample. It seemed that her severe housing difficulty, with
overcrowding, damp, mice, paraffin heaters and only one hot
water ascot, had been tolerable until she had been to stay
temporarily in a warm, clean hospital and been shown great care
and attention. On returning home the trap she was in with her
housing perhaps became much clearer to her, with the ensuing
onset of depression.

Confirmation of original findings

A review of the onset of depression in ten studies of women in the general population, using the LEDS and strict case criteria of depression, shows that all agree that the majority of affected women experience a provoking agent before the onset of illness. The actual proportion with a 'provoking agent' ranges from 62 to 94%, with an average of 83% (Brown & Harris, 1986).

Indicators of vulnerability

One of the striking findings of the Camberwell study was that the prevalence of clinical depression was higher among working-class than middle-class women, particularly if they had children at home. It was also noticeable that rates of these provoking agents were higher in just those groups. It therefore seemed possible that the differences in prevalence by class and life-stage were wholly due to these differing rates of stressful experience. However, even when only those with a provoking agent were examined, the demographic differences remained, suggesting there was something about being working class with children at home which was rendering these women more vulnerable to stress as well as more likely to experience it.

A thorough exploration of the background and social network variables suggested that four 'vulnerability factors' might be at work in this way and gave rise to a theoretical model of depressive onset which is crudely represented in Fig. 3.1.

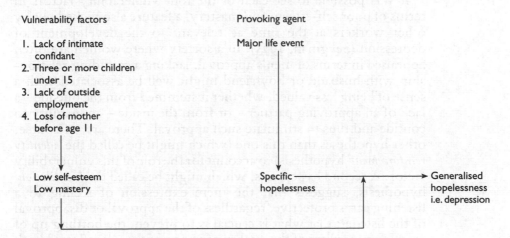

Fig. 3.1 *A model of the onset of depression in women in Camberwell.*

Vulnerability factors

Lack of an intimate confidant

'Intimate confiding' was defined in terms of the *quality* of emotional support given by close ties, the empathy forthcoming in a relationship where the respondent felt fully able to disclose her confidences. This seemed more important than the *quantity* of social contact or the amount of *practical help* given. Particularly striking was the relatively greater protection against depression afforded by intimacy with a husband or boyfriend when compared with support from a platonic male or a female friend alone, even if such a friend was seen at least once a week. But most vulnerable were those with confidant(e)s seen less than once a week or those with no confidant(e) at all. It seemed likely that the four vulnerability factors operated by increasing that sense of 'hopelessness-specific-to-the-loss' which it is assumed would develop, at least temporarily, in even the bravest heart when faced with a major loss.

A masterful approach, it was argued, would be allied with high self-esteem and would prevent the generalisation of this hopelessness reaction, through increased optimism. The vulnerability factors, it was suggested, would be linked with low self-esteem, and thus with a tendency to generalise feelings of hopelessness. This might then develop to become Beck's (1967) well-known 'cognitive triad' of clinical depression (the self seems worthless, the world seems pointless and the future hopeless) (see Chapter 17), accompanied in turn by changes in vegetative functions such as disturbances in sleep and appetite.

It was possible to see each of the four vulnerability factors in terms of poor self-esteem and mastery, a feature also picked out by other workers at the time as relevant to the development of depression (Seligman, 1975). In a society where women are often appraised in terms of men's approval, lacking a confiding relationship with husband or boyfriend might well be associated with a sense of being less valued, whether it stemmed from the outside – a lack of an approving partner – or from the inside – an inability to confide and thus to stimulate such approval. There are, of course, other hypotheses than this one (which might be called the '*identity reinforcement*' hypothesis) to account for the role of this vulnerability factor. A second hypothesis, which might be called the '*ventilation*' hypothesis, suggests that the mere expression of feeling to a listening ear is protective, regardless of the approval or disapproval of the listener; that what is crucial is to prevent the bottling up of emotion regardless of the quality of image of the self reflected back to the woman by her confidant. While this second process can be seen as more physiological than the first, with the role of physical tension possibly central in leading to the vegetative changes associated with depression, it can also be linked with feelings of self-worth: people probably feel worse about themselves when bottling up negative emotions.

Lack of alternative role identities

It seemed possible that the second and third vulnerability factors listed in Fig. 3.1 were associated with low self-esteem through the constraints they placed upon a woman trying to find a '*role identity*'. For example, women confined to the domestic role had less opportunity to win praise than those with a job (however menial or part-time) and less chance of rewarding leisure activities. Whereas a woman can often leave one child (or even two) with a neighbour while she slips out to play bingo, finding baby-minders for three children is much more of a problem.

Loss of own mother in childhood

Interpretations of the impact of the fourth vulnerability factor, loss of mother before age 11, focused less on a possible association via current constraints and more on long-term personality development. It was argued, in the tradition of Winnicott (1965) and Bowlby (1980), that healthy self-reliance and a belief in a benign environment were based on '*good-enough mothering*' early in life (see Chapter 2). Those with an early loss of mother were thought to be less likely to have received such mothering, and their long-term self-esteem would therefore be reduced. In addition, such a long-term '*cognitive set*' of low self-esteem might partly account for the association of the other three vulnerability factors with depression, even apart from their operation through current constraints upon role identity. For example, a woman with a continuing sense of inferiority might lack the confidence to take up a job or to manage contraception efficiently (thus ending up with more than two children), or she might marry someone in whom she knew she could never confide because she lacked the confidence that she would ever receive another marriage proposal. Further studies which measured self-esteem directly (Brown *et al.*, 1986) confirmed this model of the psychosocial origins of depression, based on the insight that the *generalisation* of hopelessness was the mechanism through which responses to stress became disordered.

Mediating between life event and disorder: the role of coping style

The vulnerabilities discussed so far have all involved risk factors operating before the life event occurs, although it is their role in the immediate aftermath which is proposed as crucial. In addition, the important role of both cognitive and pragmatic 'coping styles' should be considered, since these may be amenable to intervention during this critical mediating period.

Both self-blame and denial (a Pollyanna-like tendency to miss seeing the negative aspects of a situation until it is too late) have been associated with an increased risk of depression, as has helplessness in dealing with the situation (Bifulco & Brown, 1995).

Early life events and current vulnerability

As I indicated above, the fourth vulnerability factor, loss of mother either by death or by separation of at least 12 months before the age of 11, suggested that adult depression might be linked with childhood problems.

Another study, in Walthamstow, east London, expressly designed to explore experiences intervening between early loss of mother and current mental state, illuminated the process by which risk of depression in adulthood was increased over such a long time span. Two experiences closely associated with having lost a mother in this way before age 11 stood out: *poor substitute parental care* and *a premarital pregnancy* which seemed to trap women in unsupportive relationships which they might otherwise not have chosen (Harris, Brown & Bifulco, 1986, 1987). In this area of relative social mobility, such a pregnancy also seemed to have trapped them in the working class, unlike their more fortunate socially mobile contemporaries.

This study also further explored other aspects of the model of depression outlined above, by including a measure of the women's situational 'helplessness/mastery' which was found to relate both to poor substitute parental care after the maternal loss and to poor support (lack of intimate confiding) in current relationships (Harris Brown & Bifulco, 1990). It seemed as if some women had got on to a conveyor belt early in life which would carry them from one unsupportive setting to another unless they could be masterful enough to get off.

In another inner-city sample in Islington, studied in the 1980s, an index of 'childhood adversity' (defined by either the presence of marked parental rejection or neglect, violence from a member of the family, or serious sexual abuse) was an important risk factor for the development of depression later in life. Approximately a third had such experiences before the age of 17 and these women had roughly double the risk of experiencing depression during adulthood (Bifulco, Brown & Harris, 1994). However, it appeared that most of this increased risk operated through the kind of adult background variables outlined above. Indeed, without their presence the risk of depression associated with childhood adversity was not greatly different from that for other women (Brown et al., 1990). On the other hand, the probability of experiencing such unsupportive relationships in adulthood was nearly doubled among those with adversity in childhood (Harris, 1993). Box 3.2 attempts to summarise these experiences, past and present, which could suggest vulnerability to the provoking agents described.

A. Past experiences likely
  (i) Childhood adver...
      childhood loss of ...
      year or more
  (ii) premarital pregr...
       unsupportive pa...

B. Current external vul...
  Current lack of sup...
  kin or close friends

  Constrained by cos...
  children/invalids)

  Constrained by ab...
  (i) no employmer...
  (ii) inadequate financial ...

C. Current internal vulnerabilities
  Poor self-image/low self-esteem
  Tendency to self-blame
  Low mastery
  Tendency to ignore impending problems (denial)

Box 3.2 *Elements to look for in assessing background vulnerability to severe life events and major difficulties.*

Attachment theory

Childhood adversity is also associated with anxiety disorders (Brown & Harris, 1993) and, among those already depressed, with a tendency for the episode to become chronic (Brown *et al.*, 1994). These findings are in line with the predictions of 'attachment theory' (Bowlby, 1980) which suggests that each person develops their own particular internal working models of relationships on the basis of experiences with early attachment figures, and that these models will later crucially affect the quality of support available. However, a less pessimistic perspective is afforded by examples of those who had somehow disengaged themselves from the childhood pattern of unsupportiveness, either by making a fortunate marriage or by educational or professional success.

Life events, difficulties and recovery from depression

The role of loss of hope in the development of a depressive episode is underlined by recent research on clinical improvement and

...ests that events and difficulties may prove to
... a role in the course as in the onset. It also appears
...es involved may broadly mirror those leading to
...ase by changing circumstances bringing new hope to

...ery or improvement in depressive conditions that have
...for 20 weeks or more is highly related to the occurrence of
...ts that on common-sense grounds would be expected to bring
...ope, such as being rehoused, receiving a proposal of marriage
from a new boyfriend or finding a job after months without one.
However, in addition to such *'fresh-starts'*, reduction in the severity
of the ongoing difficulty and receiving support also played a part
(Brown, Adler & Bifulco, 1988).

The specificity of stressors and vulnerabilities: depression and other disorders

Depression, loss, humiliation and entrapment

The role of interpersonal support in protecting against depression is
crucial because so many provoking events involve relationships in
one way or another. The element of loss mentioned earlier included
loss of a cherished idea, and this was usually interpersonal, such as
belief in a key person's commitment, faithfulness, or trustworthi-
ness (Brown, Bifulco & Harris, 1987). A subsequent analysis
suggested that losses involving humiliation, entrapment or
bereavement carried an even higher risk of depressive onset than
other losses (Brown, Harris & Hepworth, 1994). Typical of humiliation would be, for example, a woman's discovery of a husband's
infidelity, or her finding out that a daughter has been consistently
stealing from her and lying about not going to school. Entrapment
involves events that underline the fact that the respondent is
imprisoned in a punishing situation that has already gone on for some
time: for example, a woman being told by a hospital doctor that
nothing could now be done to relieve her crippling arthritis.

Anxiety disorder, danger and vigilance

The type of events preceding pure anxiety disorders are usually
dangers rather than losses. A typical example of an event spelling
severe danger is a child's first asthmatic attack, calling for an
emergency in-patient admission: an event after which any mother
could be expected to remain constantly vigilant for a time, lest the
crisis might recur and, possibly, result in worse consequences. It is
of note that the study which first suggested this (Finlay-Jones &
Brown, 1981) was done in general practice where cases of pure
anxiety of recent origin are usually seen. Most cases encountered in
the general population of such pure anxiety (without depression)

tend to be more longstanding, while many of those with a recent onset of anxiety are 'mixed'cases. Experience of both severe loss and severe danger, either as two separate events or as a single event having both qualitative aspects, were found most often in these mixed cases, while those with pure depression tended to have experienced only loss.

The specificity of vulnerability may correspond with the specificity of stressor. Thus lack of intimate confiding was confirmed as a vulnerability factor for the depressed and mixed onsets, but not for those of pure anxiety (Finlay-Jones, 1989).

By contrast pure anxiety was associated with increased parental divorce in childhood (almost invariably involving separation from the father). It is tempting to speculate that loss of the father in childhood through divorce (often preceded by violent parental disagreement) may act as an indicator of an underlying disposition to be vigilant against dangers and violence.

Implications of life events research for prevention of mental illness in primary care

Socio-demographic factors, such as lower social class, single parenthood and inner-city residence, cannot be influenced by primary health care teams. Personal coping style, however, suggests possibilities for intervention. Dramatic and impulsive personality traits, often stemming from neglect and abuse in childhood, can themselves prove the source of severe interpersonal events as partnerships erupt or children run away from home. Other more fearful personalities are vulnerable to depression because they appraise minor events as if they were severe ones so that they are more sensitive than average. Such personalitites have often not been confident enough to create a network of supportive relationships to help them when a crisis does occur. Box 3.3 summarises the possible lines of action implied by this research.

Despite appearances something can often be done about life events

Life events are often talked about as if they are acts of God and thus knowledge about their impact will be of little use in preventive interventions.

The LEDS approach, however, has suggested that this is too simple. First, the contextual perspective shows how the degree of stressfulness is crucially related to the *meaning* of each life event, which grows out of the person's background roles and ongoing difficulties. The birth of a third child, which could in other circumstances be a joyful experience, can become a severe event in LEDS terms because it occurs in the context of marked housing or financial difficulties. There is no doubt that such difficulties could

A. Help improve existing external resources
  1. Increase ongoing support from:
      (i)   partner
      (ii) kin
      (iii) close friends

  2. Promote alternative role identities by reducing constraints from:
      (i)   other caring roles
      (ii) lack of employment
      (iii) inadequate material resources

B. Provide new sources of support to improve internal resources
  1. Counselling/psychotherapy
  2. Befriending
  3. Access to courses, e.g. on assertiveness
  4. Self-help groups
  5. Self-help booklets

C. Act directly to reduce difficulties and encourage fresh starts
  1. Contact housing departments
  2. Contact employers
  3. Encourage family reconciliations

D. Act directly to prevent patient producing further severe events, raising the severity of his/her difficulties

E. Act directly on internal resources
  1. Encourage patient not to let the event affect the totality of their self-image, i.e. discourage generalisation
  2. Make links with fortuitous nature of past to explain why self-blame is not appropriate
  3. Offer advice designed to increase masterful coping with/reduce denial of implications of severe event or difficulty

Box 3.3 *Possible measures available for primary care teams to offset the impact of severe life events.*

become the target of social policy efforts, and of individual interventions in particular medical cases (see Box 3.3, C). However, there is likely to be more opportunity for the doctor to intervene via the chain of vulnerability.

Identifying those vulnerable to severe life events
The LEDS approach has highlighted the importance of vulnerability: stressful experiences in most cases do not lead to psychiatric disorder without background vulnerability. This means that it

should be possible to identify in advance those whose specific
background experience, say early neglect or a premarital pregnancy, is likely to resonate with the specific life-event dimension
currently experienced, say separation or humiliation. Once identified, such individuals can be targeted for special attention, whether
by support from the general practitioner (Box 3.3, A), or by other
professionals (Box 3.3, B).

The primary care setting, where the primary health care team
often has knowledge of the whole family history, including separ-
tions and tribulations, may permit better assessment of such background vulnerability. Sometimes the practice will know the patient
well enough to gauge his or her interpersonal style – in the sense of
histrionic, fearful or dismissive – and will be able to anticipate, or
even prevent, the production of a new crisis or a pathological
response to it (see Box 3.3 E).

Influencing vulnerability: social support, counselling and self-help groups

Hitherto, the most usual form of intervention has been secondary
rather than primary, focusing on mediating (rather than background) vulnerability factors, particularly the provision of health
visitors or counsellors, probably because it has seemed easier to
identify the need and less costly to meet it once a severe event has
occurred and depression seems to be developing.

Corney (1987) (see Chapter 6) reported improvement in
depression after a special social worker intervention involving both
'sustaining and exploring' counselling techniques as well as practical help. However, naturalistic studies of social support suggest
that marshalling it at the last moment through professionals may
not be as effective in preventing depression as utilising an ongoing
trusted network of friends (Brown *et al.*, 1986). The development
of the *self-help group* has been one attempt to compensate for this, by
creating a continuing network rather than trying to help at the last
moment. These groups may founder without back-up support.
However where such support is available such groups can do well.
Elliott, Sanjack & Leverton, (1988) report the reduced risk of
depression after childbirth among first-time mothers offered additional group support.

Befriending

One intermediate approach which is relatively new is '*volunteer
befriending*', where a three-day training and regular group meetings
of the befrienders afford basic supervision to a new intimate
confiding relationship. This lasts for a minimum of nine months,
with weekly contacts, and often continues afterwards, at a lesser
frequency. Encouraged to be maximally available, and to particip-
ate in enjoyable activities with the befriendee as well as listening and

giving advice, these befrienders can often become genuine core contacts, unlike some health service personnel who frequently move on to other jobs. Furthermore, the organisation of befriending outside the system of medical care helps to offset the less fortunate effects upon self-esteem of the labelling process which is part of attending for psychological treatment. A befriendee will thus continue to see her doctor as well as her befriender. Full evaluation of such schemes is still awaited, but several pilot studies have had promising conclusions (Pound & Mills, 1985; Van der Eyken, 1982).

Psychotherapy and drug treatment

It is important to emphasise that some patients with depression, particularly if they have been the target of substantial early abuse, will require long-term psychotherapy rather than merely befriending or counselling. Finally, it is important to underline that none of these measures rules out a simultaneous and more traditionally medical approach through drug treatment.

Conclusion

I have attempted to highlight the importance of the personal meaning of stressful experiences across a person's lifespan and the way in which this can inform decisions about possible preventive interventions by the primary health care team. There is great scope for future research into the physiological states, genetic or acquired, which increase vulnerability to the impact of severe life events. We are only just beginning to understand how such events are mediated through the nervous, endocrine and immune systems.

Acknowledgements

The life-events research described was originally conceived by Professor George Brown, and largely supported by the Medical Research Council. I am indebted to all the colleagues who have been members of the research team over the last 20 years who participated in the data collection, to Laurie Letchford and Sheila Williams for work with the computer, and to all those who have taken the trouble to respond to our questions by telling of such painful and private experiences.

References

Beck, A.T. (1967). *Depression: Clinical, Experimental and Theoretical Aspects*, London: Staples Press.

Bifulco, A. & Brown, G.W. (1995). Coping and onset of clinical depression 2. An aetiological model. *Journal of Social Psychiatry and Psychiatric Epidemiology,* (in press).

Bifulco, A., Brown, G.W. & Harris, T.O. (1994). Childhood experience of care and abuse (CECA): a retrospective interview measure. *Child Psychology and Psychiatry*, **35**, 1419–35.

Bowlby, J. (1980). *Attachment and Loss. Vol 3: Loss: Sadness and Depression*. New York: Basic Books.

Brown, G.W. & Harris, T. (1978). *Social Origins of Depression: A Study of Psychiatric Disorder in Women*. London: Tavistock Press.

Brown, G.W., & Harris, T.O. (1986). Stressor, vulnerability and depression: a question of replication. *Psychological Medicine*, **16**, 739–44.

Brown, G.W., & Harris, T.O. (1989). *Life Events and Illness*. New York, Guilford and London: Unwin Hyman.

Brown, G.W. & Harris, T.O. (1993). Aetiology of anxiety and depressive disorders in an inner-city population. 1. Early adversity. *Psychological Medicine*, **23**, 143–54.

Brown, G.W., Andrews, B., Harris, T.O., Adler, Z. & Bridge, L. (1986). Social support, self-esteem and depression. *Psychological Medicine*, **16**, 813–31.

Brown, G.W., Bifulco, A. & Harris, T. (1987). Life events, vulnerability and onset of depression: some refinements. *British Journal of Psychiatry*, **150**, 30–42.

Brown, G.W., Adler, Z. & Bifulco, A. (1988). Life events, difficulties and recovery from chronic depression. *British Journal of Psychiatry*, **152**, 487–98.

Brown, G.W. Bifulco, A., Veiel, H. & Andrews, B. (1990). Self-esteem and depression: 2. Social correlates of self-esteem. *Social Psychiatry and Psychiatric Epidemiology*, **25**, 225–34.

Brown, G.W., Harris, T.O. & Hepworth, C. (1994). Life events and 'endogenous' depression: a puzzle re-examined. *Archives of General Psychiatry*, **51**, 525–34.

Brown, G.W., Harris, T.O., Hepworth, C. & Robinson, R. (1994). Clinical and psychosocial origins of chronic depression. 2. A patient enquiry. *British Journal of Psychiatry*, **165**, 457–65.

Corney, R. (1987). Marital problems and treatment outcome in depressed women: a clinical trial of social work intervention. *British Journal of Psychiatry*, **151**, 652–60.

Elliott, S.A., Sanjack, M. & Leverton, T.J. (1988). Parent groups in pregnancy: a preventive intervention for postnatal depression. In *Marshalling Social Support: Formats, Issues, Processes and Effects*. Gottlieb, B.H. ed. London: Sage.

Finlay-Jones, R. (1989). Anxiety. In *Life Events and Illness*. Brown, G.W. & Harris, T. eds., New York: Guilford Press.

Finlay-Jones, R. & Brown, G.W. (1981). Types of stressful life events and the onset of anxiety and depressive disorders, *Psychological Medicine*, **11**, 803–15.

Harris, T. (1993). Surviving childhood adversity: what can we learn from naturalistic studies? In *Surviving Childhood Adversity: Issues for Policy and Practice*, Ferguson, H., Gilligan, R. & Torode, R., eds., Chapter 8, pp.93–107. Dublin: Social Studies Press, Trinity College.

Harris, T., Brown, G.W. & Bifulco, A. (1986). Loss of parent in childhood and adult psychiatric disorder: the Walthamstow Study. 1. The role of lack of adequate parental care. *Psychological Medicine*, **16**, 641–59.

Harris, T., Brown, G.W. & Bifulco, A. (1987). Loss of parent in childhood and adult psychiatric disorder: the Walthamstow Study. 2. The role of social class position and premarital pregnancy. *Psychological Medicine*, **17**, 163–83.

Harris, T., Brown, G.W. & Bifulco, A. (1990). Loss of parent in childhood and adult psychiatric disorder: a tentative overall model. *Development and Psychopathology*, **2**, 311–28.

Holmes, T.H. & Rahe, R.H. (1967). The social readjustment rating scale. *Journal of Psychosomatic Research,* **11**, 213–18.

Pound, A. & Mills, M. (1985). A pilot evaluation of Newpin – home-visiting and befriending scheme in South London. *ACCP Newsletter* (4).

Seligman, M.E.P. (1975). *Helplessness: On Depression, Development and Death.* San Francisco: W.H. Freeman.

Tennant, C., Smith, A., Bebbington, P. & Hurry, J. (1979). The contextual threat of life events: the concept and its reliability. *Psychological Medicine*, **9**, 525–28.

Van der Eyken, W. (1982). *Home Start – A Four Year Evaluation*, Leicester: Homestart Consultancy.

Winnicott, D. (1965). *The Maturational Processes and the Facilitating Environment.* London: Hogarth.

[4] The prevention of postnatal depression

Deborah Sharp

Introduction

Childbirth is often assumed to be a universally happy event and for most women it is a major life event of great psychological significance. However, recent research has revealed that the months surrounding the birth bring with them the greatest lifetime risk for women of developing a mental illness (Kendell, Chalmers & Platz, 1987).

The baby blues

Postnatal depression is a term that is sometimes used to describe a variety of emotional disorders that occur in women after childbirth. However, it is more useful to reserve the term for a specific depressive illness affecting around 10% to 15% of women in the first year after birth (see Box 4.1). It must be distinguished from the 'baby blues' which affects as many as 50% of women in the first week after childbirth. The blues is characterised by tearfulness and emotional lability, usually responds to simple reassurance, is self-limiting, and is most likely to have a hormonal aetiology (Stein, 1982; Yalom *et al.*, 1968; Pitt, 1973).

Puerperal psychosis

In a very few instances the blues may herald the onset of a much rarer disorder, puerperal psychosis. This very serious illness affects only 1–2 women per thousand and has its onset in the first month after the birth (Paffenbarger, 1964; Kendell *et al.*, 1987; Brockington & Cox-Roper, 1988). Puerperal psychosis is a florid disorder which may manifest itself with signs of either mania or depression. Alternatively, there may be overt psychotic phenomena with disordered thinking, paranoia and confusion and women may even have ideas of harming themselves or the baby. It is likely to have a hormonal aetiology and occurs more often in younger women, primiparae, women with a personal or family past history of psychosis and possibly after a caesarean section.

Disorder	Prevalence	Onset
The blues	50%	3–7 days
Postnatal depression	10–15%	0–6 months
Puerperal psychosis	0.1–0.2%	1–4 weeks

Box 4.1 *Childbirth-related emotional disorders.*

Puerperal psychosis is usually best treated in hospital in a specialised mother and baby unit, where expert care can be provided. Although it usually responds well to treatment with the major tranquillisers and antidepressants, electroconvulsive therapy (ECT) is occasionally required. A full recovery is usual, but relapse after a subsequent pregnancy may occur in up to 50% of women. There is increasing interest in caring for these women in the community using aggressive outreach programmes from the secondary care sector (Oates, 1988). There are thought to be many benefits from this approach particularly with respect to the mental health of the partner and the success of the bonding of the mother and infant.

Postnatal depression

Phenomenology

In terms of severity, postnatal depression sits somewhere between the blues and puerperal psychosis, but from a public health perspective, due to its high prevalence, it is probably the most important adverse psychological outcome of childbirth. There seems to be good evidence that it affects at least 10% to 15% of women in the first postnatal year, usually beginning in the first three months and lasting in some cases for a year or more (Cox, Connor & Kendell, 1982; Kumar & Robson, 1984; Watson *et al.*, 1984).

This depression may be the start of a chronic relapsing illness or a relatively short-lived episode never to be repeated. In either case, the consequences for the woman herself, both at home and at work, for her partner and the quality of their relationship, and for her family and friends, may be irrevocable.

Postnatal depression can also have particularly adverse effects on the mother–infant relationship and subsequently on child behaviour and intellectual development (Cogill *et al.*, 1986; Caplan *et al.*, 1989; Murray, 1992; Sharp *et al.*, 1995).

Postnatal depression has attracted a lot of research interest over the last 20 years, perhaps stimulated by Brice Pitt's description in 1968 of 'atypical' depression following childbirth (Pitt, 1968). It is important at this stage to emphasise that postnatal depression is very definitely a general practice disorder and is in fact typical of the sort of depression that general practitioners see every day in their surgeries. It is hardly ever seen by psychiatrists in their hospital practice and as such does not conform to some of their rigid diagnostic criteria for major depression. This is why Pitt, a psychiatrist, described the depression he found in his study as 'atypical'.

Diagnosis

Postnatal depression is often part of the 'hidden' psychiatric morbidity which general practitioners are at present being exhorted to uncover (Goldberg & Huxley, 1992). The wide variation in symptomatology makes it difficult to diagnose, especially since some women are not aware that the symptoms from which they are suffering are due to depression (see Box 4.2). This is particularly true when somatic symptoms predominate.

The clinical features of postnatal depression are essentially those of a neurotic depression, with anxiety and irritability accompanying depressed mood. Tearfulness and tiredness contribute to a feeling of general inadequacy. Poor concentration, loss of appetite and insomnia may also be present. Loss of libido is often profound and may further damage an already strained marital relationship. Vague physical symptoms such as headache, backache and vaginal discharge for which no cause can be found are common. In a few women, obsessional thoughts about harming the baby may be present and, in a minority of women, the level of misery is so great that suicide is contemplated.

Anxiety and irritability often accompany depressed mood

Tearfulness and tiredness contribute to a feeling of general inadequacy

Poor concentration, loss of appetite and insomnia may also be present

Loss of libido is often profound and may further damage an already strained marital relationship

Vague physical symptoms such as headache, backache and vaginal discharge for which no obvious cause can be found are common

---

Box 4.2 *Symptoms of postnatal depression.*

The unhappy, irritable and exhausted mother who presents
frequently in the surgery, often on account of her children, is
familiar to us all in primary care. Hopefully, many general practitioners would recognize this woman's distress and would enquire
generally about her health but more specifically about her mood
and how she was feeling, regardless of whether the consultation
was for herself or for one of the children. However, that is just one
stereotype for postnatal depression. There are many others, and
one in particular comes to mind: the *masked depression*, the mother
who rarely consults, comes in smiling, who always looks immacu-
late, and who never consults for anything other than physical
symptoms. Suddenly her guard is down and you find that behind
the smile, is a woman overwhelmingly concerned with keeping up
the appearance of the perfect mother and wife whilst in reality there
are tears and torture: worries about her feelings for the baby,
concern about her imminent return to work, loss of libido resulting
in strain on the marriage, problems keeping the housework and
washing up to date, and generally not coping as well as she would
like. There are many other possible scenarios. The message is that
in fact any new mother can develop postnatal depression and the
concern of those working in primary care is how might we be able
to predict which women are most at risk.

Does it really exist?
Given the prevalence of depression generally in women (one month
prevalence rates between 6% and 10%) (Paykel, 1991), the question
has been posed as to whether postnatal depression exists as a distinct
syndrome. Although the existence of puerperal psychosis has been
known for well over 100 years, it is only in the last 20 or so years
that postnatal depression has been recognised as a separate diagnostic entity requiring treatment. However, it is worth noting that
neither puerperal psychosis nor postnatal depression appeared in
the International Classification of Diseases (ICD-9) (WHO, 1978)
or the Diagnostic and Statistical Manual (DSM-IIIR) (American
Psychiatric Association, 1980). Furthermore, there have always
been those, both medical and non-medical, who do not believe that
it exists and that women with young babies should stop grumbling
and just get on and cope regardless of the enormous difficulties that
some women experience.

At the other end of the spectrum, there is no doubt that the
women's movement has had a part to play in bringing postnatal
depression into the public eye. Thus voluntary organisations such
as the National Childbirth Trust (NCT), the Association for Postnatal Depression (APNI), Meet-a-Mum Association (MAMA) and
others have played a major role in bringing postnatal depression onto
the agenda of health professionals and the statutory bodies. This has
had the effect not only of educating women themselves about

a possible cause for their symptoms but also of increasing the sensitivity of health care professionals to women's psychological needs around this vulnerable period.

There have been several controlled studies whose results query whether there is in fact an increased incidence of depression after childbirth (Cooper *et al.*, 1988; O'Hara *et al.*, 1990; Cox, Murray & Chapman, 1993). None of these studies has been carried out in a primary care setting and only the Cox study used instruments appropriate to the type of morbidity commonly encountered in United Kingdom (UK) primary care. None of these studies reported a difference in the prevalence of depression in the six months following childbirth between their controls and the postnatal women. However, there was a consensus that there is indeed an increased incidence of depression in the first few weeks after birth.

At the present time, the evidence is in favour of the existence of postnatal depression, a disorder mainly seen in primary care, occurring in the first few months after delivery, but not always reaching the threshold for depression using rigid psychiatric diagnostic criteria. However, it must be recognized that this level of depression may still be extremely distressing and disabling, especially in a new mother.

Epidemiology

There has been some consensus between several studies undertaken by mental health professionals of the likely risk factors for developing postnatal depression. However, translating these predictors into a programme for prevention in primary care is hindered by the systematic bias in these studies towards a clinical psychiatric population rather than a general practice consulting population.

In terms of aetiology, the overwhelming weight of evidence supports the importance of a *history of depression* particularly during pregnancy, *marital disharmony*, and *social adversity*. For other factors such as parity, age, social class and obstetric circumstances the evidence is equivocal (O'Hara & Zekoski, 1988; Sharp, 1993).

Is it worth preventing?

The high prevalence of postnatal depression at a key point in the life of women who are in regular contact with the health service makes it an ideal candidate for primary prevention. Furthermore, the severity and duration of some episodes, often reaching criteria for major depression and lasting for at least a year, together with its potential simultaneously to adversely affect the development of the child and the marital relationship, suggests that effort put into its prevention or early detection would certainly offer health gain in the long term.

There are several studies that have provided data to counter the argument that postnatal depression is a mild and self-limiting disorder and its non-detection by general practitioners irrelevant. In a study in Edinburgh (Holden, Sagovsky & Cox, 1989) of 53 depressed women, four attempted suicide and others said that they had felt suicidal. Several studies have found that postnatal depression frequently lasts for a year or more (Pitt, 1968; Cox et al., 1982; Watson et al., 1984; Kumar & Robson, 1984). Maternal mental illness may adversely affect a child both directly through neglect, physical harm, or psychological distress, or indirectly through associated features such as marital disharmony and repeated admission to hospital.

Effects on the marital relationship

The quality of the marital relationship to a large extent determines the emotional climate in which the child develops, and many studies have found that a poor marital relationship is a risk factor for postnatal depression. In addition, one of the symptoms of postnatal depression is irritability, particularly with the partner, and marital breakdown is found to be more common after the birth of a child.

Effects on the mother–infant relationship

Postnatal depression may affect the way a mother views her child from a very early stage. Women who are depressed are less likely to breast feed their baby (Cooper, Murray & Stein, 1993). Expressing dislike, indifference, and negative feelings towards their baby at six weeks after birth, and reporting temperamental difficulties at three months have been reported more frequently in women with postnatal depression (Holden, 1991).

Several studies have shown adverse effects on the cognitive and behavioural development of the child if the mother is depressed in the first year after the birth A study in North London (Cogill et al., 1986) of a 4-year follow up of a postpartum sample, found that the children of mothers who suffered from postnatal depression were significantly delayed on a general cognitive index compared to controls. At 19 months, Stein et al. (1991) found that mother–infant interactions were less affectively positive and less mutually responsive in women with postnatal depression compared to controls. Murray found that infants of depressed mothers performed worse on object concept tasks, were more insecure and showed more mild behavioural difficulties at 18 months postnatal (Murray, 1992). Whereas Murray found that postnatal depression had no effect on general cognitive and language development, other studies have found a specific effect of depression in the first postnatal year on the cognitive development of boys (Sharp et al., 1995).

Preventing postnatal depression

Postnatal depression places an enormous burden on women and their families and although early detection and treatment can offer a good prognosis, prevention is increasingly possible. Three criteria can be used to define good practice (see Box 4.3).

First, current understanding of aetiology must be used to *define a high risk group* and a plan devised to reduce that risk. Second, the support offered in terms of mental health promotion should *help people find their own solutions*. Third, the most appropriate intervention will *draw on support from friends and relatives and voluntary groups* rather than on mental health professionals.

Principles of prevention

Jenkins offers us a useful model on which to develop our ideas for prevention of depression (Jenkins, 1992). She divides the aetiological factors into predisposing, precipitating and maintaining and then further subclassifies each factor as biological, social or psychological.

Considering postnatal depression we can use this model as follows:

1. Predisposing factors: increased vulnerability to postnatal depression in the future.
   (i)   biological: family history of depression, personal history of depression, low IQ.
   (ii)   social: emotional deprivation in childhood, loss or prolonged separation from parents or spouse, chronic work or marital difficulties, poor social support.
   (iii) psychological: poor parenting (possibly due to mental illness in parents or marital disharmony in parents), low self-esteem, learned helplessness, neurotic personality trait.
2. Precipitating factors: determine when postnatal depression occurs, i.e. after which particular pregnancy or at what particular time after delivery.
   (i)   biological: hormonal upheaval of delivery, breastfeeding, caesarian section
   (ii)   social: recent life events, especially loss events such as loss of job with consequent financial difficulties and social isolation, separation from spouse, death of a parent.
   (iii) psychological: poor adaptive response to the adversity of the above biological and social precipitating factors.
3. Maintaining factors: determine length of illness.
   (i)   biological: hormonal imbalance.
   (ii)   social: chronic social stress especially in relation to housing, finances, work, marital relationship, exacerbated in absence of close confiding relationship.
   (iii) psychological: low self-esteem, dependant personality.

Prevention can be divided into primary, secondary and tertiary (Caplan, 1964).

Primary prevention of postnatal depression

In postnatal depression this requires activity on the part of the primary care team which will allow the identification of risk factors for depression either during the pregnancy or before and thus minimise the likelihood of onset.

It would appear that, although there are well defined risk factors for postnatal depression, it is a disorder that can affect any woman in the six months after delivery. This potential universality allows us to consider some measures of primary prevention that can be directed at the whole population of pregnant women. The UK system of health care, with National Health (NHS) services available for all at the point of delivery, provides a unique opportunity for health promotion and preventive medicine (see Box 4.4).

Pre-conceptual counselling for couples contemplating pregnancy is increasingly common and provides an excellent opportunity to elicit the presence of risk factors for postnatal depression as well as to assess the current mental state of the woman. Discussion about employment and returning to work after the birth, housing, social support, the relationship with parents and in-laws, are just some of the topics which may bring to light the presence of risk factors for a childbirth-related emotional disorder. It certainly seems from recent research that a planned pregnancy, in the context of a good quality relationship, with support from friends and relatives, and the possibility of returning to work, offers the greatest likelihood of avoiding postnatal depression (Sharp, 1993).

The *antenatal clinics* that are increasingly part of every general practice's range of services can be used to provide information during pregnancy to all women about postnatal depression. With the dramatic fall in maternal and perinatal mortality that has occurred this century, together with the decrease in the average family size, there has been a tendency to assume that the adverse sequelae of childbirth are a thing of the past. In addition, the general taboo about mental illness and the suggestion that to inform

---

Define a high-risk group and plan to reduce the risk

Help people find their own solutions

Devise interventions that use friends, relatives and voluntary groups rather than mental health professionals

---

Box 4.3 *Good practice in preventing mental illness.*

women about postnatal depression could in itself cause the disorder has mitigated against the use of antenatal clinics to provide this essential service of primary prevention of a distressing emotional disorder.

Pregnancy itself is not without risk for the onset of depression and indeed some women may already be depressed at the time they become pregnant. As antenatal care moves ever further into the responsibility of the primary health care team as well as the woman herself, the continuity of care it provides lends itself ideally to discussion of such sensitive topics.

General practitioners, midwives and health visitors, who will be seeing women with enormous frequency both before and after the birth, are ideally placed to provide information about postnatal depression in an acceptable way and to monitor women's emotional well-being during the pregnancy and thereafter. If the one-to-one provision of such information is felt to be inappropriate, the use of antenatal preparation classes, leaflets, videos and informal patient-led groups may be a more useful medium.

Social support as a tool for primary prevention

It is during pregnancy that the predisposing factors for postnatal depression should be ascertained, as it is only in this way that true primary prevention can take place. Obviously it is not possible to turn back the clock and to remove the adverse life events of childhood such as the early loss of a parent, nor is it possible to offer women a quick and easy remedy to their housing and financial problems. However, it does seem to be the case that allowing the pregnant woman time to express her fears and worries about some of these social issues, in addition to providing the more usual medical model of antenatal care, is worthwhile and may result in a reduction in depression after the birth.

Several studies have looked at different forms of social support designed to provide this extra preventive aspect of antenatal care. As long ago as the late 1950s the Gordons in New Jersey reported that antenatal classes which paid specific attention to the social and psychological stresses of parenthood were effective in reducing the incidence of postpartum depression (Gordon & Gordon, 1960). It is interesting to note that, in one of the experimental groups, husbands also attended the classes and the results for this group of women revealed the lowest incidence of postpartum depression. Nearly three decades later, Elliott and her colleagues in south-east London used psychologist- and health visitor-led groups to achieve a similar objective with first and second time mothers defined as potentially vulnerable to postnatal depression (Elliott, Sanjack & Leverton, 1988).

Another study found that altering the role of midwives to provide a social intervention to women with a history of a low-birthweight baby was effective in reducing the incidence of post-natal depression (Oakley, Rajan & Grant, 1990). In a more informal fashion, many general practices and health centres provide *drop-in groups* for pregnant women, usually in association with the ante-natal clinic, which are led by health visitors and midwives and allow time for discussion of a particular topic as well as a general discussion of problems brought by members of the group. This format may allow the discussion of the emotional disorders related to childbirth with greater coverage and in a less threatening format than the one-to-one situation.

The recent government report, *Changing Childbirth* (Expert Maternity Group, 1993), placed great emphasis on the need to offer a more woman-centred type of antenatal care which provided more social support for women and their partners at this time of tran-sition in their lives. Despite the fact that one outcome of this report might be a general reduction in the total number of antenatal visits, the change in emphasis from a purely medical model to the incor-poration of a definite psychosocial agenda should result in greater attention being paid to mental health promotion in pregnant women.

Screening questionnaires

Some form of screening for emotional disorders during the preg-nancy, and for risk factors for postnatal depression, can be built into the antenatal care schedule. Knowledge of a woman's personal psychiatric history, her usual mental state, and any risk factors for depression during pregnancy or the puerperium, is the *sine qua non* for best practice in mental health promotion. Building in a routine set of questions at each antenatal visit or using a self-report ques-tionnaire are just two methods that can be used. The Edinburgh Postnatal Depression Scale (EPDS) (Cox, Holden & Sagovsky, 1987) which was originally developed for the postnatal period has now been validated for use during pregnancy (Murray & Cox, 1990), but other scales might also have a place depending on whether the intention is to screen for disorder or to confirm clinical suspicion of the presence of a psychiatric disorder.

Difficult births

It is surprising that the events of the labour and delivery themselves seem to have very little relation to the later development of postnatal depression. Thus there appears to be no real benefit to be gained from offering extra support to women who have had a particularly unpleasant or traumatic birth. However, studies have been reported that show that just as women who have a companion in labour have a better obstetric outcome (Sosa *et al.*, 1980; Klaus *et al.*, 1986), they are also less likely to have lower scores on anxiety and depression inventories at six weeks postnatal (Wolman *et al.*, 1993).

Secondary prevention

If risk factors are assessed during pregnancy, the question then arises as to how best to ensure that women identified as high risk receive the appropriate health or social care. Studies of secondary prevention of postnatal depression suggest that increased health visitor intervention in the early weeks after delivery might offer one way of diminishing the likelihood that a woman at risk will become a 'case'.

The best evidence for this comes from the work of Holden and colleagues in Edinburgh who found that, when health visitors made special visits to women suffering from postnatal depression, (defined by a score of 12 on the EPDS), to offer six sessions of mother-centred counselling, the women were less likely to be ill than women who had received routine care (Holden *et al.*, 1989). This use of health visitors in a different role, i.e. mother-centred rather than baby-centred, has gained wide approval and training programmes for them to be able to extend their role in this way are now being reported (Gerrard *et al.*, 1993).

In a similar vein, a study of highly anxious postpartum women in Australia found that a professional intervention from a social worker was more effective than a non-professional intervention or no intervention at all in lowering anxiety state levels (Barnett & Parker, 1985).

Screening for psychiatric disorder, in both primary and secondary care service settings, is increasingly being used to improve detection rates. Instruments which have been used in this context include the General Health Questionnaire or GHQ (Goldberg & Williams, 1988), the Hospital Anxiety and Depression scale, or HADS (Zigmond & Snaith, 1983) and the Beck Depression Inventory, or BDI (Beck *et al.*, 1961). An assessment of the relative merits of the different rating scales available to screen for postnatal depression has been undertaken by Harris and colleagues in Cardiff (Harris *et al.*, 1989).

It has been shown time and again that the clinical judgement of primary health care professionals is *not* sufficiently sensitive to pick up more than about half the cases of depression (Freeling *et al.*, 1985) and postnatal depression is no exception (Briscoe, 1986). It is likely that a combination of asking appropriate questions about the risk factors for depression, followed by the judicious use of a standardised questionnaire, offers the greatest likelihood of early detection of depression during pregnancy and in the postnatal period. The use of a self-report questionnaire such as the EPDS may have the effect not only of increasing physician awareness of postnatal depression (Webster *et al.*, 1994), but might also increase the likelihood of a woman discussing her distress with that physician (Schaper *et al.*, 1994).

Conclusion

Improving the ability of general practitioners and other primary care professionals involved in antenatal and postnatal care to detect the signs of depression during pregnancy or the early puerperium would most certainly help shorten the time that women suffer with their symptoms, and ensure that appropriate treatment was instituted at a much earlier stage. There is plenty of evidence in the literature about the efficacy of skills training to improve the mental health skills of general practitioners (Gask, McGrath & Goldberg, 1987) and the postgraduate education of midwives and health visitors is paying increasing attention to this important area (Gerrard *et al.*, 1993; Lepper, Dimatteo & Tinsley, 1994).

There is a case to be made for a much greater emphasis to be paid to all aspects of mental health in the training of health professionals involved in the care of the pregnant woman and the newly delivered mother. In accordance with the current fashion for developing guidelines to inform 'best practice' and also clinical audit which form part of general practitioners' terms of service under their 1990 contract, a joint initiative between psychiatrists and general practitioners for secondary prevention is underway in Nottingham to try to improve the care of women with postnatal depression by improving detection and offering appropriate treatment with antidepressants (M. Oates, personal communication).

Postnatal depression is a common and distressing illness and provides health professionals with an excellent paradigm for developing packages of preventive care that might be used in other areas of mental health promotion. It is a disorder that is characteristically rather difficult to diagnose and one that is unlikely to be amenable to a preventive programme that relies solely on primary prevention. It is therefore vitally important that general practitioners, midwives and health visitors keep up to date in this rapidly moving field in order that they make the most of their unique position (Box 4.4), and whilst providing continuity of care to an at-risk group, constantly monitor the mental state of the pregnant and newly delivered mother.

Mental illness is one of the five key areas in the government's Health of the Nation strategy (Department of Health, DOH, 1991). Prevention is one of the cornerstones of its longer-term success, and postnatal depression is identified as an area in which there is a compelling case to be made for all professional groups to develop the appropriate skills for its care and treatment.

In summary, the predictors for postnatal depression are perhaps

Pre-conceptual counselling
Antenatal clinics
Postnatal visit
Baby clinics
Family planning clinics
Routine surgery consultations

Box 4.4 *Opportunities for prevention: primary and secondary.*

not surprising . . . an unplanned pregnancy, a poor marriage, financial difficulties, housing problems . . . enough to make any of us depressed. And a new baby on top of all that. A reasonable explanatory model for this illness fits very closely with that put forward by Brown and Harris in their work *Social origins of depression* (Brown & Harris, 1978, Chapter 2). Postnatal depression seems to occur in those women who possess certain *vulnerability factors* and in whom the pregnancy acts as a *provoking factor* for the onset of depression. It is 'the straw that breaks the camel's back'.

Summary

To prevent postnatal depression, we need first to dispel the myth that it is an uncommon disorder which invariably requires referral to a psychiatrist. Secondly, women need to be provided with more information during their pregnancy about both normal and abnormal psychological reactions to childbirth, so that they can ask for help when necessary. Thirdly, the primary care team needs to be able to predict who is most likely to succumb so that preventive measures and treatment can be instituted. Fourthly, general practitioners and health visitors need to acquire the skills that will allow more accurate recognition and treatment of psychological morbidity during the first postnatal year. Such treatment will often entail effective liaison between members of the primary care team as well as improved communication with their colleagues in the hospital and the community (Sharp, 1992).

References

American Psychiatric Association (1980). *Diagnostic and Statistical Manual of Mental Disorders* (3rd ed). Washington, DC.

Barnett, B. & Parker, G. (1985). Professional and non-professional intervention for highly anxious primiparous mothers. *British Journal of Psychiatry*, **146**, 287–93.

Beck, A.T., Ward C.H., Mendelson, M. Mock, J. & Erbaugh, J. (1961). An inventory for measuring depression. *Archives of General Psychiatry*, **34**, 1229–35.

Briscoe, M. (1986). Identification of emotional problems in postpartum women by health visitors. *British Medical Journal*. **292**, 1245–47.

Brockington, I. & Cox-Roper, A. (1988). The nosology of puerperal mental illness. In *Motherhood and Mental Illness (2)* Kumar, R. & Brockington, eds. England: Wright.

Brown, G.W. & Harris, T. (1978). *Social Origins of Depression*. London: Tavistock.

Caplan, G. (1964). *Principles of Preventive Psychiatry*. New York: Basic Books.

Caplan, J., Cogill, S., Alexandra, H., Robson, K., Katz, R. & Kumar, R. (1989). Material depression and the emotional development of the child. *British Journal of Psychiatry*, **154**, 818–23.

Cogill, S., Caplan, H., Alexandra, H., Robson, K. & Kumar R. (1986). Impact of maternal postnatal depression on cognitive development of young children. *British Medical Journal*, **292**, 1165–7.

Cooper, P., Campbell E., Day, A., Kennerley, H. & Bond, A. (1988). Non-psychotic psychiatric disorder after childbirth. A prospective study of prevalence, incidence, course and nature. *British Journal of Psychiatry*, **152**, 799–806.

Cooper, P.J., Murray, L. & Stein, A. (1993). Psychosocial factors associated with the early termination of breast-feeding. *Journal of Psychosomatic Research*, **37**, 171–6.

Cox, J., Connor, Y. & Kendell, R. (1982). Prospective study of the psychiatric disorders of childbirth. *British Journal of Psychiatry*, **140**, 782–6.

Cox, J., Holden, J. & Sagovsky, R. (1987). Detection of postnatal depression: development of the 10-item Edinburgh postnatal depression scale. *British Journal of Psychiatry*, **150**, 782–6.

Cox, J.L., Murray, D. & Chapman, G. (1993). A controlled study of the onset, duration and prevalence of postnatal depression. *British Journal of Psychiatry*, **163**, 27–31.

DOH. (1993). Key Area Handbook–Mental Illness, London: HMSO.

Elliott, S.A., Sanjack, M. & Leverton, T.F. (1988). Parents' groups in pregnancy – a preventive intervention for postnatal depression? In *Marshalling Social Support: Formats, Processes and Effects*, Gottlieb, B. H., ed., pp. 87–111, Sage Publications.

Expert Maternity Group (1993). *Changing Childbirth*. London: HMSO.

Freeling, P., Rao, B.M., Paykel, E.S., Sireling, L.I. & Burton, R.H. (1985). Unrecognised depression in general practice. *British Medical Journal*, **290**, 1880–83.

Gask, L., McGrath, G. & Goldberg, D. (1987). Improving the psychiatric skills of established general practitioners; evaluation of group teaching. *Medical Education*, **21**, 362–8.

Gerrard, J., Holden, J.M., Elliott, S.A., McKenzie, P., McKenzie, J. & Cox, J.L. (1993). A trainer's perspective of an innovative programme teaching health visitors about the detection, treatment and prevention of postnatal depression. *Journal of Advanced Nursing*, **18**, 1825–32

Goldberg, D. & Huxley, P. (1992). *Common Mental Disorders: A Bio-Social Model*. London: Routledge.

Goldberg, D. & Williams, P. (1988). *The General Health Questionnaire: A User's Guide*. Windsor: NFER. Nelson.

Gordon, R.E. & Gordon, K.E. (1960). Social factors in the prevention of postpartum emotional problems. *Obstetrics and Gynecology*, **15**, 433–8.

Harris, B., Huckle, P., Thomas, R., Johns, S. & Fung, F. (1989). The use of rating scales to identify postnatal depression. *British Journal of Psychiatry*, **154**, 814–16.

Holden, J. (1991). Postnatal depression: its nature, effects and identification using the Edinburgh Postnatal Depression Scale. Birth, **18**, 211–21.

Holden, J., Sagovsky, R. & Cox, J. (1989). Counselling in a general practice setting: controlled study of health visitor intervention in treatment of postnatal depression. *British Journal of Psychiatry*, **298**, 223–6.

Jenkins, R. (1992). Depression and anxiety: an overview of preventive strategies. In *The Prevention of Anxiety and Depression: The Role of the Primary Care Team*. London: HMSO.

Kendell, R., Chalmers, J.C. & Platz, C. (1987). Epidemiology of puerperal psychosis. *British Journal of Psychiatry*, **150**, 662–73.

Klaus, M.H., Kennel, J.H., Robertson, S.S. & Sosa, R. (1986). Effects of social support during parturition on maternal and infant morbidity. *British Medical Journal*, **293**, 585–7.

Kumar, R. & Robson, K. (1984). A prospective study of emotional disorders in childbearing women. *British Journal of Psychiatry*, **144**, 35–47.

Lepper H.S., Dimatteo, M.R. & Tinsley, B.J. (1994). Postpartum depression: how much do obstetric nurses and obstetricians know? *Birth*, **21**, 149–54.

Murray, D. & Cox, J.L. (1990). Screening for depression during pregnancy with the Edinburgh depression scale (EPDS). *Journal of Reproductive and Infant Psychology*, **8**, 99–107.

Murray, L. (1992). The impact of postnatal depression on infant development. *Journal of Child Psychology and Psychiatry*, **33**, 543–61.

O'Hara, M. & Zekoski, E. (1988). Postpartum depression – a comprehensive review. In *Motherhood and Mental Illness (2)*. Kumar, R. & Brockington, I. eds. England: Wright.

O'Hara, M., Zekoski, E., Philipps, L. & Wright, E. (1990). Controlled prospective study of postpartum mood disorders: comparison of childbearing and non-childbearing women. *Journal of Abnormal Psychology*, **99**, 3–15.

Oakley, A., Rajan, L. & Grant, A. (1990). Social support and pregnancy outcome. *British Journal of Obstetrics and Gynaecology*, **97**, 155–62.

Oates, M. (1988). The development of an integrated community-orientated service for severe postnatal mental illness. *In Motherhood and Mental Illness (2)*. Kumar, R. and Brockington, I., eds. England: Wright.

Paffenbarger, R. (1964). Epidemiological aspects of postpartum mental illness. *British Journal of Preventive Social Medicine*, **18**, 189–95.

Paykel, E.S. (1991). Depression in women. *British Journal of Psychiatry*, **158**, 22–9

Pitt, B. (1968). Atypical depression following childbirth. *British Journal of Psychiatry*, **114**, 1325–35.

Pitt B. (1973). Maternity blues. *British Journal of Psychiatry*, **122**, 431–3.

Schaper, A.M., Rooney, B.L., Kay, N.R. & Silva, P.D. (1994). Use of the Edinburgh postnatal depression scale to identify postpartum depression in a clinical setting. *Journal of Reproductive Medicine*, **39**, 620–3.

Sharp, D. (1992). Predicting postnatal depression. In *The Prevention of Depression and Anxiety: The Role of the Primary Care Team*. London: HMSO.

Sharp, D. (1993). Childbirth related emotional disorders in primary care: a longitudinal prospective study. Unpublished PhD Thesis. University of London.

Sharp, D., Hale, D., Pawlby, S., Schmücker, G., Allen, H. & Kumar, R. (1995). The impact of postnatal depression on boys' intellectual development. *Journal of Child Psychology and Psychiatry*, **36**, 8.

Sosa, R., Kennell, J., Klaus, M., Robertson, S. & Urrutia, J. (1980). The effect of a supportive companion on perinatal problems, the length of labour, and mother–infant interaction. *New England Journal of Medicine*, **303**, 597–600.

Stein, A., Gath, D.H., Bond, A., Day, A. & Cooper, P.J. (1991). The relationship between postnatal depression and mother–child interaction. *British Journal of Psychiatry*, **158**, 46–52.

Stein, G. (1982). The maternity blues. In *Motherhood and Mental Illness (1)*. Brockington, I. and Kumar R. eds. London: Academic Press.

Watson, J., Elliott, S., Rugg, A. & Brough, D. (1984). Psychiatric disorder in pregnancy and the first postnatal year. *British Journal of Psychiatry*, **144**, 453–62.

Webster, K.L., Thompson, J.M.D., Mitchell, E.A. & Werry, J.S. (1994). Postnatal depression in a community cohort. *Australian and New Zealand Journal of Psychiatry*, **28**, 42–9.

Wolman, W-L., Chalmers, N., Hofmeyr, J. & Nikodem, V.C. (1993). Postpartum depression and companionship in the clinical birth environment: a randomised, controlled study. *American Journal of Obstetrics and Gynecology*, **168**, 1388–93.

World Health Organisation (1978). *Mental Disorders: Glossary and Guide to their Classification in Accordance with the Ninth Revision of International Classification of Diseases*. Geneva: WHO.

Yalom, I. Lunde, D., Moos, R. & Hamburg, I. (1968). Postpartum blues syndrome. *Archives of General Psychiatry*, **18**, 16–27.

Zigmond, A. & Snaith, R. (1983). The hospital anxiety and depression scale. *Acta Psychiatrica Scandinavica*, **67**, 361–70.

[5] Bereavement

Colin Murray Parkes

Introduction

Bereavement is a prime example of a major stress which carries with it a risk to physical and mental health. There is now reason to believe that this risk can be reduced by appropriate action before or at the time of the bereavement. The primary health care team are in an ideal position to assess the risk and, when it is necessary, to intervene. The chapter which follows highlights some of the major issues and the reader is referred to *Bereavement: Studies of Grief in Adult Life* (Parkes, 1986) and to the other volumes referenced here for a more detailed account of a field that has developed a great deal in recent years.

Effects of bereavement on physical and mental health

The effects of bereavement on health have been attested in numerous studies many of which have been reviewed by the American Medical Association (Osterweiss, Solomon & Green, 1984). They showed increases in use of health care services, particularly in countries where fees are not charged to the user. Mortality rates are increased and the risk of certain specific medical disorders, notably hyperthyroidism, is increased. Suicide rates are increased as is the risk of affective disorders and other psychiatric conditions (Box 5.1).

Further research has begun to explain some of the links between the psychological and physical effects of bereavement. There is evidence that the immune response system is impaired during the early months of bereavement. This impairment correlates with the intensity of depression and it seems likely that it would be reduced by any action which reduces depression. The effects on mortality are largely explained by an increase in the death rate from myocardial infarction. This is likely to result from autonomic effects on an already damaged myocardium. The risk is much greater in men than in women and this suggests that it may relate to the masculine tendency to repress grief rather than to its expression. Effects of

Increased use of health care systems

Increased mortality (particularly heart disease and suicide)

Psychosomatic disorders (e.g. hyperthyroidism)

Aggravation of pre-existing disorders (e.g. muscle and joint conditions)

Psychiatric disorders
  (a) *non-specific stress disorders (e.g. reactive anxiety and depression, post-traumatic stress disorder)*
  (b) *pathological grief (chronic grief, delayed grief, inhibited grief and identification reactions)*

Box 5.1 *Effects of bereavement on health.*

bereavement on the neuro–endocrine system are complex and the only ones which may be specific to bereavement are changes in prolactin and growth hormone levels. These seem to correlate with the intensity of separation distress rather than with depression but not to the point where they could be used as a biological measure of grief (see Jacob's 1993 book for a full review of recent research).

The psychiatric disorders which complicate bereavement include *affective disorders*, particularly anxiety and depressive reactions, *post-traumatic stress disorder*, disorders resulting from *abuse of alcohol or other drugs*, and a wide variety of other reactions which reflect the personal vulnerability of the person rather than the bereavement. Some reactions are specific to bereavement: the so-called pathological grief reactions. These include *chronic grief* (an unusually intense and protracted grief), *delayed or inhibited grief* (in which the normal expression of grief is absent or minimal but partial or full expression then occurs at inappropriate times or in ways which interfere with normal functioning) and *identification reactions* (hypochondriacal disorders closely resembling the illness of the dead person). The causes of these psychiatric complications will be considered in conjunction with the factors which determine risk.

Normal grief

Many of those who seek help from the primary health care team are not 'sick' in any real meaning of the word. Certainly, grief is not an illness requiring treatment and it is important for professionals not to label bereaved people as suffering from 'depression' or other psychiatric disorders when in fact they are simply grieving. We should not refuse help to people simply because they do not have a psychiatric diagnosis. Offering help to people at crisis points in their lives can prevent psychiatric disorders.

Although there is individual, familial and cultural variation in the response to bereavement, there is a pattern to grieving. The typical reaction to a major loss, such as the death of a husband, will first be described as will the normal range of response seen in western societies.

Patterns of grieving

Grief can best be seen as the outcome of a conflict between a deeply felt need to cry aloud and to search for the one who is gone, and a counter-urge to maintain control. The adult knows very well that crying for a dead person will not bring them back, but we have a powerful impulse to do just that. What emerges is a compromise.

At the moment of death there is often a reaction of *acute distress* often including anger. People may hit out irrationally and say things that they later regret. Usually, within a few minutes, they are back in control and there often follows a period of *numbness* or blunting of emotions which may last for a few hours or days.

This is followed by the 'pangs of grief', episodes of *intense pining* or yearning for the lost person, which alternate with *periods of apathy*. The pangs are triggered by any reminder of the loss. People oscillate back and forth between approaching and avoiding these painful pangs.

In the early stage of bereavement people may find it difficult to take in and fully realise the implications of the death. They spend a long time thinking about the events leading up to the loss as if, even now, they could find out what went wrong and put it right. In their search for an explanation they may accuse something or someone whom they see as to blame. Often, this is someone close to them, or it may be a doctor or nurse who did or did not do something which might have contributed to the death. Many of these accusations are irrational, reflecting the intensity of the rage that may be a part of grieving. Unfortunately this can lead to estrangement from the very people whom the bereaved need to support them. Carers who recognise this reaction for what it is, a part of grieving, are unlikely to be hurt by it.

The urge to search is typically accompanied by a vivid mental image of the dead person who is often felt to be near at hand. At times people misidentify sights or sounds as indicators of the presence of the lost person. A widow will see her husband in the street, then, as the other person gets closer, she realises her mistake. Vivid hallucinations in which the dead person appears nearby may occur at times when people are in a drowsy state of mind. They are reported by up to 50% of bereaved people and are not a sign of psychosis. Sometimes these hallucinations continue for great lengths of time but more often they fade away as time passes. A similar phenomenon is the bereavement dream in which the dead person is alive again. Even in the dream, however, there is usually some sign that the person is not fully alive. These dreams are characteristically very vivid, so much so that the bereaved may feel that the real world is less real than the dream world.

So great is the intensity of anxiety during these early stages that the bereaved commonly suffer minor symptoms reflecting the repeated arousal of the sympathetic nervous system and inhibition of the parasympathetic. The ability to concentrate is impaired and this affects short-term memory to a minor degree. People find it difficult to get to sleep at night and their sleep is restless. Others find themselves sleeping excessively. Appetite is impaired and many people lose weight during the first month or so. By three months, normal appetite has usually been regained and by a year many bereaved people have put on too much weight.

While bereaved people seldom disbelieve the fact of the death, it takes a long time to discover just what this means. Loved people are a part of our 'assumptive world', the world which we assume to exist on the basis of our experience up to now. This internal model of the world enables us to recognise the world that we meet and plan our behaviour accordingly. It includes everything that we take for granted, habits of thought built up over many years that are not easy to change. A widow, out of habit, will lay the table for two, then realise that there are no longer two people to eat breakfast. Every chain of thought seems to lead to a blind alley. Perhaps the person who died was the person to whom we naturally turned at times of trouble. Now that we are faced with the biggest trouble we have ever experienced, we find ourselves repeatedly turning toward someone who is not there. Each time we do this we experience another pang of grief.

The term *'grief work'* was coined by Sigmund Freud for the work which has to be done in the course of grieving. The bereaved need to seal off the blind alleys of thought and develop new and different ways of coping with life. As they do this their view of themselves and their world changes. At first people tend to feel inadequate. Their accustomed supports are gone, they find it hard to cope, and the familiar world seems to have become a very unsafe place. Gradually, however, they become aware that they are not as weak and helpless as they had thought. They may be surprised to find themselves taking on roles and tasks of the one now dead and succeeding at them. This leads to a gradual *restoration of confidence*. As the pangs of grief die down it becomes easier to 'accept' the full reality of the loss. As the appetite returns, people become aware that they have not lost every good thing that came with the dead person.

When people say *'He (or she) lives on in my memory'* they are saying something that is true for, just as the growing child eventually becomes independent of its parents because it has learnt to be like them, so each love relationship leaves us permanently changed. Two years or so after bereavement people look back and say, '*I am tougher than I ever dreamed*'. Interestingly, they are often also more caring and sensitive to the sufferings of others. Bereavement teaches us some hard lessons.

There is no clear end point to grief. In building a new view of the world and of one's own place in it, one does not lose the old. Years later the discovery of a photograph in a drawer or a visit from an old friend can trigger another pang of grief so that people say, '*You don't get over it, you learn to live with it*'. For this reason the picture of grief as a series of phases through which one passes only once on the road to recovery is unsatisfactory. Even so there is a process to grief and, although people travel back and forth many times across the so-called 'phases of grief', like corks on the ocean, they gradually realise that there is a ground swell or tide which transcends these moment to moment fluctuations. In the end most people recognise that they have 'recovered'.

The rate of *recovery* varies as does the style of grieving. Old age is often a time of multiple bereavements, yet old people often seem to cope with these rather better than younger people, perhaps because they have come to expect them. But one should not be misled by their relative lack of overt distress into thinking that old people do not grieve. Their grief often takes a more gradual form and they may take longer than young people to find their way into a new life. In fact, for the very old, who are coming close to their own death, to begin again may not be a reasonable thing to expect. Bereavement is one of the commoner causes of depression in old age and loneliness, which can be a form of grief, is the besetting problem.

Bereaved children

The reaction of children to bereavement is determined partly by the stage of development that they have attained and partly by the support which they now receive. Adults, for the best of motives, often try to protect children by telling them nothing about the risk to a sick parent or other relative. Even after bereavement the dead person is not mentioned in the hope that the children will not grieve. In later life, people who have lost a parent in childhood regularly report their confused and frightened feelings at having been left out of family mourning.

Contrary to popular belief, children think a great deal about death. This is hardly surprising when so many children's games and entertainments involve the subject. Since it is not possible to protect children from the painful realisation that a family member has died, it is more helpful if adults join in the games and communicate with the children in whatever language they understand. When it is a parent who has died, it is also most important that the child receives 'parenting' that is good enough to ensure that their security is not seriously undermined.

The necessity of grief

People who come from societies in which overt emotional grieving is expected and encouraged often seem to come through the process of grieving faster and with less liability to depression than do people from societies in which the 'stiff upper lip' is the rule. This confirms the impression of psychotherapists that grief needs to be expressed and that we neglect it at our peril.

Risk factors

Prospective studies of bereaved people followed up for several years after bereavement have enabled us to identify people before, or at the time of a bereavement, who are at special risk and likely to benefit from the help of a counsellor or other carer from outside the family. They also shed light on the causal mechanisms that can lead to psychiatric and other problems in bereavement. Risk factors can be divided into unusually traumatic circumstances and unusually vulnerable people (Box 5.2).

Unusually traumatic circumstances

Some bereavements are more traumatic than others, thus, the death of a spouse and the death of a child carry a greater risk than the death of a sibling or grandparent. Mothers losing children are at greater risk than fathers, and the death of a parent carries particular risk to young or adolescent children.

These factors contribute to risk but none of them, on their own, make it necessary for a person to receive counselling if they are being well supported by their families. On the other hand the other risk factors listed in Box 5.2 are so traumatic that counselling should be offered to most people who experience them. This is most obvious in disaster areas where there is a good case for offering proactive counselling to all affected families.

Sudden, unexpected and untimely bereavements, particularly if they are also associated with horrific memories or images, commonly give rise to a type of reaction that has many of the features of post-traumatic stress disorder. High levels of anxiety and hyperalertness are associated with a tendency to be 'haunted' by painful memories or imagined images of the traumatic death. These intrude into consciousness and are triggered by any sight or sound which brings the death to mind. At night, they may appear in the form of recurrent dreams or nightmares.

So painful are these images that people will often go to great lengths to avoid situations that will remind them of the loss. They may shut themselves up at home, refuse to allow their family to

Traumatic circumstances
  Death of a spouse or child
  Death of a parent (particularly in early childhood or adolescence)
  Sudden, unexpected and untimely deaths (particularly if associated
    with horrific circumstances)
  Multiple deaths (particularly disasters)
  Deaths by suicide
  Deaths by murder or manslaughter

Vulnerable people
  Insecure attachment to parents in childhood (particularly 'learned
    fear' and 'learned helplessness')
  Low self-esteem
  Low trust in others
  Ambivalent attachment to deceased person
  Dependent or interdependent attachment to deceased person
  Previous psychiatric disorder
  Previous suicidal threats or attempts
  Absent or unhelpful family

Box 5.2 *Factors increasing the impact of bereavement.*

speak of the dead person and put away photographs and other reminders. Despite this they usually have a strong feeling that the person is not really dead, that he or she sees and hears everything that they do, and may walk in through the door at any moment. Even years later they will say, '*I can't believe it's true, it doesn't seem real*'. This feeling of unreality makes it difficult for them to enter into new relationships and to replan their lives.

Other types of traumatic bereavement such as deaths by suicide or murder give rise to complex reactions which are often complicated by feelings of intense anger or self-reproach or both. Whenever a death is attributable to human action, issues of blame and justice arise. It is important for justice to be seen to be done and the bereaved will take an interest in all legal proceedings which follow a death. Compensation claims often have more to do with a wish for justice than with financial reward and bereaved people will readily acknowledge that no amount of money can compensate them for the loss. Counselling may be needed if people are to work through feelings of rage to the point where they can be creative rather than destructive.

Personal vulnerability

Vulnerability to bereavement, like personal vulnerability to other stresses often goes back a long way. The attachments we make to our parents in childhood form the blue prints of future attachments and colour the way we react when these attachments end. Two particular kinds of problem follow types of parenting which evoke 'learned fear' or 'learned helplessness'. (See Parkes, 1991 for a more thorough exposition of these problems.)

In order to survive, we must all learn what to be afraid of, and for this reason small children are very sensitive to the fears of their parents. If the parents are abnormally fearful, either because they see the world as very dangerous or because they see their child as very frail, we should not be surprised if the child comes to view the world in the same way. Such children grow up very insecure and may develop close but dependent relationships with others to whom they become attached. When these relationships come to an end, they become exceedingly anxious and may suffer from chronic grief.

Most children learn, sooner or later, how to cope, either by standing on their own two feet or by relying on others. But children whose parents are only intermittently present or who are inconsistent in their responses to their child leave the child feeling helpless and unable to cope. When, later in life, they are faced with major demands on their coping ability as is likely to happen if they are bereaved, they easily slip into a state of depression. (Seligman has provided much evidence for this in his book *Helplessness*, 1975.)

Whether or not problematic relationships in adult life have been preordained, they are likely to affect the way people react when those relationships come to an end. Ambivalent relationships regularly give rise to complicated grief. Self-reproaches may then lead to self-punitive grieving (*'Why should I be happy when he (or she) is dead?'*). Similarly, relationships in which one person has come to rely excessively on the other often lead to chronic grief. Interestingly, it is not always the 'weak' person in the 'strong/weak' relationship who breaks down when the relationship ends. Often it takes a bereavement to reveal the extent to which the 'strong' partner needed the 'weak' one to reassure them of their own strength. These relationships are best thought of as 'interdependent'.

The first line of support for most people at times of trouble is their own family. In fact, families exist to provide security to their members. Unfortunately, in the world today, the traditional supportive function of the family often fails, either because people have moved away from their families or because existing families are unsupportive. In Raphael's studies (1984) of bereaved families in Australia, she found that people who rate their family as 'unsupportive' had more problems after bereavement than people who rate their families as 'supportive'. She also found that it was *this* group who obtained the greatest benefit from bereavement counselling. This suggests that what counselling does is to provide the sort of help which most people need and get from their own families.

In assessing bereavement risk, all of the above factors need to be taken into account. In addition, a previous history of heart disease, mental illness or suicidal threat is further grounds for regarding someone as likely to need help. Members of the primary health care team often possess much of this information and any that they do not have can easily be obtained by tactful questioning. Bereaved people, far from resenting such questions, are usually grateful for any interest which we take and we may be surprised to find that we are the only people to whom they have been able to talk about their bereavement.

Helping the bereaved

Counselling organisations

Having established that someone is 'at risk' the next step is to decide who is the best person to help. Sometimes this is likely to be a member of the team, at others it will be a clergyman or an accredited counsellor working for *Cruse – Bereavement Care,* or one of the other organisations for the bereaved. *Age Concern* offers help to elderly bereaved people in many areas and other organisations focus on other types of loss. Thus *Gay Bereavement,* as the name implies, provides special help to bereaved homosexuals, *The Compassionate Friends* is a self-help group run by and for bereaved parents and *SANDS,* The Society for Antenatal and Neonatal Deaths, helps this group of bereaved parents. A complete and up-to-date list of organisations for the bereaved in the United Kingdom is kept by The National Association of Bereavement Services (1992).

The primary health care team

Ideally, help for the bereaved begins before bereavement. As we have seen, sudden and unexpected bereavements are more traumatic than those that have been anticipated, yet most bereavements do cast their shadow before. Members of the primary health care team are often in a position to warn people about a coming bereavement but, because it is a task we all hate, we often fail to do it either by adopting an absurdly optimistic attitude or by leaving it to someone else to break the news. As a result, people are often unprepared for the losses that take place in their lives. When someone has an illness that is likely to end fatally, the general practitioner is often the only person in a position to provide continuity of care to the family as well as the patient. Time spent on this task will often reap dividends later and the family will remember with gratitude the support which they received when they most needed it.

The death of a loved person can be an inspiring or an horrific event. Unnecessary suffering in the patient, uncaring staff or failure to involve the family in decisions and care which affect the patient, can all leave indelible memories in the minds of the survivors. By the same token, a little kindness to patient or family will be remembered. The moment of death is an awesome time for us all and the professionals may be tempted to step back feeling that we have failed in our task to keep the patient alive and that '*There is nothing else we can do*'. Yet, this is the time when the family need us most, to stay close and to provide them with emotional support. This means very much more than providing a shoulder to cry on.

Giving permission to grieve

Almost the first thing that a mother tells her baby to do is to '*Stop crying*'. In western society the pressure to keep a 'stiff upper lip' is very great and people imagine that, if they do not keep a strict control over their feelings at all times they will 'break down'. This is reflected in the lay view of the 'nervous breakdown' which is assumed to result from losing control of dangerous feelings. At times of intense grief, it is very difficult to maintain this degree of control and people may need permission to vent their feelings and reassurance that, when they do this, they are not going to go mad.

Anxiety symptoms

Many of the symptoms which people bring to their doctors in the early stages of bereavement are reflections of anxiety and tension. While we all know that disasters happen they happen to other people not to me. Most of us go through life blissfully ignoring the fact that, despite all the advances of modern science, 100% of people still die. When, on the other hand, someone close to us dies, we not only lose that sense of invulnerability but we may go to the other extreme of expecting more disasters. In this circumstance it should not surprise us if a widow, lying in bed, notices that her heart is beating faster than usual. It occurs to her that her husband died of a heart attack, has she too got heart trouble? The more she worries, the faster her heart beats, and the faster her heart beats, the more she worries. In no time she has worried herself into an attack of paroxysmal tachycardia. In this way, normal symptoms of anxiety may aggravate and perpetuate themselves.

It is vital to make an accurate diagnosis in such cases for, as we have seen, bereavement *can* cause or aggravate real heart disease. In most instances, a careful history and examination makes it perfectly clear what kind of problem we are dealing with. Explanation and reassurance, perhaps coupled with instruction in relaxation exercises, which leave the bereaved person with something they can do when they begin to panic, may be all that is needed to cure the symptom.

What of the person who *has* heart disease and suffers a bereavement? In such cases everyone may tiptoe around the bereaved person fearing that anything which upsets them will cause their death. Patients themselves may be frightened to grieve. Yet the evidence indicates that inhibition of grief may be more hazardous to the heart than its expression. When people grieve they usually feel better for a 'good cry'. This means that it is not necessarily a good idea to over-protect people with known heart disease. On the other hand, it is quite logical to use beta-blocking drugs such as propranolol to reduce the nervous input from the cortex to the heart and, although no conclusive research has demonstrated this at the present time, it is reasonable to prescribe such medication to protect a damaged heart from the effects of a bereavement.

Psychotropic medication

This is more controversial. A few years ago every bereaved person could expect to be given diazepam to relieve the pangs of grief, but many people became 'hooked' and, at one drug withdrawal clinic, bereavement was found to be the commonest life event leading to benzodiazepine abuse. While the evidence for other damage is inconclusive, there are many who believe that tranquillisers inhibit the grieving process and delay recovery. There is no reason to believe that single doses of diazepam or other benzodiazepines given at irregular intervals do any harm, but regular doses for more than a week are not recommended.

Less controversial is the use of antidepressants. These are indicated when there are clear symptoms of major depression. They are less habit forming than the benzodiazepines, but the tricyclic group is cardiotoxic and one of the commonest causes of suicidal death is an overdose of tricyclics. On the other hand, the selective serotonin re-uptake inhibitors, such as fluoxetine, are much safer and have been successfully used in the treatment of panic syndromes and anxiety states as well as depression. At this time, no trials of their use for the treatment of normal or pathological grief have been published and until this is done they should be used with caution in this group of patients.

Counselling

Counselling for bereaved people needs to be flexible in order to meet the wide range of needs that may exist. In the early stages, people are likely to need permission to express grief and all the turmoil of emotions that well up. Hypnagogic hallucinations or illusions of the presence of the dead person near at hand are very common, and people may need reassurance that they are not a sign of madness.

As time passes, people may also need permission and encouragement to stop grieving and get on with the tasks of replanning their lives. Some cling to their grief as an excuse to remain withdrawn and will benefit from introduction to social or other groups.

Because bereaved people feel very insecure, it is important for us to attempt to provide them with a secure base, i.e. a place and a relationship in which they will feel safe enough to talk and think about the things that feel very unsafe. Intrusive memories and images are an example. It takes courage and trust to talk about these yet the very act of sharing horrific thoughts diminishes the horror and helps the patient to regain control. The more people try to control their frightening thoughts by avoiding them, the more they tend to sneak up when least expected. The best way of regaining control is by choosing to think the thoughts that haunt you. This makes it easier subsequently to set the thoughts aside.

Similarly, recurrent dreams, which may be so bad that people are afraid to go to sleep, occur *because* people expect them to occur. Most people feel as if their dreams are done to them and are unaware of the extent to which we control our own dreams. It helps to explain to people that our dreams are simply the thoughts we think while we are asleep. Like waking thoughts, they can be controlled up to a point but, like waking thoughts, they tend to sneak up on us if we over-control them.

The secret of treating recurrent dreams is not to try to stop them altogether, but to suggest to the sufferer that they think of a different ending. Most recurrent dreams end with an horrific happening; if the end can be changed, the person will stop dreading the beginning, and as soon as they stop dreading them the dreams will stop.

Suicidal ideas

Whenever bereaved people seem unusually agitated or depressed we should not hesitate to ask, '*Has it been so bad that you have wanted to kill yourself?*'. This simple question will almost always get an honest answer. Most people will say, '*Well I wouldn't care if I died tomorrow but I've got the family to think of . . ., etc.*' This does not constitute a serious suicidal risk. The person who is at risk for suicide will not only admit this but will have a plan of action. It is most important to find out what this plan is if we are to prevent it. Most often, people at risk of suicide will indicate that they have a hoard of medication which they have thought of taking. The hoard is a kind of 'emergency exit' ('*If things get too bad I can always take the tablets*') and, while it is important to remove the temptation, we need to put something else in its place. The telephone number of the local branch of Samaritans is one alternative for people can phone if their grief becomes intolerable. Others will be greatly reassured to know that their general practitioner will not be angry if they call in 'for a chat'.

Psychiatric treatment

The prescription of a non-toxic antidepressant is a wise precaution in such cases but we must remember that all of these take two or three weeks to produce their full benefit, and extra support will be needed until the patient is out of danger. This can often be obtained from the family, supported by the primary health care team, but psychiatric admission should always be considered if the risk is thought to be immediate. Referral to a psychiatrist does not mean that the primary health care team should withdraw, rather it sets the scene for liaison and collaboration between primary and secondary carers.

Box 5.3 summarises the types of interventions the primary health care team should consider for any bereaved person.

Support for team members

Emotional support given to families at times of bereavement can be one of the most rewarding but also one of the most taxing activities in the lives of the caring professions. It is all too easy for caring but busy people to offer more than they can reasonably give or to become 'over-involved' to the point where we lose our objectivity and good judgement. The best way to guard against this risk is to share the burden of care within and, if necessary, outside the team. Regular team meetings are essential not only to enable a planned

---

Be available to discuss the person's feelings before and after bereavement

Give 'permission' to grieve if necessary

Treat anxiety symptoms with very short-term benzodiazepines or beta-blockers

Expect physical symptoms, but take them seriously

Treat depression if it is severe enough to interfere with the person's day to day functioning, with antidepressants

Counselling for those at higher risk, either in the practice or through a counselling organisation

Ask about suicidal thoughts

Psychiatric referral for those developing pathological grief

Box 5.3 *Possible primary care interventions to prevent pathological grief reactions.*

programme of care to be worked out but also to enable those most involved to share their own feelings. If it is all right for families to cry, it should be alright for carers to do the same, and we have no need to feel ashamed if we too, at times, need to lean on other members of the team. The team member who is brave enough to share grief with other members of the team often gives them permission to do the same. This makes for a much closer and mutually trusting team and it is salutary to see the way in which teams who are helping families through these major turning points in their lives often themselves benefit.

In the end we all have to face the fact of our own mortality and that of those we love. Each time we succeed in helping someone else to face up to, and cope with, these awesome facts of life, we are also, indirectly, helping ourselves.

References

Jacobs, S. (1993). *Pathologic Grief: Maladaptation to Loss*. Washington, DC., and London: American Psychiatric Press.

National Association of Bereavement Services. (1992). *National Directory of Bereavement and Loss Services*. National Association of Bereavement Services, 20 Norton Folgate, London E1 6DB.

Osterweiss, M., Solomon, F. & Green, M. (eds.) (1984). *Bereavement: Reactions, Consequences and Care*. Washington, DC: National Academy Press.

Parkes, C.M. (1986). *Bereavement, Studies of Grief in Adult Life*. 2nd edn, New York: Pelican, Harmondsworth, Middlesex and International Universities Press.

Parkes, C.M. (1991). Attachment, bonding and psychiatric problems after bereavement in adult life. In *Attachment Across the Life Cycle*. Parkes, C. M., Stevenson-Hinde J. and Marris P., eds. London and New York: Routledge.

Raphael, B. (1984). *The Anatomy of Bereavement*. London: Hutchinson.

Seligman, M.E.P. (1975). *Helplessness*. San Francisco, California: Freeman.

[6] Preventing mental illness amongst people of ethnic minorities

Sangeeta Patel

Introduction

Research on the ethnic minorities has concentrated upon those who do not describe their origins as white. Much of this chapter also concentrates upon these groups: in Britain, the majority originate from the African–Caribbean countries and South Asia. The uneven distribution of these groups can have marked effects upon the lists of general practitioners (Gillam *et al.*, 1989). This chapter aims to outline the important factors which need to be taken into account by general practitioners considering mental illness in people of ethnic minorities.

Terminology

Description of people of different racial and ethnic origins is a complex area; as a source of discrimination, it is also a sensitive one which warrants a short explanation. In this chapter, I have used terms in common current usage in Britain: 'black people' as a broad category to describe all those people whose origins are not 'white' who, although different in many respects, share the exposure to racism: 'African–Caribbean' to describe those people who originate from Africa and the Caribbean of African descent, 'Asian' or more correctly 'South Asian' to describe those people who originate from the Indian subcontinent, and other self-explanatory terms, e.g. 'Chinese'.

Race and ethnicity

There are differences between the terms 'race' and 'ethnicity'. The historical development of the word 'race' sheds light upon the complexities of its interpretation. 'Race' was a term coined in the sixteenth century to describe the lineage of people connected by common descent or origin. With the rise of imperialism and Darwinism by the eighteenth century, different races of people were thought of as subspecies (Banton, 1987). The biological theories which suggest that racial and genetic characteristics are responsible for attitudes and patterns of behaviour have been disproved (Spuhler & Lindzey 1967; Osborne 1971; Jones, 1981), but the term 'race' still carries connotations of inferiority (Fernando 1991; Rex, 1986).

'Ethnicity' is not simply another term which has yet to develop pejorative overtones, but is used to describe as a group those who 'are thought by themselves and/or others to share a common origin and to share important segments of a common culture' (Yinger, 1981). This 'sense of belonging' comes from a mixture of shared origin, cultural values, and social pressures. It is therefore sensitive both to changes in cultural values as a result of marginalisation from, or assimilation into, the majority culture and to social pressures contingent upon racial characteristics. All of these will vary widely between individuals as well as between groups (Fernando, 1991).

Ethnic minority groups in Britain

Classification

Only recently has there been an accepted classification of ethnic minority groups. The decennial census data from England and Wales usually included questions relating to ethnic minorities: from 1851 onwards there was a question on 'place of birth' and later 'nationality' until 1961; the 1971 census contained a question on 'parents' place of birth'; however, in 1981 the then Secretary of State considered a question on ethnic origin 'too sensitive' to be included in the census (Donaldson & Parsons, 1990). The census of 1991 asked 'To which ethnic origin do you consider yourself to belong' with the options of White, Black–Caribbean, Black–African, Black–Other, Indian, Pakistani, Bangladeshi, Chinese, and Other. They were coded into 35 categories (OPCS, 1992).

Other commonly used sources of data include the General Household Survey, a continuous interview survey of people at 10 000 addresses, which includes a question on ethnic group (OPCS, annually); the Labour Force Survey, a continuous survey of 1 in 350 households since 1973 (OPCS, 1986) which has contained a question on self-reported ethnic origin since 1983; the fourth morbidity survey in general practice which looked at every consultation in 60 practices (OPCS, 1992); and more recently the Health Education Authority survey of 1994 (HEA, 1994).

There are problems in using a self-reported description of ethnic origin: many people are uncertain how to classify themselves.

The categories used are broad and are often inadequate for research into characteristics which may vary between subgroups. Nevertheless, ethnic monitoring has begun within the health service, using the same classifications as the decennial census and there are plans to expand this throughout the health service (Health and Ethnicity Programme, 1991).

Distribution of ethnic minority groups

The 1991 census showed that 5.9% of the 49.9 million people living in England and Wales considered themselves to be of non-white ethnic origin (Balarajan & Soni Raleigh, 1992). The percentages in each ethnic group are shown in Box 6.1. The census showed uneven distribution of the ethnic minorities, with clusters in some cities, particularly London, constituting 26% of Inner London and 17% of Outer London. The Black–Caribbean, Black–African, and Black–Other groups tended to share the same geographical areas, with 60% of the Black–Caribbean group and 80% of the Black–African group living in London. The Indian, Pakistani and Bangladeshi groups tended to live in different districts and boroughs from each other: half of the Bangladeshis lived in predominantly inner London, one-third of the Indians lived in predominantly outer London and one-fifth of the Pakistanis lived in the West Midlands and West Yorkshire. One-third of the Chinese lived in London, and tended to be more evenly distributed than the other groups (Balarajan & Soni Raleigh, 1992).

Social and family factors

Inequalities in social class and gender affect the mental health of disadvantaged groups (Brown & Harris, 1978). Ethnic minority status compounds this disadvantage (Kessler & Neighbors, 1986; Atkin & Rollings, 1993; Ahmad, 1992; Ulbrich, Warheit & Zimmerman, 1989). Ethnic minorities are over-represented in the lower social classes. In general, black people have lower incomes than white people, they are less likely to be employed, and live in poorer quality housing (Brown, 1984).

Black Caribbean	1.0%
Black African	0.4%
Black Other	0.4%
Indian	1.7%
Pakistani	0.9%
Bangladeshi	0.3%
Chinese	0.3%
Other Asian	0.4%
Other	0.6%

Box 6.1 *Ethnic minorities in England and Wales (OPCS, 1992).*

Migration

Migration can affect mental health in different ways. A lower prevalence of mental illness in migrants than in the native culture may arise by virtue of migrants coming from a country with low prevalence; self-selection of the most mentally stable for migration; the subsequent improvement of real income; and the underdiagnosis of mental illness using criteria inappropriate for that culture (Kleinman, 1987). Alternatively, a higher prevalence of mental illness in migrants can arise by virtue of their coming from a country with higher prevalence; self-selection of the mentally unstable for migration; the frustration of expectations (Fenton, 1985); the displacement into a society where their own cultural beliefs may no longer be the norm (Halpern, 1993); and the over-diagnosis of mental illness using inappropriate (western) criteria (Rack, 1986). A combination of these factors will affect any group of migrants.

Migration factors include those that 'pull' people towards another country for social and economic reasons and ones that 'push' people out, such as political situations (Murphy, 1977; Rack, 1982). Social class change is often an accompaniment of migration (Robinson, 1992).

Active postwar recruitment from the 'New Commonwealth' countries in the 1940s and 50s resulted in people coming to England expecting to improve their social status. An increase in their actual income did not prevent the drop in social class status relative to the British community and has often led to black people feeling as though they are treated like second class citizens. They may have expected to rise in the social classes with time and hard work, but population studies have shown that this is not the case with the African–Caribbeans and the Pakistanis (Robinson 1992), amongst whom a sense of disappointment is prevalent.

People who have been forced to leave their country of previous residence to come to Britain as refugees may have the initial security from refuge replaced by discrimination (Littlewood & Lipsedge, 1978). Their social situation in their previous country of residence may have been satisfactory and they will be faced with the prospect of rebuilding it, often in middle-age, with little emotional or financial preparation, and no recognition of their previous experience.

Studies of the mental health of migrants have often utilised standardisation of social class (Cochrane & Stopes-Roe, 1981). However, standardisation of social class between migrants and the native British made on the basis of income, occupation and housing have been criticised for (mistakenly) assuming that these bear the same conceptual significance in both cultures (London, 1986; Helman, 1990).

Family structure, roles and carers

There tend to be two conflicting stereotypes of ethnic minority families. One stresses 'the great strength of extended family ties' amongst African–Caribbean and Asian groups whilst the other suggests that they are 'families broken, divided, weak and themselves responsible for any difficulties they face' (Fenton, 1985). The extended family is more common amongst Asians, but there is still a significant proportion who live alone with few relatives in this country (Atkin et al., 1989). The extended family is uncommon among African–Caribbean families (Barker, 1984). One-third of the African–Caribbean elderly have been reported to be living alone and a further third with their spouse only (Fenton, 1985). However, among 100 South Asians and 100 West Indians interviewed in inner-city Bristol, 35% of both groups reported that their family 'had been able to keep together for the most part', whilst 13% of South Asians and 32% of Afro-Caribbean interviewees spoke of their family as 'mostly separated', and 10% said their families were 'divided between the UK and abroad' (Fenton, 1985).

Maintaining traditional roles within families may not be so easy in Britain where women face social and economic pressures to gain employment, in a climate where men have more difficulty doing so (Brown, 1984). Much of the care of the ill and disabled does, however, continue to be provided by the family. The disadvantage associated with ethnicity appears to increase the burden. The emotional strain is added to by isolation particularly amongst women, who have difficulties with access to health care and communication (McAvoy & Sayeed, 1990). The economic costs further prevent educational opportunities and advancement at work, which prevent improvement to poor housing (Farrah, 1986). Both the demographic characteristics of the black population and their traditional patterns of caring are changing in a way which will further increase the strain upon the carers and cared for (Atkin & Rollings, 1993).

Community support

To some extent, the members of ethnic minorities may be protected from the effects of social pressures to change towards the majority culture by being surrounded by other members of their groups (Halpern, 1993). However, black communities in Britain may not be able to provide the support required by their members: few black residents have been reported to attend any community groups or associations, except of a religious kind and these did not prevent their feeling of isolation (Fenton, 1985; Atkin & Rollings, 1993).

Statutory and voluntary services

With the exception of their general practitioner, the knowledge and use of statutory health and community services by ethnic minorities is limited (Donaldson & Odell, 1986; Atkin *et al.*, 1989). Black people often are not aware of services they may have, and when they are made aware, many express a wish to use them but are often limited by the feeling that these services do not cater for their needs. Unfortunately, the practice and policy of statutory community service provision often ignores the needs of black people or marginalises them by focusing upon the difference in their cultural practices from the white 'norm' (Atkin, 1991; Pearson, 1988).

Voluntary service provision for the black community is provided, on the whole, by black people, with less secure funding, since at present the mainstream voluntary sector does not seem to cater for the black community (Bowling, 1990; Confederation of Indian Organisations, 1993). This situation is likely to be aggravated by the present government policy of contracting out community services, which will increase the relative importance of the mainstream voluntary sector.

Culture and mental illness

Culture has been described as 'systems of shared ideas, systems of concepts and rules and meanings that underlie and are expressed in the ways that humans live' (Kessing, 1981), and as 'a set of guidelines (both explicit and implicit) which individuals inherit as members of a particular society, and which tells them how to view the world, how to experience it emotionally, and how to behave in it in relation to other people, to supernatural forces or odds, and to the natural environment. It provides them with a way of transmitting these guidelines to the next generation' (Helman, 1990). Cultures have profound influences upon the beliefs and behaviour of individuals, their moral and religious views, their expectations of good health, and their beliefs about the causality of illness (Fabrega, 1984; Helman, 1990; Foster & Anderson, 1978; Fernando, 1991).

Goals such as spiritual enlightenment, financial or educational achievement, and marriage and childbirth are ascribed different levels of importance in different cultures (McQueen, 1978; Kakar, 1984): the frustration of these goals will lead to distress in those cultures which value them highly (Helman, 1990).

Normality within cultures

Which beliefs and behaviours are considered normal and which ones abnormal will vary from culture to culture, and will depend upon the role and status of the person concerned as well as the context of their behaviour (Horwitz, 1982). Whether certain beliefs or behaviours are considered to be outside the normal range for members of minority cultures can only be adequately ascertained by someone with an understanding of the values of that culture (Adebimpe, 1984; Coulter, 1979).

Help-seeking behaviour

Communication of distress to other members of the same culture and those outside it is expected to elicit a range of given responses (Beliappa, 1991; Bal, 1987). It has been argued that minority cultures need to behave in the same ways as the majority cultures for their distress to be recognised and helped. Preferred sources of help, such as general practitioners, psychotherapists, gurus or shamans, and expectations of these healers are also culturally determined and will have been influenced by the previous exposure to and impact of these (Dow, 1986; Kakar, 1984; Obeyeskere, 1977).

Somatisation and psychologisation

It has been reported that many of the ethnic minority cultures 'somatise' their mental illness (Kirmayer, 1984; Mumford *et al.*, 1991): that is, they ascribe a physical symptom to a physical illness, when it is attributable to a psychological illness (Goldberg & Huxley 1980, 1992). Somatisation is common in all ethnic groups (Bhatt, Tomenson & Benjamin, 1989; Mayou, 1976; Teja, Narang & Aggarwal 1971; Kirmayer, 1984). It may be seen to represent a view held by doctors of cultural inferiority (Fernando, 1988).

'Psychologisation' has been described by anthropologists as the ascribing of symptoms to a psychological illness. This has been encouraged by health education campaigns, such as the 'defeat depression campaign' (Priest, 1991), which aims to decrease the stigma of mental illness. Much health education is designed for the majority culture and does not reach the ethnic minority groups as effectively (HEA report, 1994). 'Psychologisation' has been reported amongst the white middle-classes (Helman, 1990).

The tendency to 'somatise' and 'psychologise' is also culturally determined. Even the distinction assumes (mistakenly) that the Western biomedical mind–body dualism applies universally (Bracken, 1993; Fernando, 1991).

Culture and psychiatry

The concept of abnormal beliefs and behaviours as mental illness, to be treated by psychiatrists or other doctors, is also culturally bound. Psychiatric diagnoses have been developed in the west and are often (wrongly) accepted as universal (Fabrega, 1984; Fernando, 1991). The use of western diagnostic categories to describe diseases in other cultures where they may not be applicable has been described as 'category fallacy' (Kleinman, 1987). The validation of these categories worldwide using 'gold standards' also developed in the west has been criticised for being only a method of replication of observations (of western illness) rather than a true description of mental illness within those cultures. This does make research into mental illness in different cultures difficult to interpret (Jones & Gray, 1986). It has been argued that the findings of such research should not be ignored, if cultural contexts have been taken into consideration (Leff, 1990). The development and use of psychiatric diagnoses and research, like other medical research, is subjected to bias in the choice of areas to study, the models used, and which findings are reported which makes it more likely that currently fashionable ideas will be published.

In the past, those studies that reinforced stereotypes were more readily accepted. Anthropological work, based on scanty evidence, suggesting that non-Caucasians had smaller brains which made them of inferior intelligence was widely accepted at one time. Cannabis psychosis was regarded as more prevalent amongst West Indians although, in fact, cannabis use was equally prevalent amongst corresponding white groups (Littlewood, 1988; Onyango, 1986; Lipsedge, 1993).

Current trends in cross-cultural psychiatry
Three main features have been identified in current cross-cultural psychiatry; research concentrates on black rather than white immigrants (of more than 150 papers, only a handful deal with the Irish mentally ill); published work tends to show increased rates of mental illness in ethnic minorities rather than decreased rates; and most research has been conducted on hospitalised psychotic patients. The emphasis in the literature on psychosis in African–Caribbeans (Harrison et al., 1988; McGovern & Cope, 1987) and parasuicide and eating disorders in young Asian women (Merrill & Owens, 1986; Mumford & Whitehouse, 1988) has been said to reflect popular stereotypes of West Indians as out of control and Asians as too controlled (Townsend, 1979). This has the effect of raising awareness amongst health care workers of these conditions, which may interfere with their appreciation of other more common aspects of mental health, such as those coping strategies which prove effective amongst the ethnic minority groups, and their awareness of adjustment disorders, anxiety, and depression which are much more common than the more severe conditions in these communities.

The politics of cross-cultural psychiatry are complex and represent a wide range of views ranging from those of western psychiatrists as overtly or covertly racist to those of psychiatrists as (misguidedly) ethnocentric (Burke, 1984; Rack, 1982, Fernando, 1991, Littlewood, 1990).

Prevalence of mental illness amongst ethnic minorities

There are usually limitations which must be taken into account when interpreting studies of the prevalence of mental illness amongst ethnic minority groups (Ineichen, 1990; Shaunuk *et al.*, 1986; Giggs, 1986; London, 1986). These include differences in classification of the ethnic minority groups, using classifications which are too broad to yield meaningful results, limitations in matching patients with controls of native British origin, and the use of western psychiatric categories in groups where they may not be applicable (Pasamanick, 1963; Jones & Gray, 1986; Adebimpe, 1984; Loring & Powell, 1988).

There remains controversy as to whether the raw experience of mental illness is the same in all ethnic groups (Littlewood, 1990). Many cross-cultural psychiatrists argue that it is the same fundamental disease that affects us all, with different ethnic and cultural wrappings (Birnbaum, 1923; Singer, 1975; Bebbington, 1978; Sartorious, Jablensky & Shapiro, 1977; Sartorius *et al.*, 1986). Others would argue that the form, and not merely the content, of mental illness is itself a cultural construct (Bracken, 1993; Littlewood, 1990; Marsella, 1978, 1984; Yap, 1974). Given these limitations, for those ethnic groups where the psychiatric illness is less influenced by social factors and where the groups which are being compared are not so culturally diverse, the results reported may yet be valid (Leff, 1990; Littlewood, 1990). Even when care has been taken to develop instruments which take into account cultural differences in symptomatology, however, the meaning and context of the illness may not be comparable (Krause, 1994; Fabrega, 1984; Fernando, 1991).

Bearing in mind these limitations, the rate of prevalence of mental illness amongst the South Asians has been reported to be lower than that of the British population in some studies (Cochrane & Stopes-Roe, 1977, 1981; Ineichen, 1990; Ebrahim *et al.*, 1991) and the same in others (Murray & Williams, 1986). Suicide rates among the ethnic minorities have generally been reported to be lower than that of the native British (Health & Ethnicity Programme, 1991) with the notable exception of young Asian women, in whom it may be higher (Merrill and Owens, 1988). Among those of African–Caribbean origin, rates of psychosis have been reported to be higher than among the native British population (Giggs, 1986; Harrison *et al.*, 1988; McGovern & Cope, 1987; Dean *et al.*, 1981), whilst rates of anxiety and depression seem to be lower (Lloyd, 1993). However, anxiety and depression are still much more likely than psychosis among African–Caribbean people. There is concern that increasing awareness of the rarer culture-bound disorders which affect ethnic minorities detracts from the important message that all mental illness is profoundly influenced by culture. These reports must be appreciated in the context of current trends in

British society and those of the ethnic group studied. Attempts to generalise about mental illness in ethnic minorities often emphasise the differences between them and the British and risk reinforcing stereotypes and further marginalising those of different ethnic origin. For general practitioners treating individual patients, they need to remain mindful of their symptoms in the wider context of their illness.

Presentation of mental illness

The expression of symptoms of mental illness is influenced by the sufferer's interpretation of them, the significance of that interpretation for the sufferer, and their expectations of society (Helman, 1990; Foster & Anderson, 1978). For patients, their general practitioner is one part of the network of social relationships which make up their own health care system (Kleinman, 1980). For ethnic minority groups, as in western society, much mental illness is treated without involvement of formal health care services. There has been emphasis upon the use of alternative practitioners by ethnic minority groups, but the actual proportion who do consult alternative practitioners is low (Bhopal, 1989; HEA, 1994).

Symptoms presented to general practitioners are part of a complex set of beliefs and values of which general practitioners may be unaware (Fernando, 1991). Worldwide, 'soul loss' is a more common symptom than 'depression' (Shweder, 1985). Presentation of somatic symptoms has been reported amongst South Asians (Krause *et al.*, 1990; Bal, 1987; Mumford *et al.*, 1991), African–Caribbeans (Lloyd, 1993), the Chinese and others, but particular somatic symptoms vary between cultures, subcultures and individuals. Examples of somatic symptoms commonly reported amongst the South Asians include 'sinking heart' (Krause, 1989), fatigue, and dizziness (Mumford, *et al.*, 1991), and amongst the Africans 'heat', 'peppery' and 'crawling' sensations (Ohaeri & Odejide, 1994). However, the variation within such broad subgroups has been raised. Studies reporting symptoms of depression in India found differences in the somatic symptoms expressed between those of North India and those of South India (Mumford *et al.*, 1991; Bhugra, 1994; Teja, Narang & Aggarwal, 1971).

Patient–doctor communication

Language, interpretation and advocacy

Language difficulties are often cited as the major barriers to communication. The percentage of people who do not speak English is decreasing: in 1994 the rates amongst Indians were 15% (8% of men), amongst Pakistanis 28% and amongst the Bangladeshi community 41% (HEA, 1994). Generally, language problems tend to be dealt with *ad hoc*, using family members, friends or neighbours, or another worker on-site who speaks the same language. These strategies may not be appropriate because of issues of confidentiality, the shift in the balance of power between the patient and their translator, which is particularly important if the translator is a family member or close friend, and the tendency of the untrained to interpret rather than just translate. It has been suggested that Asian women need advocates and not interpreters (Parsons & Day, 1992). The employment of staff sharing the same racial or ethnic background as the patient does not necessarily solve the problem of cultural difference: many black employees have assimilated the culture of their profession and are often uncomfortable in their roles as 'race experts'. They may not have the skills and confidence to work from an antiracist and multicultural perspective (Atkin & Rollings, 1993; Pearson, 1988). In addition, they often face tensions by having to choose between being loyal to the agencies that employ them or becoming advocates for their clients (Ahmad, 1988; Owusu-Bempah, 1990). General practitioners working in areas where they do not share the same language as many of their patients can acquaint themselves with the use and limitations of interpreters and advocates.

Access to general practitioners and communication

Clearly, if there is no understanding of verbal communication, then assessment of mental health will be very limited, but the emphasis upon language as the chief inhibitor to communication has been criticised (Bowes & Domokos, 1995; McAvoy & Sayeed, 1990). Among those from ethnic minorities who speak the same language as their general practitioner, a higher proportion report problems with communication than among the English, suggesting wider problems of communication (Brewin, 1980; Bowes & Domokos, 1995; Jain *et al.*, 1985; HEA, 1994). These communication difficulties may reflect wider differences in status or power between doctors and their ethnic minority patients.

The accessibility and approachability of general practitioners both before and during the consultation will affect patients' perceptions of these power differences. General practitioners can make themselves more accessible to their ethnic minority patients by appropriate adjustment of the barriers to access, such as appointment systems, telephone access and receptionist behaviour (Farooqi, 1993). During consultations, general practitioners can encourage patients to give cues to mental illness by demonstrating interest and concern (Marks, Goldberg and Hillier 1979; MIND, 1986). It is this aspect that has been the greatest source of dissatisfaction with their general practitioners expressed by ethnic minority patients.

Detection of mental illness

Factors important in the detection of depression by the general practitioner have been well documented (Chapter 10). Some of these factors will be particularly applicable to ethnic minority patients (Box 6.2). General practitioners are less likely to diagnose depression in those who do not seem overtly depressed, those who have concurrent physical illness and those who present with somatic symptoms.

General practitioners have been reported to perceive consultations with their ethnic minority patients to take longer and to be less satisfying (Ahmad, 1992). This may prevent them from allowing patients to express the verbal and vocal cues which would enable them to diagnose mental illness (Davenport, Goldberg & Millar, 1987). General practitioners may have difficulty judging from their patient's demeanour whether this is within normal limits appropriate to their culture. Expression of emotion is, to an extent, culturally determined (Fernando, 1991; Coulter, 1979). However, one's cultural beliefs determine how one should behave and not how one may actually behave (Helman, 1990), so generalisations may not apply to individuals. This is particularly true of members of minority cultures, who will assimilate and integrate into the majority culture to varying degrees. General practitioners may ascribe to culture what is actually abnormal, or may interpret as abnormal a culturally normal reaction to social, political, or economic pressure. The views of other people close to the patient will usually enlighten the general practitioner.

Concurrent physical illness is more prevalent in ethnic minority groups. It has been reported that they are less likely to take part in healthy activities and in health promotion (HEA, 1994). Ethnic minorities tend to have lower levels of employment, lower

---

Greater tendency to present with physical symptoms

Varying expressions of distress

Concurrent physical illness more likely

Inhibition of cues of depression from patient

Difficulty judging the patient's demeanour

Ascribing abnormal behaviour to cultural factors

Misinterpreting culturally appropriate behaviour

Box 6.2 *Difficulties in detecting psychological distress in patients of ethnic minorities.*

incomes, and poorer housing all of which have been shown to be associated with poorer physical health. Differences in consultation rates by disease category among ethnic groups have been reported (Johnson, Cross & Cardew, 1983; Gillam et al., 1989). In one practice it was found that the Irish and West Indians consulted less than the native British, while the Asians consulted more, but all three ethnic groups had lower rates for consulting for mental disorder. There were higher rates for Asians in the category of 'symptoms and ill-defined conditions' and back pain, and for West Indians more consultations for back pain. It is possible that these reflected misdiagnoses of physical rather than mental disorders by general practitioners (Gillam et al., 1989; Bal, 1987).

Cross-cultural management in general practice

When assessing the mental health of people of ethnic minorities their symptoms should be viewed in as much of the cultural context as is possible for the health worker to ascertain, without reducing their culture to symptoms and causes of pathology, e.g. attributing mental health problems to 'culture conflict' or to a 'fatalistic attitude' (Lawrence, 1982; Parmar, 1981). Patients' cultural backgrounds will determine their expectations of health, their perceptions of their current state of health and the factors needed to change it, what they consider to be medical problems, and their expectations of their healers. The doctor will have his or her own ideas of a patient's beliefs, determined by the doctor's cultural views and experience. These may be very different from the patient's actual beliefs. In negotiating further management, the doctor must be aware of both views and attempt to ensure that future treatment is culturally acceptable for the patient.

Treatment

It has been reported that Asian patients require lower doses of antidepressants to avoid side-effects (Lewis et al., 1980; Allen, Rack & Vaddadi, 1977). African–Caribbean patients tend to receive higher doses of neuroleptic and depot treatments in hospitals, although a difference in sensitivity to neuroleptic medication has not been reported. Depressed Asian patients are more likely to receive electroconvulsive therapy (Littlewood 1986; Chen, Harrison & Standon 1991). Reasons cited for this include doctors' perception of mentally ill black and Asian patients as poorly compliant with oral treatment (Lipsedge, 1993; Harrison et al., 1984), and that, like much of British society, doctors fear the black mentally ill, or perceive them to be more likely to be violent (Fernando, 1988; Lewis, Croft-Jeffreys & David, 1990). In fact, black mentally ill offenders have been reported to be less violent than comparable white patients (Lawson, Yesavage & Werner,

1984). Black patients will be aware of these perceptions of them by society and will be sensitive to them from their health carers. General practitioners must be aware that these views do not affect their treatment of their own black mentally ill patients.

Psychotherapy

In Britain, patients from ethnic minorities are rarely referred for psychotherapy (Cole & Pilisuk, 1976; Kareem & Littlewood, 1992). This may be because of the assumption by psychiatrists and general practitioners that they lack the psychological mindedness, verbal sophistication or capacity for psychological insight (Lipsedge, 1993; Campling, 1989). Alternatively, it may reflect the controversy about the extent to which psychoanalysis and other western therapies have been found appropriate outside the middle-class white context in which they were elaborated, and that individual psychotherapy is inappropriate for those of South Asian and African–Caribbean culture because of the western emphasis on the autonomous self.

The quantitative measurement of the outcomes of intercultural therapy is confounded with methodological issues. Taking these into consideration, racially sensitive psychotherapy has been reported to be effective (Moorhouse, 1992). Racially sensitive therapy does not necessarily have to be from a therapist of the same ethnic background, but from one aware of racial and cultural factors within therapy (Thomas, 1992).

Referral

It has been reported that race is one factor affecting referral (Brewin, 1980; Yamamoto, James & Palley, 1968). Black people are less likely to be referred for further psychiatric or psychological treatment (Yamamoto et al., 1968). African–Caribbeans are less likely to be referred for mental illness by their general practitioner at an early stage of illness (Owens, Harrison & Boot, 1991) and are more likely to be admitted to hospital by the police or social services under a section of the Mental Health Act (Moodley & Perkins 1991; McGovern 1987; Rogers & Faulkner, 1987). Referral is a complex process influenced by views of both patient and doctor (Morgan, 1989; Goldberg & Huxley, 1980; Littlewood, 1986). Certain aspects of the patient can deter the doctor from referring them on – it may be that they fail to present their problem in a way that the general practitioner recognises it, or they present later (Harrison et al., 1989), or that they deter the general practitioner from referring them on. It has been suggested that psychiatric treatment carries more stigma in the communities of ethnic minorities than among the native British. This has been disputed and cited as a source of blame upon the minority community for their own problems (Lipsedge, 1993).

Follow-up

Black patients are less likely to leave a consultation with their general practitioner with an appointment for follow-up (Gillam et al., 1989). Their attendance for follow-up to psychiatric services to monitor treatment, relapse or recurrence is lower than the native British (Yamamoto et al., 1967; Campling, 1989). This may be a result of understandably negative views of psychiatric services, of which the general practitioner needs to be aware.

Conclusions

A chapter is only enough to highlight factors to consider when considering mental illness in the many groups that contribute to a multiethnic Britain. Attempts to make generalisations in such a complex field carry the danger of reinforcing stereotypes, which only does a disservice to the rapidly changing minority cultures and to those who care for them. Care must be taken that although those from ethnic minorities do suffer problems, they are not viewed as the problems themselves. General practitioners need to be particularly attentive to their patients from ethnic minorities, to permit them to express the cues which reveal their distress, to attend to these specifically in spite of concurrent physical symptoms, assess them in the patient's cultural context, and negotiate treatments which will be culturally acceptable. In all of these aspects, the general practitioners need to be aware of their own prejudices and to accept as the first point of access to the health service that they have a responsibility not to perpetuate the individual and institutional discrimination that many of those from ethnic minorities have to face.

References

Aakster, C.W. (1986). Concepts in alternative medicine. *Social Science and Medicine*, **22**, 265–73.

Adebimpe, V.R. (1984). American blacks and psychiatry. *Transcultural Psychiatric Review* **21**, 83–111.

Ahmad, B. (1988). Community social work: sharing the experience of ethnic groups. *Social Work Today*, **19**, 13.

Ahmad, W.I.U. (1992). *Race and Health in Contemporary Britain*. Milton Keynes: Open University Press.

Ahmad, W.I.U., Baker, M.R. & Kernohan, E.E.M. (1990). Race, ethnicity and general practice. *British Journal of General Practice*, **40**, 223–4.

Ahmad, W.I.U., Baker, M.R. & Kernohan, E.E.M. (1991). General practitioners' perceptions of Asian and non-Asian patients. *Family Practice*, **8**. 52–6.

Allen, J., Rack, P. & Vaddadi, K.S. (1977). Differences in the effects of clomipramine on English and Asian volunteers: preliminary report on a pilot study. *Postgraduate Medical Journal*, **53**, 79.

Atkin, K. (1991). Health, illness, disability and black minorities: a speculative critique of present day discourse. *Disability, Handicap and Society*, **6**, 37–47.

Atkin, K. & Rollings, J. (1993). *Community Care in a Multi-Racial Britain: A Critical Review of the Literature*. London: HMSO.

Atkin, K., Cameron, E., Badger, F. & Evers, E. (1989). Asian elders' knowledge and future use of community social and health services. *New Community*, **15**, 439–46.

Bal, S.S. (1987). Psychological symptomatology and health beliefs in Asian patients. In *Clinical Psychology, Research and Development*. Dent, H., ed. London: Croom Helm.

Balarajan, R. & Soni Raleigh, V. (1992). The ethnic population of England and Wales: the 1991 census: *Health Trends*, **24**, 113–16.

Balarajan, R., Yuen, P. & Raleigh Soni, V. (1989). Ethnic differences in general practice consultation. *British Medical Journal*, **299**, 958–60.

Banton, M. (1987). *Racial Theories*. Cambridge: Cambridge University Press.

Barker J. (1984). *Black and Asian old people in Britain*. Mitcham: Age Concern Research Unit.

Bebbington, P.E. (1978). The epidemiology of depressive disorder. *Culture, Medicine and Psychiatry*, **2**, 297–341.

Beliappa, J. (1991). *Illness or Distress? Alternative Models of Mental Health*. London: Confederation of Indian Organisations.

Bhatt, T.A., Tomenson, B. & Benjamin, S. (1989). Transcultural patterns of somatisation in primary care. *Journal of Psychosomatic Research*, **33**, 671–80.

Bhopal, R.S. (1989). Inter-relationships between folk, traditional and western medicine within an Asian community in Britain. *Social Science and Medicine*, **22**, 99–105.

Bhugra, D. (1994). Cultural differences within depressive disorder. Presentation to conference 'Depression, its diagnosis, its diversity and its treatment', St George's Hospital Medical School, London, November 1994.

Birnbaum, K. (1923). Der Aufbau der Psychosen (the making of a psychosis). In *Themes and Variations in European Psychiatry*. Bristol: Wright.

Bowes, A.M. & Domokos, T.M. (1995). South Asian women and their general practitioners: some issues of communication. *Social Sciences in Health*, **1**, 22–33.

Bowling, B. (1990). *Elderly People from Ethnic Minorities: A Report on Four Projects*. London: Age Concern Institute of Gerontology.

Bracken, P. (1993). Post-empiricism and psychiatry: meaning and methodology in cross-cultural research. *Social Science and Medicine*, **36**, 265–72.

Brewin, C. (1980). Explaining the lower rates of psychiatric treatment among Asian immigrants to the United Kingdom. *Social Psychiatry*, **15**, 17–19.

Bridges, K.W. & Goldberg, N.P. (1985). Somatic presentation of DSM-III psychiatric disorders in primary care. *Journal of Psychosomatic Research*, **29**, 563–9.

Brown, C. (1984). *Black and White Britain: The Third PSI Survey.* London: Heinemann.

Brown, G.W. & Harris, T. (1978). *Social Origins of Depression: A Study of Psychiatric Disorder in Women.* London: Tavistock Press.

Burke, A.W. (1984). Racism and mental illness. *International Journal of Social Psychiatry*, Special Issue, **30**, 1 and 2.

Campling, P. (1989). Race, culture and psychotherapy. *Psychiatric Bulletin*, **13**, 550–1.

Carpenter, L. & Brockington, I.F. (1980). A study of mental illness in Asians, West Indians and Africans in Manchester. *British Journal of Psychiatry*, **137**, 201–5.

Carter, J.H. (1994). Racism's impact upon mental health. *Journal of the National Medical Association*, **86**, 543–7.

Chen, E.Y.H., Harrison, G. & Standon, P. (1991). Management of first episode of psychotic illness in Afro-Caribbean patients. *British Journal of Psychiatry*, **158**, 517–22.

Cochrane, R. & Stopes-Roe, M. (1977). Psychological and social adjustment of Asian immigrants in Britain: a community survey. *Social Psychiatry*, **12**, 195–206.

Cochrane, R. & Stopes-Roe, M. (1981). Psychological symptom levels in Indian immigrants: a comparison with the native English. *Psychological Medicine*, **11**, 319–27.

Cole, J. & Pilisuk, M. (1976). Differences in the provision of mental health services by race. *American Journal of Psychiatry*, **46**, 519–25.

Community Relations Commission (1976) *Aspects of Mental Health in a Multicultural Society. Notes for the Guidance of Doctors and Social Workers.* London: CRC.

Confederation of Indian Organisations (1993). *Enquiry into Health Information Activity in the Asian Voluntary Sector.* London.

Coulter, J. (1979). *The Social Construction of the Mind: Studies in Ethnomethodology and Linguistic Philosophy.* London: Macmillan.

Cruikshank, J.K. & Beevers, D.G. (1990). *Ethnic Factors in Health and Disease.* London: Wright.

Davenport, S., Goldberg, D. & Millar, T. (1987). How psychiatric disorders are missed in primary care. *Journal of Psychosomatic Research*, **29**, 563–9.

Dean, G., Walsh, D., Downing, H. & Shelley, E. (1981). First admissions of native-born and immigrants to psychiatric hospitals in South east England, 1976. *British Journal of Psychiatry*, **139**, 506–12.

Donaldson L. & Johnson, M. (1990). Elderly Asians. In *Health Care for Asians*. McAvoy, B. and Donaldson, L., eds. Oxford: Oxford University Press.

Donaldson, L.J. & Odell, A. (1986). Aspects of the health and social services of elderly Asians in Leicester: a community survey. *British Medical Journal*, **293**, 1079–82.

Donaldson, L. & Parsons, L. (1990). Asians in Britain, the population and its characteristics. In *Health care for Asians*. McAvoy, B and Donaldson, L. eds. Oxford: Oxford Medical Publications.

Donovan, J. (1984). Ethnicity and race: a research review. *Social Science and Medicine*, **19**, 663–70.

Dow, J. (1986). Universal aspects of symbolic healing: a theoretical synthesis. *American Anthropologist*, **88**, 56–8.

Ebrahim, S., Patel, N., Coats, M. *et al.* (1991). Prevalence and severity of morbidity among Gujarati Asian elders: a controlled comparison. *Family Practice*, **8**, 57–62.

Fabrega, H. (1984). Culture and psychiatric illness: biomedical and ethnomedical aspects. In *Cultural Conceptions of Mental Health and Therapy*. Marsella, A.M. and White, G.M. eds. pp. 29–68. Dordrecht: Reidel.

Farooqi, A. (1993). How can family practice improve access to health care for black and ethnic minority patients? In *Access to Health Care for People from Black and Ethnic Minorities*. Hopkins, A. and Bahl, V., eds. pp. 57–62. London: Royal College of Physicians.

Farrah, M. (1986). Black elders in Leicester: an action research report on the needs of black elderly people of African descent from the Caribbean. *Social Services Research*, **1**, 47–9.

Fenton, S. (1985). *Race, Health and Welfare: Afrocaribbean and South Asian People in Central Bristol: Health and Social Services*. Bristol: University of Bristol.

Fernando, S. (1988). *Race and Culture in Psychiatry*. London: Croom Helm.

Fernando, S. (1991). (ed.) *Mental Health, Race and Culture*. London: Macmillan.

Foster, G. & Anderson, B.G. (1978). *Medical Anthropology*. Chichester: John Wiley.

Francis, E., David, J., Johnson, N. and Shashidharan, S. (1989). Black people and psychiatry in the UK. *Psychiatric Bulletin*, **13**, 482–5.

Furnham, A. and Sheik, S. (1993). Gender, generational and social support correlates of mental health in Asian immigrants. *International Journal of Social Psychiatry*, **39**, 22–33.

Giggs, J. (1986). Ethnic status and mental illness in urban areas. In *Health, Race and Ethnicity*. Rathwell, T. and Phillips, D., eds. London: Croom Helm.

Gillam, S.J., Jarman, B., White, P. & Law, R. (1989). Ethnic differences in consultation rates in urban general practice. *British Medical Journal*, **299**, 958–60.

Goldberg, D. & Huxley, P. (1980). *Mental Illness in the Community: The Pathway to Psychiatric Care*. London: Tavistock.

Goldberg, D. & Huxley, P. (1992). *Common Mental Disorders: A Bio-social Model*. London: Routledge.

Halpern, D. (1993). Minorities and mental health. *Social Science and Medicine*, **36**, 597–607.

Harrison, G., Ineichen, B., Smith, J. & Morgan, H.G. (1984). Psychiatric hospital admissions to Bristol II: social and clinical aspects of compulsory admission. *British Journal of Psychiatry*, **145**, 605–11.

Harrison, G., Owens, D., Holton, A., Neilson, D. & Boot, D. (1988). A prospective study of severe mental disorder in Afro-Caribbean patients. *Psychological Medicine*, **18**, 643–57.

Harrison, G., Holton, A., Neilson, D., Owens, D., Boot, D. & Cooper, J. (1989). Severe mental disorder in Afro-Caribbean patients: some social, demographic and service factors. *Psychological Medicine*, **19**, 683–96.

Health and Ethnicity Programme (1991). North East & North West Thames Regional Health Authorities, London.

Health Education Authority (HEA) (1994). *Black and Minority Ethnic Groups in England, Health and Lifestyles*. London: HEA Publications.

Helman, C., ed. (1990). *Culture, Health and Illness*. London: Wright.

Horwitz, A.V. (1982). *The Social Control of Mental Illness*. New York: Academic Press.

Ineichen, B. (1990). The mental health of Asians. *British Medical Journal*, **200**, 1669–70.

Jain, C., Narayan, N., Narayan, P. *et al.* (1985). Attitudes of Asian patients in Birmingham to general practitioner services. *Journal of the Royal College of General Practitioners*, **35**, 416–18.

Johnson, M.R.D., Cross, M. & Cardew, S.A. (1983). Inner city resident ethnic minorities and primary health care. *Postgraduate Medical Journal*, **59**, 664–7.

Jones, B.E. & Gray, B.A. (1986). Problems in diagnosing schizophrenia and affective disorder in American blacks. *Hospital and Community Psychiatry*, **37**, 61–5.

Jones, J.S. (1981). How different are human races? *Nature,* **293**, 188–90.

Kakar, S. (1984). *Shamans, Mystics and Doctors: A Psychological Inquiry into India and its Healing Tradition.* London: Unwin Paperbacks.

Kareem, J. & Littlewood, R. (1992). *Intercultural Therapy: Themes, Interpretations and Practice.* Oxford: Blackwell.

Karseras, P. & Hopkins, E. (1987). *British Asians: Health in the Community.* Chichester: John Wiley.

Kessing, R.M. (1981). *Cultural Anthropology: A Contemporary Perspective.* New York: Holt, Rinehart and Winston.

Kessler, R. & Neighbors, H. (1986). A new perspective on the relationships among race, social class and psychological distress. *Journal of Health and Social Behaviour,* **27**, 107–15.

Kirmayer, L.T. (1984). Culture, affect and somatisation. Part I. *Transcultural Psychiatric Review,* **21**, 159–87.

Kleinman, A. (1980). Major conceptual and research issues for cultural (anthropological) psychiatry. *Culture, Medicine and Psychiatry,* **4**, 3–13.

Kleinman, A. (1987). Anthropology and psychiatry: the role of culture in cross-cultural research on illness. *British Journal of Psychiatry,* **151**, 447–54.

Krause, E.B., Rosser, R.M., Khiani, M.L. & Lotay, N.S. (1990). Psychiatric morbidity among Punjabi medical patients measured by the general health questionnaire. *Psychological Medicine,* **20**, 711–19.

Krause, I.B. (1989). The sinking heart: a Punjabi communication of distress. *Social Science and Medicine* **29**, 563–75.

Krause, I.B. (1994). Numbers and meaning: a dialogue in cross-cultural psychiatry. *Journal of the Royal Society of Medicine,* **87**, 278–82.

Lawrence, E. (1982). In the abundance of water the fool is thirsty: sociology and black 'pathology'. In *The Empire Strikes Back.* London: Centre of Contemporary Cultural Studies.

Lawson, W.B., Yesavage, J.A. & Werner, P.D. (1984). Race, violence and psychopathology. *Journal of Clinical Psychiatry,* **45**, 284–92.

Leff, J. (1990). The 'new cross-cultural psychiatry' a case of the baby and the bathwater. *British Journal of Psychiatry,* **156**, 305–7.

Lewis, G., Croft-Jeffreys, C. & David, A. (1990). Are British psychiatrists racist? *British Journal of Psychiatry,* **151**, 410–15.

Lewis, P., Vaddadi, K.S., Rack, P.H. & Allen, J.J. (1980). Ethnic differences in drug response. *Postgraduate Medical Journal,* **56**, 46–9.

Lipsedge, M. (1993). Mental health: access to care for black and ethnic minority people. In *Access to Health Care for People from Black and Ethnic Minorities*. Hopkins, A. and Bahl, V., eds. pp. 169–183. London: Royal College of Physicians.

Littlewood, R. & Lipsedge, M. (1978). Migration, ethnicity and diagnosis. *Psychiatrica Clinica*, **11**, 15–22.

Littlewood, R. & Lipsedge, M. (1979). *Aliens and Alienists*. London: Unwin Hyman.

Littlewood, R. (1986). Ethnic minorities and the Mental Health Act: patterns of explanation. *Bulletin of the Royal College of Psychiatrists*, **10**, 306–8.

Littlewood, R. (1988). Community initiated research. A study of pyschiatrists' conceptualisations of cannabis psychosis. *Bulletin of the Royal College of Psychiatrists*, **12**, 486–8.

Littlewood, R. (1989). Cannabis psychosis. *Psychiatric Bulletin*, **13**, 148–9.

Littlewood, R. (1990). From categories to contexts: a decade of the 'new cross-cultural psychiatry'. *British Journal of Psychiatry*, **156**, 308–27.

Lloyd, K. (1993). Depression and anxiety among Afro-Caribbean general practice attenders in Britain. *International Journal of Social Psychiatry*, **39**, 1–9.

London, M. (1986). Mental illness among immigrant minorities in the United Kingdom. *British Journal of Psychiatry*, **149**, 265–73.

Lopez, S. & Hernandez, P. (1976). How culture is considered in evaluations of psychotherapy. *Journal of Mental Diseases*, **176**, 598–606.

Loring, M. & Powell, B. (1988). Gender, race and DSM III, A study of the objectivity of psychiatric diagnostic behaviour. *Journal of Health and Social Behaviour*, **29**, 1–22.

McAvoy, B. & Sayeed, A. (1990). Communication. In *Health Care for Asians*. McAvoy, B. and Donaldson, L., eds. Oxford: Oxford University Press.

McGovern, D. & Cope, R. (1987). The compulsory detention of males of different ethnic groups, with special reference to offender patients. *British Journal of Psychiatry*, **150**, 505–12.

McQueen, D.V. (1978). The history of science and medicine as the theoretical sources for the comparative study of contemporary medical systems. *Social Science and Medicine*, **12**, 69–74.

Marks, J., Goldberg, D. & Hillier, V. (1979). Determinants of the ability of general practitioners to detect psychological illness. *Psychological Medicine*, **9**, 337–53.

Marsella, A.J. (1978). Thoughts on cross-cultural studies on the epidemiology of depression. *Culture, Medicine and Psychiatry*, **2**, 343–57.

Marsella, A.J. (1984). Culture and mental health: an overview. In *Cultural Conceptions of Mental Health Therapy*. Marsella, A.J. and White, G.M., eds. pp. 359–388. Dordrecht: Reidel.

Mayou, R. (1976). The nature of bodily symptoms. *British Journal of Psschiatry*, **129**, 55–60.

Merrill, J. & Owens, J. (1986). Ethnic differences in self-poisoning: a comparison of Asian and White groups. *British Journal of Psychiatry*, **148**, 708–12.

Merrill, J. & Owens, J. (1988). Self poisoning among four immigrant groups. *Acta Psychiatrica Scandinavica*, **77**, 77–80.

MIND (1986). *Mental Health Services in a Multiracial Society: Statements by the MIND Black and Ethnic Minorities Mental Health Working Party*. London: Mind Policy paper II.

Moodley, P. & Perkins, R. (1990). Blacks and psychiatry: a framework for understanding access to psychiatric services. *Psychiatric Bulletin*, **14**, 538–40.

Moodley, P. & Perkins, R. (1991). Routes to psychiatric in-patient care in an inner-London borough. *Social Psychiatry and Psychiatric Epidemiology*, **26**, 47–51.

Moodley, P. & Perkins, R. (1994). Perception of problems in psychiatric inpatients: denial, race and service users. *Social Psychiatry and Psychiatric Epidemiology*, **28**, 189–93.

Moorhouse, S. (1992). Quantitative research in intercultural therapy. In *Intercultural Therapy*. Kareem, J. and Littlewood, R. eds. Oxford: Blackwell.

Morgan, D. (1989). Psychiatric cases: an ethnography of the referral process. *Psychological Medicine*, **19**, 743–53.

Mumford, D.B. & Whitehouse, A.M. (1988). Increased prevalence of bulimia nervosa among Asian schoolgirls. *British Medical Journal*, **297**, 278.

Mumford, D.B., Bavington, J.T., Bhatnagar, K.S., Hussain, Y., Mirza, S. & Naraghi, M.M. (1991). The Bradford Somatic Inventory: a multi-ethnic inventory of somatic symptoms reported by anxious and depressed patients in Britain and Indo-Pakistan subcontinent. *British Journal of Psychiatry*, **158**, 379–86.

Murphy, H.B. (1977). Migration, culture and mental health. *Psychological Medicine*, **7**, 677–84.

Murray, J. & Williams, P. (1986). Self-reported illness and general practice consultations in Asian-born and British-born residents of West London. *Social Psychiatry*, **21**, 139–45.

Nayani, S. (1989). The evaluation of psychiatric illness in Asian patients using the HAD scale. *British Journal of Psychiatry*, **155**, 545–7.

Obeyeskere, G. (1977). The theory and practice of psychological medicine in the Ayurvedic tradition. *Culture, Medicine and Psychiatry*, **1**, 155–81.

Ohaeri, J.U. & Odejide, O.A. (1994). Somatisation symptoms among patients using primary health care facilities in a rural community in Nigeria. *American Journal of Psychiatry*, **151**, 728–31.

Onyango, R.S. (1986). Cannabis psychosis in young psychiatric inpatients. *British Journal of Addiction*, **81**, 419–23.

OPCS. (1986). *Labour Force Survey 1985: Ethnic Group and Country of Birth, OPCS Monitor*. London: HMSO.

OPCS. (1992). *Office of Population Censuses and Surveys: County Monitors*. London: OPCS.

Osborne, F. (1971). Races and the future of man In *The Biological and Social Meaning of Race*. Osborne, F., ed. pp. 149–157. San Francisco: Freeman.

Owens, D., Harrison, G. & Boot, D. (1991). Ethnic factors in voluntary and compulsory admissions. *Psychological Medicine*, **21**, 185–96.

Owusu-Bempah, J. (1990). Toeing the white line. *Community Care*, **838**, 16–17.

Parmar, P. (1981). Young Asian women: a critique of the pathological approach. *Multiracial Education*, **3**, 19–25.

Parsons, L. & Day, S. (1992). Improving obstetric outcomes in ethnic minorities: an evaluation of health advocacy in Hackney. *Journal of Public Health Medicine*, **14**, 183–91.

Pasamanick, B. (1963). Some misconceptions concerning difference in the racial prevalence of mental disease. *American Journal of Orthopsychiatry*, **33**, 72–86.

Pearson, R.M. (1988). *Social Services in a Multi-racial Society*. London: Social Services Inspectorate, Department of Health.

Priest, R.G. (1991). A new initiative on depression (editorial). *British Journal of General Practice*, **41**, 487.

Rack, P.H. (1982). *Race, Culture and Mental Disorder*. London: Tavistock.

Rack, P.H. (1986). Migration and mental illness. In *Transcultural Psychiatry*, Cox, J., ed. pp. 59–75. London: Croom Helm.

Rashid, A. & Jagger, C. (1992). Attitudes to and perceived use of health care services amongst Asian and non-Asian patients in Leicester. *British Journal of General Practice*, **42**, 197–201.

Rex, J. (1986). Sociological concepts and the field of ethnic and race relations. In *Race and Ethnicity*. Rex, J., ed. Milton Keynes: Oxford University Press.

Robinson, V. (1992). Move on up: the mobility of Britain's Afro-Caribbean and Asian populations. In *Migration Processes and Patterns. Vol 2, Population Redistribution in the UK*. Stillwell, J., Rees, P. and Baden, P., eds. London: Bellhaven Press.

Rogers, A. & Faulkner, A. (1987). *A Place of Safety: MIND's Research of Police Referrals to Psychiatric Services*. London: MIND.

Rogler, L. (1993). Culturally sensitising psychiatric diagnosis: a framework for research. *Journal of Nervous and Mental Diseases*, **181**, 401–8.

Sartorius, N., Jablensky, A. & Shapiro, R. (1977). Two year follow-up of the patients included in the WHO international pilot study of schizophrenia. *Psychological Medicine*, **7**, 529–41.

Sartorius, N., Jablensky, A., Korten, A. *et al.* (1986). Early manifestations and first contact incidence of schizophrenia in different cultures. *Psychological Medicine*, **16**, 909–28.

Shaikh, H.A. (1985). Cross-cultural comparison of psychiatric admissions of Asian and indigenous patients in Leicestershire. *International Journal of Social Psychiatry*, **31**, 3–11.

Shaunuk, S., Lakhani, S.R., Abraham, R. & Maxwell, J.D. (1986). Differences among Asian patients. *British Medical Journal*, **293**, 1169.

Shweder, R.A. (1985). Menstrual pollution, soul loss and the comparative study of emotions. In *Culture and Depression*. Kleinman, A. and Good, B., eds. Berkeley: University of California Press.

Singer, K. (1975). Depressive disorders from a transcultural perspective. *Social Science and Medicine*, **9**, 289–301.

Soni Raleigh, V., Bulusu, L. & Balarajan, R. (1990). Suicides among immigrants from the Indian sub-continent. *British Journal of Psychiatry*, **156**, 46–50.

Spuhler, J.N. & Lindzey, G. (1967). Racial differences in behaviour. In *Behaviour: Genetic Analysis*. Hirsch, J., ed. pp. 367–414. New York: McGraw-Hill.

Sundquist, J. (1993). Ethnicity as a risk factor for mental illness. A population-based study. *Acta Psychiatrica Scandinavica*, **87**, 208–12.

Teja, J.S., Narang, R.L. & Aggarwal, A.K. (1971). Depression across cultures. *British Journal of Psychiatry*, **119**, 253–60.

Thomas, L. (1992). Racism and psychotherapy: working with racism in the consulting room. In *Intercultural Therapy: Themes, Interpretations and Practice*. Kareem, J. and Littlewood, R., eds. Oxford: Blackwell.

Townsend, J.M. (1979). Stereotypes and mental illness: a comparison with ethnic stereotypes. *Culture, Medicine and Psychiatry*, **3**, 205–30.

Tylee, A. & Freeling, P. (1989). The recognition, diagnosis and acknowledgement of depressive disorders by general practitioners. In *Depression, An Integrative Approach*. Paykel, E. and Herbst, K., eds. London: Heinemann.

Ulbrich, P.M., Warheit, G.J. & Zimmerman, R.S. (1989). Race, socioeconomic status and psychological distress: an examination of differential vulnerability. *Journal of Health and Social Behaviour*, **30**, 131–46.

Webb, P. (1981). Health problems of London's Asians and Afro-Caribbeans. *Health Visitor*, **54**, 141–7.

Webb-Johnson, A. (1991). *A Cry for Change: An Asian Perspective on Developing Quality Mental Health Care*. UK: Confederation of Indian Organisations.

Wessely, S., Castle, D., Der, G. & Murray, R. (1991). Schizophrenia and Afro-Caribbeans: a case control study. *British Journal of Psychiatry*, **159**, 795–881.

Westermeyer, J. (1990). Working with an interpreter in psychiatric assessment and treatment. *Journal of Nervous and Mental Diseases*, **178**, 745–9.

World Health Organisation (1979). *Schizophrenia: An International Follow-up Study*. Chichester: John Wiley and Sons.

Wright, C.M. (1983), Language and communication problems in an Asian community. *Journal of the Royal College of General Practitioners*, **33**, 101–4.

Yamamoto, J., James, Q.C., Bloombaum, M. & Hatten, J. (1967). Racial factors in patient selection. *American Journal of Psychiatry*, **124**, 630–6.

Yamamoto, J., James, Q.C. & Palley, N. (1968). Cultural problems in psychiatric therapy. *Archives of General Psychiatry*, **19**, 45–9.

Yap, P.M. (1974). *Comparative Psychiatry: A Theoretic Framework*. Toronto: University of Toronto Press.

Yinger, M. (1981). Toward a theory of assimilation and dissimilation. *Ethnic and Racial Studies*, **4**, 3.

[7] The prevention of mental illness in people with learning disability

Jenny Curran and Sheila Hollins

Definition and prevalence of learning disability

Learning disability is the term adopted by the Department of Health to describe what has previously been termed mental handicap, and while controversy remains as to the most appropriate terminology (Gath, 1992), we will use learning disability in this chapter. The essential elements of learning disability include intellectual and other associated impairments arising during the developmental period, most frequently around the time of birth, and resulting in long-term disability in performing some or all of the major life activities which require intellectual and social function. Learning disability is often divided into moderate, and severe or profound. Such broad terms tend to obscure the individual's mix of abilities and disabilities, often concentrating on the deficits in a negative way. However, it is important to recognise that the label covers a very wide range of abilities, and this in turn will affect both the manifestation and management of mental illness in people with learning disability.

Estimating the prevalence of learning disability is difficult. A variety of different methods of identification have been used, as well as differing definitions, so that figures will vary with the age profile, and location of a particular population. The estimated lifetime prevalence of mild learning disability is about 3% in the United Kingdom, and the more disabled group, including moderate to profound learning disability, is ten times less common, occurring in about 3 per 1000 at school age (Fryers, 1984). In an average general practitioner's practice with a list size of 2000 patients, there may be four to six people with severe learning disability, and 20 to 30 people with mild learning disability (Box 7.1).

In an average general practitioner practice of list size 2000, there may be 4 to 6 people with severe learning disability, and 20 to 30 people with mild learning disability.

Box 7.1 *Prevalence of learning disability.*

33% to 66% of community samples of people with learning disability show a significant degree of psychopathology (Bregman, 1991).

Box 7.2 *Prevalence of psychopathology in learning disabled people.*

Prevalence of mental illness in people with learning disability

Numerous surveys have shown that people with learning disability have high rates of mental illness (Corbett, 1979). There are many methodological problems with the surveys, not least because most of the studies surveyed people with learning disability who were living in large institutions. Prevalence rates of 40% or more were assumed to be due to the fact that institutionalised patients belonged to a subgroup of people with learning disability. However, several community studies have also found high rates. The Swedish Community Survey, which studied adults aged 20–60 years, found that 33% of those with mild learning disability and 71% of those with severe learning disability showed evidence of psychiatric disturbance (Gostason, 1985). In Rutter's Isle of Wight study, 30–42% of learning disabled nine to eleven year-olds had signs of mental and behavioural problems (Rutter *et al.*, 1976). The current consensus is that between one- and two-thirds of learning disabled people in community samples exhibit a significant degree of psychopathology (Bregman, 1991) (Box 7.2).

Aspects of mental illness in people with learning disability

All the common psychiatric problems seen in general psychiatric services are also seen in the psychiatry of learning disability, and a brief discussion of the main diagnostic groups is summarised by Bernal and Hollins (1995). However, the forms that mental illness can take in people with learning disability are more various than in the general population. There is wide scope for psychiatric illness to be distorted in its presentation by the co-existence of learning disability (Bicknell, 1983; Vitiello & Behar, 1992).

There may be behavioural changes which suggest disturbed mental functioning. For example, a severely learning disabled man who is distressed by a change in carers may develop problems of incontinence, having previously been continent. Researchers have attempted to standardise assessment of people with severe and profound learning disability by developing checklists and scales (Aman *et al.*, 1985; Matson *et al.*, 1991) which include a wide variety of behaviours that can indicate mental illness. The important clinical point is to consider a symptom in the context of the individual's overall developmental level.

'Problem' behaviour

Behavioural changes in people with learning disability can also result in disruption to the surrounding environment, and this is sometimes called challenging behaviour. There are several definitions of challenging or problem behaviour. One that is widely used is defined as follows:

> Behaviour of such an intensity, frequency or duration that the physical safety of the person or others is likely to be placed in serious jeopardy, or behaviour which is likely to seriously limit or deny access to the use of ordinary community facilities (Emerson *et al.*, 1988).

The relationship between challenging behaviour and mental illness is complex, but a proportion of those people with learning disability who exhibit challenging behaviour are mentally ill and require specialist assessment and treatment (Holland & Murphy, 1990).

Pitfalls in the recognition of mental illness in people with learning disability

Psychiatric illness is often missed when presenting to general practitioners (Goldberg & Huxley, 1980), and general practitioner characteristics that increase recognition of such disorders are currently under investigation (Millar & Goldberg, 1991). Patient characteristics, and the manner in which the psychiatric problem is presented, are also relevant. No research has been done on the presentation and diagnosis of psychiatric disorder in general practice by patients who have a learning disability. It would seem a reasonable hypothesis that a proportion of such psychiatric disorder is misdiagnosed.

A further hypothesis is that a proportion of more severely disabled people with learning disability who are experiencing symptoms of illness, but are not able to present themselves for treatment, are not taken to the general practitioner by their carer either. In terms of Goldberg & Huxley's (1980, Chapter 1) pathways to care, for many people with learning disability, there is an extra stage within the first filter (illness behaviour) between illness in the community (level 1) and illness presented to primary care services (level 2), which is *recognition by the carer of illness behaviour*. There is no research that examines this hypothesis at present, but at a clinical level it seems that neither general practitioners nor carers are particularly adept at recognising signs of possible mental illness in people with learning disability.

Diagnostic overshadowing

Symptoms of mental illness may be wrongly attributed to co-existing learning disability.

For example, a young woman with a moderate learning disability had episodes of irritability and tearfulness over several years. The staff who worked in her home believed that such 'moodiness' was a part of her disability and had not remarked on this to the general practitioner. When a new staff member joined the staff team and wondered whether the behavioural changes could be a sign of mental or physical illness, the young woman was taken to see the general practitioner who diagnosed a recurrent depressive illness and successfully treated her with antidepressants.

This process of misattribution has been termed 'diagnostic overshadowing' (Reiss, Levitan & Szyszo, 1982).

Diagnostic overshadowing also commonly occurs when symptoms of physical illness are wrongly interpreted as being due to the learning disability. Untreated physical morbidity can contribute to mental illness and behavioural problems, particularly when pain or sensory impairment occurs and remains unrecognised. A number of surveys have shown that physical problems are often missed in people with learning disability (Beange & Bauman, 1990). The commonest conditions affecting people with learning disability are sensory impairment, epilepsy and other neurological disorders such as cerebral palsy, skin disorders, musculoskeletal disorders and psychiatric problems. Between 30% and 55% of people with learning disability have daily prescribed medicine, and many suffer with poor dental care and hygiene (Welsh Health Planning Forum, 1992). Clinicians require a low threshold of suspicion for mental illness in people with learning disability, and should exclude physical pathology.

Community teams – the potential for specialist help

Traditionally the majority of people with learning disability, including many with severe and multiple problems, have lived at home with their families. Parents have looked to their general practitioner for access to health care for their sons and daughters, with specialist health care being provided directly only for long-stay hospital inpatients. Since the late 1970s, community health care teams have been developed to support people with learning disability being resettled from institutions or already living in community settings. These multidisciplinary teams have varied in the extent to which they have met health or social care needs, and they are still evolving differently in different parts of the country.

Some trends are apparent, however. Psychiatrists have developed a subspeciality in the community, working with this client group and their carers. Some psychiatrists have developed special expertise in the forensic psychiatry of learning disability, or in psychotherapy, and many have considerable expertise in the management of epilepsy. Some work with the whole age range, whilst others work only with adults, or in a few instances only with children. A new type of community nurse has developed with expertise in supporting skills development for people with learning disability, and usually with counselling experience, but with a very limited general or psychiatric nursing background. Teams include speech, occupational and physiotherapists and may include an attached general practitioner clinical assistant.

The work of these teams has tended to be somewhat ideologically driven, with a commitment to the principles of 'normalisation' (Tyne, 1981), and more recently of 'social role valorisation' (Wolfensberger, 1983). One consequence has been the determination to help people with learning disability to use generic mainstream health care rather than to provide separate segregated services. Such a service may, however, be too dependent on the client or carer for its initiation.

With respect to the mental health of people with learning disability, the debate continues about the extent to which people should have access to general psychiatric services and the extent to which specialist learning disability services are required. People who, despite learning disability, can communicate and who present with more typical symptoms of mental illness, are likely to be served adequately within either a mainstream psychiatric service or a specialist learning disability service. When a patient has severe communication problems, or challenging behaviour, making a diagnosis is complex, and a specialist service will usually be required.

Primary and secondary prevention of mental illness in people with learning disability

A child born with a developmental disability whose parents are supported and encouraged in making healthy attachments is probably both protected from developing mental health problems (primary prevention), and also more likely to have early access to diagnosis and treatment of any mental health problems (secondary prevention). As many people with learning disability are cared for by their families, this preventive approach will have implications in adult life as well as childhood. It is also possible that healthy emotional attachments developed in childhood may facilitate the process of the adult person with learning disability leaving home, in addition to the provision of acceptable alternative placements.

One stated reason for deinstitutionalisation programmes and the development of 'community care' for people with learning disability has been to prevent environmental problems adding to their disability. Numerous studies have shown increases in adaptive behaviour among people with learning disability following resettlement from institutions, even among older people (Fine, Tangeman & Woodward, 1990). However, there is little evidence that mental illness or behavioural problems can be prevented in total by living in the 'community', and further research is needed to identify which social and environmental factors have a positive impact on the mental health of people with learning disability.

A number of strategies for the secondary prevention of mental illness in people with learning disability will be discussed. It is necessary for such strategies to be carefully evaluated, with cost–benefit analyses (Hafner & An Der Heiden, 1991). The suggested strategies are based on some early evaluation work, but further research and audit is needed in all these areas.

Promoting healthy attachments

Certain groups of people with learning disability are at higher risk of abuse, for example, those who experience communication difficulties. Long-term effects of abuse, including sexual abuse, in people with learning disability are currently under research. Case studies suggest harmful effects on emotional and cognitive functioning (Sinason, 1986). Prevention of all forms of abuse of children and adults with learning disability requires multi-agency action to foster healthy emotional attachments and identify families at risk of abusing (e.g. where a parent has a substance abuse problem) (Sobsey, 1994), as well as teaching assertiveness skills and giving sex education to people with learning disability (Craft & Hitching, 1989). Early recognition of abuse will prevent it continuing long term and affecting personality development. Specially designed picture books are now available to support professionals and carers working with adults with learning disability who have been sexually abused (Hollins & Sinason, 1992).

Primary health care teams are well placed to identify high risk situations, and so must be included in any prevention strategies. A collaborative study in Oxford involved midwives referring mothers of sick or handicapped babies, to a special service (Ounstead et al., 1982). The service, in turn, usually involved the general practitioner and health visitor, fully informing them of the midwife's worries and alerting them to the possible need for considerable support. Health visitors are well situated to provide family support and to liaise with other services.

There is disagreement about the nature of the response of parents to the birth of a child with a severe disability. One hypothesis is that parents have to grieve the loss of the perfect baby they were expecting before they can fully accept the disabled child (Bicknell, 1983; Hollins, 1985). Others reject this bereavement model, stressing instead the importance of attachment theory in understanding parental adjustment (Sobsey, 1994). Damrosch & Perry (1989) asked mothers and fathers to describe their emotions prospectively and found that they had quite different reactions from each other, with mothers typically experiencing periods of good adjustment alternating with periods of depression or despair. Fathers showed a gradual improvement in adjustment over time, but without the setbacks experienced by their wives. The adjustment of parents is assumed to have some impact on the experience of the child. Early intervention has been recommended but is more often aimed at promoting skills development for the child, rather than assisting the development of a healthy emotional relationship between parent and child (Cunningham & Davis, 1985).

Screening for sensory impairment
Up to half of people with learning disability have one sensory impairment (visual defects in 25% to 55% and hearing loss in 5% to 25%), while 18% of people with learning disability have two sensory impairments. Behavioural problems are 50% more frequent in people with learning disability with additional sensory impairment (Welsh Health Planning Forum, 1992). Challenging behaviour in people with Down's Syndrome may be associated with unrecognised deafness, which is easily missed by parents and carers (Yeates, 1989). Hearing loss contributes to poor speech, impaired social skills and attention deficits. Poor vision can similarly seriously disrupt social development, particularly in young children. Of people with severe learning disability, 75% have refractive errors, and the majority of people with Down's Syndrome suffer with eye problems. Many of these needs remain unrecognised (Howells, 1986).

Prevention and early treatment of these conditions is likely to reduce behavioural difficulties in people with learning disability. One approach adopted by the Welsh Health Planning Forum is to define clear health gain targets and related service targets. The health targets should influence District Health Authorities and Family Health Service Authorities, in partnership with appropriate others, to develop policies to determine prevalence levels and improve access to screening for the target disorders. Purchasers of services for people with learning disability should include preventive work in their specifications, and informed providers should collaborate in defining priority health gain targets. General practitioners and their primary health care team colleagues have a central

Health gain targets
Ensure that no one with a learning disability has:
- *an unmanaged refractive error*
- *an untreated hearing deficit*
- *an unassessed combined visual and hearing deficit (by 1997)*

Service targets
In partnership with ophthalmic opticians, audiometricians, and specialists in deafness and blindness, district health authorities and family health service authorities should ensure that clear policies exist to determine the prevalance of visual defects, hearing defects and combined visual/hearing defects among people with learning disability, including encouragement of sight and hearing tests and ready access to special techniques for the management of deaf and blind people.

Box 7.3 *Example of health gain targets and associated service targets from the Protocol for Investment in Health Gain. (Welsh Health Planning Forum, 1992.)*

role in the development of such services as purchasers, and also as providers, since some sensory impairment can be screened in primary care, although others require specialist assessment. An example of the health gain approach is given in Box 7.3.

Communication difficulties
Communication problems are also a commonly encountered difficulty for people with learning disability. Often simple skills on the part of the professional are all that are required to minimise the handicapping aspects of the communication difficulty. Attention to the professional's own style of communication, with appropriate rate, sentence length and construction and vocabulary, combined with a respectful attitude and willingness to spend the time needed to put the person with learning disability at ease, are often the key to a successful consultation. More serious communication difficulties will require specialist assessment and management, such as the use of augmented communication. The Makaton Vocabulary is an example of augmented communication, and is a language programme involving the use of symbols and signing designed to encourage language development in children and adults with communication difficulties (Grove & Walker, 1990). There are other complex problems, such as the presence of autistic features, or neurological deficits which may also contribute to communication difficulties. A recent study found that 60% of those with a learning disability living at home had a speech and language problem, with 30% having little or no speech, and research shows that behavioural

problems are commoner in people with learning disability with communication difficulties (Welsh Health Planning Forum, 1992).

The prevention of behavioural and emotional difficulties in people with learning disability requires both early assessment and management of communication difficulties where they occur, because these difficulties can be a predisposing or maintaining factor, or both, for the mental or behavioural problem.

Specialist speech and language therapists are frequently members of the community team for people with learning disability, and have a vital role to play in both assessment and treatment strategies. Parents and carers as well as other professionals benefit from the specialist advice. The Welsh Office has prioritised assessment and augmentation of communication skills for people with learning disability, their carers, and staff working and living with people with learning disability in the form of health gain targets and service targets (Welsh Planning Forum, 1992).

Improving access to primary care

The role of the primary health care team is pivotal, in preventing, detecting and managing mental illness (provider role) and in referring to specialist services (purchaser role). Many people with learning disability must rely on the observation and intervention of another person, usually though not necessarily, the primary carer. While no research has been done on this process in people with learning disability, the World Health Organisation studies on the pathways to care (Gater *et al.*, 1991) have shown that other groups may use more complex routes to reach the general practitioner services. In some parts of the world, the primary health care service is frequently bypassed, and referral direct to specialist mental health services occurs. This may often occur with people with learning disability, when a social worker or other member of the community team for people with learning disability refers to the psychiatrist on the team. Referral can then bypass the general practitioner with the risk that the general practitioner may be unaware of the details of the referral. Even when communications between the primary health care team and community team for people with learning disability are good, general practitioners may miss important aspects of preventive care, which may involve education of the carers.

The role of carers

This requires better understanding. It is widely acknowledged that mental illness is a stigmatising label. In our experience, families and care workers are often reluctant to entertain the idea of the person with learning disability receiving the additional stigma of a mental illness. Indeed, for some the learning disability is denied also. Carers may fear that the person with learning disability will receive medication without the necessary monitoring. Indeed, research shows that, at least some people with learning disability (those who have severe learning disability and challenging behaviour), are not infrequently prescribed psychotropic medication for long periods without regular review (Hubert, 1992). Such fears may inhibit the carer from involving the general practitioner when needed. The primary health care team can attempt to minimise this potential block in the pathway to care by encouraging carers to use their services, and by educating them to the possibility of emotional difficulties in people with learning disability. The community team for people with learning disability can aid in this process by liaising with carers and their families to encourage use of primary health care services, by accompanying the person with learning disability to see the general practitioner if this is appropriate, and by education of the primary health care team towards good practice in a variety of areas, including medication review, family support and disability awareness.

Improving the detection of mental illness

Training is the key issue in helping primary health care teams to detect mental illness in people with learning disability. The basic psychiatric skills of history taking and mental state examination are now taught to trainee general practitioners. However, many doctors have had little or no formal training about learning disability, and may have some difficulty in applying their basic psychiatric skills to people with learning disability. Here are some guidelines for assessing possible mental illness, which are based on the brief but informative handout entitled *Psychiatric Illness and Learning Disability* available from the Department of Psychiatry of Disability, St George's Hospital Medical School (Bernal & Hollins, 1995).

The history

Assessment involves careful enquiry into the social setting, and into the concerns of the family, carers or other professionals. Who is most concerned about the problem? Often a variety of agencies may be involved, with differing perspectives. A history should be obtained from the person with learning disability if communication skills permit, and from an informant or informants. It is important to gain a picture of the person's highest level of functioning and developmental level and it is a common pitfall to assume that a low level of functioning is caused by the learning disability *per se*. Mental illness often results in loss of skills in people with learning disability. Identification of autistic features is also important, as people with learning disability have higher rates of autistic disorder and autistic symptoms (Wing, 1994), which may overshadow an additional problem of mental illness.

Altered sleep pattern	Overactivity, restlessness
Change in appetite	Irritability and aggression
Social withdrawal	Self-injury
Loss of skills	Sexual disinhibition
Loss of interest	Bizarre movements, abnormal postures

Box 7.4 *Changes in behaviour which may be due to mental illness.*

The presenting problem

Some common behavioural changes which may reflect an under-lying mental illness are listed in Box 7.4.

It is not unusual to find behavioural changes associated with loss of a familiar carer or routine. Bereavement reactions may be missed, presenting either some time after the death, or in an atypical form. People with learning disability are sometimes excluded from funerals of very close relatives and friends, and occasionally from the fact of the death itself. Depression can present with typical biological features, with irritability, or other behavioural changes. *Feeling Blue* is a picture book about depression for adults with learning disability and their carers, which is designed to help recognise and seek help for this common mental health problem (Hollins & Curran, 1995).

Unacknowledged grieving might be prevented through educa-tion of families, carers and professionals about the emotional needs of people with learning disability (Hollins & Sireling, 1991, 1994). Oswin's (1991) book *Am I Allowed to Cry?* is a powerful testimony to the widespread social responses which foster pathological grief in people with learning disability.

Medication history

Medication, particularly anticonvulsants and psychotropics, may precipitate behavioural problems, so a careful drug history should be taken. Those with brain damage are particularly susceptible to the disinhibiting effects of benzodiazepines. People with learning disability may also be more susceptible to the motor side-effects of neuroleptics. If the patient has limited communication skills, or a pre-existing neurological disorder, such side-effects will be more difficult to recognise. Epilepsy is more common in people with learning disability, and neuroleptics and many tricyclic antidepres-sants lower the seizure threshold, thus increasing the required dose of anticonvulsant when both types of drug are needed. Given their sensitivity to neuroleptics and the potential for drug interactions, the threshold for 'high dose' antipsychotics should be lower for people with learning disability (Thompson, 1994). Rational prescribing of psychotropics in people with learning disability should follow the guidelines of Einfeld (1990), which state that the precise symptoms for which the drug is prescribed should be defined and a rationale for the choice of drug should be given; a reliable and valid method of monitoring changes in the target symptoms is required, and following reduction in those symptoms, an attempt to reduce the dose should be made and withdrawal should follow a planned regime.

Physical causes

Physical examination may reveal a cause of distress, such as a dental abscess, or a painful foot condition that has been overlooked. Constipation is a not infrequent cause of discomfort. People with Down's Syndrome are at risk of becoming hypothyroid and investigations, including sensory assessment, are particularly important in those who cannot complain. A protocol for primary health care is discussed in the Royal College of General Practitioners' paper *Primary Care for People with Mental Handicap* (Howells, 1990). A number of possible medical causes for behavioural symptoms are discussed in detail in the paper by Kastner and colleagues (Kastner *et al.*, 1990).

Examination of the mental state

A brief mental state examination is helpful and possible even in someone with no functional language. Bernal and Hollins (1995) suggest that mental state examination in people with learning disability should include observation of dress, posture, communication style, behaviour at interview, and response to particular people or subjects of conversation. It should involve an informant who knows the patient well.

Use of screening tools to identify mental illness in people with learning disability

Specialists in the field of learning disability may use checklists as part of the assessment process when a mental illness or behavioural problem is suspected (Sturmey, Reed & Corbett, 1991). There are many problems with reliability and validity of the tools, but they can be used in conjunction with the usual assessment methods of full history-taking and examination (Hurley & Sovner, 1992). Researchers are developing the equivalent of the extensively used standardised psychiatric interview the *Present State Examination* for people with learning disability, called PAS ADD (Psychiatric Assessment Schedule Adapted for Developmentally Delayed), which is primarily a research tool at present (Moss *et al.*, 1993).

In the main, early detection of mental illness in primary care currently relies on clinical acumen without the aid of any screening tool. Proactive services which are committed to a preventive approach would be required to screen all individuals with learning disability. The instrument would therefore have to be robust enough for a variety of users, including parents, teachers, workers in day care and residential services to use reliably. To be useful it would also have to achieve reasonable levels of specificity and sensitivity for treatment-responsive disorders. In the absence of such an instrument, training of carers and primary health care workers in the recognition of mental illness in people with learning disability must become a training priority.

The role of the community team

The assessment of such complex, often inter-related aspects of an individual's functioning is time consuming, and may involve multidisciplinary assessment by the community team for people with learning disability. The team has a central role in secondary prevention by virtue of its much larger client group with learning disability, by comparison with a single-handed general practitioner or even a group practice of five to six general practitioners, who might have 20 to 30 people between them with severe or profound learning disability. However, many of the community team members may not have had the benefit of a dual training in mental illness and learning disability and may not be experienced in the assessment and treatment of mental illness. In addition, a significant proportion of people with mild learning disability are not in active contact with the community team, yet are at increased risk of developing mental illness.

Nurses working in the community team for people with learning disability should be trained in mental illness assessment and treatment. Community psychiatric nurses and their psychiatric colleagues can also offer training to carers in residential homes and day care services. Purchasers should include such training in the service specifications. Training packs are now available on a wide variety of issues related to learning disability, including mental illness (Bouras *et al.*, 1995). Training sessions are also a regular feature of many community teams' work.

Such services require continued backing at managerial level, and a recognition that many people may need intensive support in the longer term. This has important implications for staff support, in order to prevent or minimise staff 'burn-out'. Though small in total number, the service demands of this group can be great, including their demands on primary care. Box 7.5 summarises important points for the primary health care team.

Summary points for primary health care teams

Learning disability covers a wide range of abilities and each problem requires individual assessment.

Health visitors should devote more time to parents of disabled children.

Between one-third and two-thirds of people with learning disability will have psychological problems.

Suspect psychological problem when behavioural changes occur, or the level of functioning deteriorates.

Exclude physical illness when behaviour changes.

Assess the person with an informant who knows them well.

Have a clear end point in mind before prescribing psychotropic medication.

Consider involving the community team for people with learning disability, for long-term shared care.

Box 7.5 *Important points to remember.*

References

Aman, M., Singh, N., Stewart, A. & Field, C. (1985). The Aberrant Behaviour Checklist: a behaviour rating scale for the assessment of treatment effects. *American Journal of Mental Deficiency*, **89**, 485–91.

Beange, H. & Bauman, A. (1990). Health care for the disabled: Is it necessary? In *Key Issues in Mental Retardation Research*. Fraser, W. I., ed. London: Routledge.

Bernal, J. & Hollins, S. (1995). Psychiatric illness and learning disability: a dual diagnosis. *Advances in Psychiatric Treatment*, **1**, 138–45.

Berney, T. (1990). Psychiatric aspects of well-established syndromes. *Current Opinion in Psychiatry*, **3**, 575–80.

Bicknell, J. (1983). The psychopathology of handicap. *British Journal of Medical Psychology*, **56**, 167–78.

Bouras, N., Kon, Y., Murray, B. & Joyce, T. (1995). *Mental Health in Learning Disabilities. A Training Pack*. Brighton: Pavilion Publishing.

Bregman, J. (1991). Current developments in the understanding of mental retardation Part II: psychopathology. *Journal of the American Academy of Child and Adolescent Psychiatry*, **30**, 861–72.

Corbett, J.A. (1979). Psychiatric morbidity in mental retardation. In *Psychiatric Illness and Mental Handicap*. Snaith, P. and James F. E., eds. London: Gaskell.

Craft, A. & Hitching M. (1989). Keeping safe: sex education and assertiveness skills. In *Thinking the Unthinkable: Papers on Sexual Abuse and People with Learning Difficulties.* Brown, H. and Craft, A. pp. 29–38. London: FPA Education Unit.

Cunningham, C. & Davis, H. (1985). Early parent counselling. In *Mental Handicap* Craft M., Bicknell, J. and Hollins, S., eds. London: Baillière Tindall.

Curran, J. & Hollins, S. (1994). Consent to medical treatment and people with learning disability. *Psychiatric Bulletin* **18**, 691–3.

Damrosch, S. & Perry, L. (1989). Self-reported adjustment, chronic sorrow, and coping of parents of children with Down's syndrome. *Nursing Research*, **38**, 25–30.

Department of Health. (1994). *Advisory Group on Behavioural Disturbance and Mental Health Service Developments for People with Learning Disabilities: Specialist Mental Health Services for People with Learning Disabilities.* London: HMSO.

Einfeld, S. (1990). Guidelines for the use of psychotropic medication in individuals with developmental disabilities. *Australia and New Zealand Journal of Developmental Disabilities*, **16**, 71–3.

Emerson, E., Cummings, R., Barrett, S., Hughes, H., McCool, C. & Toogood, A. (1988). Challenging behaviour and community services: who are the people who challenge services? *Mental Handicap*, **16**, 16–19.

Fine, M., Tangeman, P. & Woodward, J. (1990). Changes in adaptive behaviour of older adults with mental retardation following deinstitutionalization. *American Journal of Mental Retardation*, **6**, 661–8.

Fryers, T. (1984). *The Epidemiology of Severe Intellectual Impairment.* London: Academic Press.

Gater, R., de Almeida e Sousa, R. & Caraveo, J. *et al.* (1991). The pathways to psychiatric care: a cross-cultural study. *Psychological Medicine*, **21**, 761–74.

Gath, A. (1992). Terminology and learning disability. *British Journal of Hospital Medicine*, **48**, 357–9.

Goldberg, D. & Huxley, P. (1980). *Mental Illness in the Community: The Pathways to Psychiatric Care.* London: Tavistock.

Goldberg, D. & Huxley, P. (1992). *Common Mental Disorders: A Bio-social Model.* London: Routledge.

Gostason, R. (1985). Psychiatric illness among the mentally retarded: a Swedish population study. *Acta Psychiatrica Scandinavica*, 71 Suppl. **318**, 1–117.

Grove, N. & Walker, M. (1990). The Makaton vocabulary: Using manual signs and graphic symbols to develop interpersonal communication. *Augmentative and Alternative Communication*, 15–28.

Hafner, H. & An Der Heiden, W. (1991). Methodology of evaluative studies in the mental health field. In *Evaluation of Comprehensive Care of the Mentally Ill*. Freeman, H. and Henderson, J., eds. Royal College of Psychiatrists, London: Gaskell.

Holland, A. & Murphy, G. (1990). Behavioural and psychiatric disorder in adults with mild learning difficulties. *International Review of Psychiatry*, **2**, 117–36.

Hollins, S. (1985). Families and handicap. In *Mental Handicap* Craft, M., Bicknell, J. and Hollins, S., eds. London: Baillière Tindall.

Hollins, S. & Curran, J. (1995). *Feeling Blue. Beyond Words*. London: Sovereign Series.

Hollins, S. & Sireling, L. (1991). *When Dad Died. Working Through Loss with People who have Learning Disabilities. A Professional Learning Resource*. Windsor: NFER-Nelson.

Hollins, S. & Sireling, L. (1994) *When Mum Died – A Counselling Picture Book. Beyond Words*. 2nd ed. London: Sovereign Series available from St George's Hospital Medical School, London SW17 0RE, UK.

Hollins, S. & Sinason, V. (1992). *Jenny Speaks Out, Bob Tells All. Beyond Words*. London: Sovereign Series.

Howells, G. (1986). Are the medical needs of mentally handicapped people being met? *Journal of the Royal College of General Practitioners*, **36**, 449–53.

Howells, G. (1990). Drug therapy of mental disorders. In *Primary Care for People with a Mental Handicap*. London: Royal College of General Practitioners.

Hubert, J. (1992). *Too Many Drugs, Too Little Care: Parents' Perceptions of the Administration and Side-Effects of Drugs Prescribed for Young People with Severe Learning Difficulties*. London: Values Into Action.

Hurley, A. & Sovner, R. (1992). Inventories for evaluating psychopathology in developmentally disabled individuals. *The Habilitative Mental Healthcare Newsletter*, **11**, 7–8.

Kastner, T., Freidman., D. O'Brien, D. & Pond, W. (1990). Health care and mental illness in persons with mental retardation. *Habilitative Mental Healthcare Newsletter*, **9**, 3.

Matson, J., Gardner. W., Coe, D. & Sovner, R. (1991). A scale for evaluating emotional disorders in severely and profoundly mentally retarded persons: development of the diagnostic assessment for the severely handicapped (DASH) scale. *British Journal of Psychiatry*, **159**, 404–9.

Millar, T. & Goldberg, D. (1991). Determinants of the ability of general practitioners to manage common mood disorders. *Journal of the Royal College of Practitioners*, **41**, 305, 357–9.

Moss, S., Patel P., Prosser H., Goldberg, D., Simpson, N., Rowe, S. & Lucchino, R. (1993). Psychiatric morbidity in older people with moderate and severe learning disability. I: development and reliability of the patient interview (PAS-ADD). *British Journal of Psychiatry*, **163**, 471–80.

Oswin, M. (1991). *Am I Allowed to Cry? A Study of Bereavement Amongst People with Learning Difficulties*. London: Souvenir Press.

Ounstead, C., Roberts J., Gordon, M. & Milligan, B. (1982). Fourth goal of perinatal medicine. *British Medical Journal*, **284**, 879–82.

Reiss, S., Levitan, G. & Szyszo, J. (1982). Emotional disturbance and mental retardation: diagnostic overshadowing. *American Journal of Mental Deficiency*, **86**, 567–74.

Rutter, M., Tizard, J., Yule, W., Graham, P. & Whitmore, K. (1976). Isle of Wight studies 1964–1974. *Psychological Medicine*, **6**, 313–32.

Sinason, V. (1986). Secondary mental handicap and its relationship to trauma. *Psychoanalytic Psychotherapy*, **2**, 131–54.

Sobsey, D. (1994). *Violence and Abuse in the Lives of People with Disabilities: The End of Silent Acceptance?* Baltimore: Brookes.

Sturmey, P., Reed, J., & Corbett, J. (1991). Psychometric assessment of psychiatric disorders in people with learning difficulties (mental handicap): a review of measures. *Psychological Medicine*, **21**, 143–55.

Thompson, C. (1994). The use of high dose antipsychotic medication: consensus statement. *British Journal of Psychiatry*, **164**, 448–58.

Tyne, A. (1981). *The Principle of Normalisation: A Foundation for Effective Services*. London: Campaign for Mentally Handicapped People.

Vitiello, B. & Behar, D. (1992). Mental retardation and psychiatric illness. *Hospital and Community Psychiatry*, **43**, 494–9.

Welsh Health Planning Forum (1992). *Protocol for Investment in Health Gain: Mental Handicap (Learning Disabilities)*. Welsh Office: NHS. Directorate.

Wing, L. (1994). The autistic continuum. In *Mental Health in Mental Retardation. Recent Advances and Practices*. Bouras, N., ed. Cambridge: Cambridge University Press.

Wolfensberger, W. (1983). Social role valorisation: a proposed new term for the principle of normalisation. *Mental Retardation*, **21**, 234–9.

Yeates, S. (1989). Hearing in people with mental handicaps: a review of 100 adults. *Mental Handicap*, **17**, 33–7.

[8] The role of counselling in primary prevention

Roslyn Corney

Introduction

In this chapter, we will consider the role of counselling for those presenting with acute and chronic social problems. We will also include the role of counselling for those with physical ill health, with its major role in the prevention of anxiety and depression resulting from illness. The counselling skills of primary care professionals will be considered as well as those offered by trained counsellors.

The development of mental illness is the result of a combination of factors including individual characteristics (biological, heredity, childhood experiences) and the individual's perception of their current environment. Aspects of the individual's environment known to be associated with an increased high risk of developing mental illness have been discussed in Chapter 3. We need to consider the role of acute and chronic social stressors, including relationship difficulties and social problems such as unemployment, poor housing and financial difficulties. The role of social support is also important. Providing social support reduces the likelihood of mental distress resulting from life events and social problems, although controversy remains as to whether it has a direct positive effect upon health or whether it acts only as a 'buffer', modifying the effects of stressors (Murray, 1992).

The primary health care team can try to reduce social stresses directly: reducing the stress imposed by marital disharmony by offering marital counselling, for example. The team may also try to reduce the subjective impact of life events. This could include interventions such as preparing a wife for the death of her husband who has a chronic illness. Finally, the team might offer social support either directly or through the development of other supportive networks, such as self-help groups.

The role of the primary health care team

A number of studies have shown that patients with psychological or social problems are more likely to contact their general practitioner for help than any other agency (Goldberg & Huxley, 1992). The pivotal role of the general practitioner was shown in a study of 281 individuals of all ages who admitted to a personal or emotional problem (Corney, 1990); 43% of the women and 27% of the men in this sample had discussed their personal problems with their general practitioner. Health visitors were also important as confidant(e)s for women; 10% of the women in the sample, and 3% of the men indicated that they had discussed their problem with the health visitor. Other agencies were mentioned by smaller percentages of the sample; approximately 8% had contacted a psychiatrist, 7% a social worker, 6% a counsellor or psychotherapist and 6% a priest.

This study found that general practitioners were contacted for every type of problem and, in order of frequency, these were: depression/anxiety, bereavement, coping with chronic illness, marital problems, problems with children and practical problems. Of those with marital problems, 71% had contacted their general practitioner – the only professional contacted in most cases. Other studies of individuals with marital difficulties have also shown that the general practitioner is more likely to be approached than any other professional (Chester, 1971; Mitchell, 1981).

Since this study was conducted, there have been considerable changes in staffing in primary care. It is now likely that other health professionals such as the practice nurse are either approached for help with a wide range of problems or find out about their patients' social problems during a consultation for other reasons.

It follows that, as the general practitioner and other members of the primary health care team are often the only professionals approached by patients, their response may determine patients' future help-seeking and confiding behaviour as well as the outcome of the immediate problem. Developing the skills of the general practitioner, practice nurse and health visitor in identifying psychosocial problems, and in responding, showing empathy, giving support and knowing when to refer are therefore very important.

Reducing mental problems resulting from physical ill-health

The primary health care team has a crucial role in dealing with the psychological problems of patients suffering from physical illness. When individuals become ill, their concerns, preoccupations and worries have been shown to change dramatically, focusing around the illness and the effect it may have on their daily activities, their work and their family life.

The most common reactions of patients to illness are distress and anxiety. Overall estimates suggest that between 30% and 60% of general hospital patients suffer significant levels of psychological distress at the time of hospitalisation and during the first year afterwards (Nichols, 1984).

Distress is also common among relatives which in turn affects the patient. In a study conducted by Mayou and colleagues of patients suffering from coronary heart disease, four out of five patients and half of their spouses revealed mild or moderate distress while in hospital and approximately half of the patients and spouses still felt distressed two months later (Mayou, Foster & Williamson, 1978).

Recognising the patient's feelings and concerns is important in medical terms not only as a preventive measure in terms of mental health but also because the presence of psychological distress has been found to have a negative effect on recovery from illness. In a large scale survey, Querido studied 1630 patients admitted to a hospital in Amsterdam. Six months after discharge, 70% of patients who were classified as distressed whilst in hospital were in an unsatisfactory condition medically, in comparison with only 30% of those classified as non-distressed. While 1128 of the 1630 patients had been given a favourable medical prognosis, only 660 had lived up to this expectation. The majority of those who failed to improve had been classified as distressed while in hospital (Querido, 1959).

Distress at all phases of an illness can usually be reduced by providing information about the illness and treatment. For example, giving adequate information and preparation before surgery has been shown to reduce postoperative pain and symptoms, the time taken to recover, and anxiety levels (Ley, 1988).

It is often the period of uncertainty, of not knowing, which patients state as the most difficult period to bear. Ley in his review of the literature suggests that there is no evidence of increased anxiety or depression when patients are told of their diagnosis (1988). Even studies of cancer patients suggest that the majority of patients would prefer to be informed, although there is still some debate whether all patients should be told. Surveys indicate that most patients wish to know as much as possible about their illness, its causes, treatments and outcome.

Other studies have also indicated that emotional distress can be reduced by actively involving patients in treatment and in decisions regarding treatment. Patients then regard themselves as being actively involved in treating or fighting the illness and exercising choice rather than feeling passive and helpless. Findings such as these indicate the need for all professionals working with ill patients to use counselling skills. It is important to acknowledge and respond to any distress arising, to convey information in a way in which the patient understands, and to help them in their decision-making where appropriate.

The role of the counsellor in general practice

The work of the general practitioners and other members of the primary health care team has always included counselling, whether this is seen as the application of counselling skills in the consultation or 'the informed use of the counselling process with selected patients' (McCleod, 1992). The skills and techniques of counselling are an important and necessary part of the work of all general practitioners. 'Listening sensitively to the patient and helping to make sense of his distress, the use of explanation, guidance and informed reassurance are all "tools of the trade"' (McCleod, 1992). However, the majority of doctors enter general practice with little training in counselling. This lack of preparation for counselling, together with the very real constraints of time has 'limited the capacity of many general practitioners to recognise patients' needs adequately and to respond effectively to these needs' (McCleod, 1992).

In most cases, the general practitioner's, and other members of the primary health care team's, ability to offer support or sympathy may be adequate or all that is needed. However, with some patients, more time and expertise may be considered necessary to improve the situation or prevent further difficulties arising.

In previous years, there was little in the way of outside help available except through voluntary agencies such as the Marriage Guidance Council (now Relate) or referral to a psychiatrist or a clinical psychologist (usually with a long waiting list).

It is therefore not surprising that the employment of counsellors by general practitioners is now a major growth area in general practice. This is not only due to the increasing recognition of the importance of counselling and psychotherapy in medical care but also because recent legislative changes make it more easy for general practitioners to employ counsellors. Since the new general practitioner contract was introduced in 1990, the range of staff eligible for reimbursement through the ancillary staff scheme has been extended, and some Family Health Service Authorities have been willing to fund counsellors working in general practice using this scheme. In addition, general practitioner fundholders can now pay for counselling sessions out of their mental health services budget.

What is counselling?

There has been much confusion regarding what counselling is and what takes place within the 'counselling session'. The large variety of professionals and others who consider that they offer support, understanding and care in their interactions with clients or patients are understandably confused on how this differs from the treatment or therapy offered by a counsellor.

Counsellors vary in the techniques they use and the underlying theories of human behaviour they believe in. In Britain, many models of counselling exist (Herink in 1980 listed over 250) and the range and diversity of approach and the claims made about their effectiveness can be confusing for those seeking counselling, those seeking to employ a counsellor, or those seeking counselling training (Sutton, 1987). In addition, the majority of counsellors would describe themselves as eclectic, mixing the methods that they consider most appropriate to the particular situation and client. Thus, for example, some counsellors might employ behaviour therapy for the treatment of phobic symptoms (see Chapter 11) in a similar manner to psychologists or behaviour therapists. Therefore, there is no standardised counselling intervention; it is likely that no two counsellors operate in quite the same way (Tyndall, 1985).

The variety of counselling models can be broadly grouped into two different schools: directive and non-directive counselling. Active or directive counsellors tend to interpret, instruct and direct their clients, and reflective, or non-directive counsellors tend to elicit and reflect, guide and support their clients (Irving & Heath, 1989).

The most widely practised counselling model is non-directive counselling. Non-directive counsellors are trained not to advise clients but to help them make decisions for themselves. The counsellor respects the client as an equal, and assumes that the client can, with help, resolve his or her difficulties. The counsellor aims to develop a therapeutic alliance with the client and to convey acceptance and understanding of the client and empathy with his or her situation. The counsellor structures the process to allow the client time and freedom to explore thoughts and feelings in an atmosphere of trust and respect. The process aims to deepen the client's understanding of the situation and ways of dealing with it and thus enables choices and decisions to be based on personal insights gained rather than the advice and direction of others (Irving & Heath, 1989).

Irving and Heath categorised counselling interventions into three categories: crisis work, remedial work and developmental/educational work (Box 8.1). Crisis work is likely to include incidents of violence, child battering, suicide attempts and sudden loss. Remedial work tends to deal with relationship problems, bereavement, sexual dysfunction, low self esteem, low income, unemployment, anxiety and depression. Developmental work will focus on the management of stress, strengthening self-assertiveness, problems with control of teenagers and looking after elderly relatives, pre-marital counselling and behavioural problems associated with eating and smoking.

Some counsellors prefer to work with individuals or couples, while others may also work with families and groups (Box 8.2).

Crisis work
Sudden loss
Violence
Suicide attempts
Bereavement or impending bereavement

Remedial work
Relationship difficulties
Social problems
unemployment
financial difficulties
poor housing
isolated young mothers
Acute physical illness
impending hospitalisation
difficult treatment choices
Coping with chronic illness
Sexual dysfunction

Developmental work
Stress management
Assertiveness training
Eating problems and smoking

Box 8.1 *Counselling interventions.*

Group counselling can be a useful adjunct to one-to-one counselling for clients with similar or related problems and counselling small groups of clients with similar needs may be as effective as individual work (Irving & Heath, 1989).

The techniques used by counsellors differ from those of psychoanalysts and psychotherapists in a number of ways although they may overlap to an extent. Psychoanalysts use specific techniques such as free association, interpretation and transference. Transference occurs when clients respond to the therapist in ways which echo their responses to other meaningful figures in their lives. Psychotherapists, in general, also focus on the transference relationship between patient and therapist, although they use a variety of other methods which distinguish it from psychoanalysis. In counselling there is less emphasis on, though not necessarily less awareness of, the transference between counsellor and client. Counselling tends to be shorter-term and problem-centred, focusing on current difficulties and life problems, rather than analysis of the deep-seated longer-term personal problems dealt with in

---

Counselling clients
Individually
Couples
Groups

Helping other members of the primary health care team
Giving support, listening, advising
Supervising counselling by other team members
Leading discussions on patient-centredness
Sharing the care of long-term intractable problems
Developing good practice guidelines
  For breaking bad news
  For offering patients a choice of treatments

Evaluating the effectiveness of the counselling
Finding out which patients benefit most

Box 8.2 *Potential roles of the practice counsellor.*

psychoanalysis and psychotherapy. While there is a great deal of overlap particularly with psychotherapy, it might be argued that short-term, problem-centred counselling is better suited to general practice settings (Rowland, 1992).

Counselling and counselling skills
Some of the skills used by counsellors are desirable in all consultations, such as using open-ended and reflective questioning, or observing inconsistencies between verbal and non-verbal cues (Harris, 1987). In addition, the core skills of listening, reflecting and showing empathy are not the exclusive property of counsellors and are necessary in the majority of helping situations. Counsellors would argue, however, that there is a difference between using counselling skills within the confines of a surgery consultation, for example, and counselling in the formal sense outlined above.

Whether or not doctors and others should offer 'formal' counselling is open to some debate (Rowland, Irving & Maynard, 1989; Kelleher, 1989). Counsellors have argued that, although counselling skills help the general practitioner in his or her consultations, the focus of the doctor's work is different from that of the counsellor (Rowland *et al.*, 1989). In general, the aim and function of a counsellor is to help clients to help themselves, to clarify their own difficulties and attempt to resolve them themselves. The general practitioner's role is often different; he or she can be viewed as an expert, whose job is to diagnose disorders and prescribe treatment (Noon, 1992). Even those general practitioners who have trained as counsellors do not always find it easy to enter into this sort of counselling relationship or to have the time or emotional resources to do so (Rowland *et al.*, 1989).

Advantages of locating counsellors in primary care

The value of counselling attachments to general practice is that the patients who need counselling can be referred on without too much delay. Studies of such attachments have found that they facilitate referral and feedback between the counsellor and other members of the primary health care team if communications are good. This is particularly important in prevention, as counselling may be accepted by clients at an earlier stage.

Clients can see a practice-based counsellor in a familiar environment and are likely to feel less stigmatised than if they were referred to a specialist service off-site. The fact that their own doctor has suggested counselling may overcome clients' fear or initial scepticism of its value. Take-up of appointments for counselling in general practice is higher than that at a marriage guidance clinic or in a psychiatric outpatient clinic. One of the problems of referring patients to psychiatrists is that many patients fail to turn up for the first appointment (Illman, 1983).

Developing skills and offering support

A successful placement of a counsellor in general practice should not only benefit the individual patients seen by the counsellor but also benefit other members of the primary health care team. In a survey of general practitioners working with marriage guidance counsellors (Corney, 1986), respondents felt that the counsellor's main task was counselling clients, but a third of the doctors mentioned that the counsellor also provided support to other team members.

General practitioners who work with counsellors appear to value their work with patients and appreciate the opportunity to share and discuss their own feelings about patients and their relationships with them (McCleod, 1992). Employing a counsellor in the primary health care team seems to heighten other team members' awareness of their own reactions to patients, and encourages them to improve their own counselling skills. Time needs to be invested by the counsellor in supporting and developing the skills of other team members who are interested in taking on a role in this area. McLeod points out that a counsellor who builds up a good relationship with a practice and who finds time for case discussion provides a new and useful resource in primary care. Very few team members have the luxury of time to reflect on their practice, and yet offering such time could enable them to function more effectively and feel more supported.

Some members of the primary health care team may not wish to become more involved in counselling, but it is still important to develop their skills of identification so that they know when to refer on to others when necessary. Counsellor support to other members of the team may enable them to undertake some of the counselling work themselves. Sharing the care of patients with long-term intractable problems may help reduce the stress imposed by these patients. While workers in other caring professions, such as counselling and social work, have supervision sessions built into their work, few health professionals have these opportunities. There may be no forum where they can be given support and help to disentangle their own feelings, avoidances, prejudices, and emotional responses. Counsellors may be able to supply this type of support and supervision.

Counsellors may also suggest ways in which a more 'patient-centred' approach is adopted. A patient-centred health professional learns to seek out the 'real' problem by attending to a variety of verbal and non-verbal cues presented by the patient, rather than simply attending to the presenting complaint, which may not represent their most major problem (Byrne & Long, 1976). A doctor who attends to the patient's concerns, worries and own theories about the illness is more likely to find out what is wrong (Tuckett *et al.*, 1986). Thus many of the communication skills needed by health professionals are similar to those used by counsellors in their daily work with clients. Studies have consistently demonstrated that patients prefer doctors who show sensitivity, warmth and concern to those who appear detached and unconcerned (DiMatteo, 1985). Discussions of particular patients or joint consultations can be important ways of developing the skills and confidence of all staff members, including those of the counsellor.

Although counsellors may see their role as enabling other staff to take on some of the emotional and psychological problems of their patients, it is also important that medical staff are aware that problems (and harm) can ensue when untrained staff attempt to counsel disturbed clients who need more experienced help. It can be dangerous when unsupported staff are left dealing with complex and difficult emotional problems on their own. A counsellor working closely with the team can advise staff on their management of patients as well as when to refer elsewhere.

Help for those with physical illness

Although studies of counsellor attachments (Corney & Jenkins, 1992) indicate that the majority of their referrals are patients with psychosocial problems, there may still be an important role for the counsellor in terms of patients whose major problem is that of a physical illness.

Helping clients manage their chronic illness, discussing options for treatment or being involved in health promotion are all important areas in which the counsellor can have a role. Patients who need to make a decision over treatment may find it helpful to discuss the alternatives with a counsellor. This is becoming more common with the increasing recognition of the importance of allowing the patient a choice of treatment. This may often need the involvement of a counsellor to help ensure that the information given has been understood and assimilated.

A counsellor may also have an important role in improving compliance with treatment. It has been estimated that one-third of all patients do not co-operate with short-term treatments and half or more do not co-operate with long-term treatments (DiMatteo & DiNicola, 1982). Patients bring their own ideas about their illness (Tuckett et al., 1986), and failure to discuss these ideas has been shown to leave the patient confused which, in turn, has been shown to reduce compliance with treatment and satisfaction with the consultation (Korsch, Gozzi & Francis, 1968).

In primary care in the United States, counsellors are involved in the treatment of a wide range of conditions. The Hawaii Medicaid Project (Cummings, 1990) found that targeted, focused psychological treatment produced a dramatic and significant reduction in patients' subsequent medical needs and consumption of medical resources. This six-year study included patients with heart disease, hypertension, diabetes and even substance abuse. At the present time, a similar clinical trial is planned for this country although it may be more difficult to show a reduction in the use of resources as average health expenditure per patient is lower in this country than in the USA.

The need for the evaluation of counselling

Evaluative studies are essential for a number of reasons. First, some patients may be helped more than others. In a time of limited resources, it is essential to focus on those individuals who can benefit most from counselling. Evaluative studies should aim to identify these patients.

Secondly, in training and manpower consideration, it is important to know what level of skill is necessary for benefit to occur. Would a young harassed single mother benefit more from a self-help group of other single mothers, or from advice on childrearing from a health visitor, or from individual therapy from a counsellor? Some clients may benefit most by the setting up of a self-help group, while the more seriously disturbed or damaged client will probably need skilful and knowledgeable handling.

Thirdly, there is a wide range of therapies from behaviour therapy to psychoanalysis. It is important to find out which therapies are more acceptable to patients and which benefit them most. At the present time, research suggests that it is not the methodology that is important but the qualities of the counsellor. Counsellors who offer warmth, genuineness and empathy have been shown to be consistently effective regardless of their theoretical approach (Truax & Carkhuff, 1976; Howe, 1993).

Subjective accounts

These suggest that counsellor attachments work well, with much consumer, counsellor and general practitioner satisfaction. Waydenfeld and Waydenfeld (1980) found that 44 out of the 47 clients who completed a client questionnaire felt they had been helped. Anderson and Hasler (1979) sent questionnaires to the first 80 patients referred to the counsellor. of which 55 (69%) returned them. Of this group, 47 agreed that counselling should be available in general practice, 43 would use the counselling service again and 46 would recommend it to their relatives or friends.

Subjective accounts are valuable, but need to be treated with caution. It may be very difficult to criticise a service especially when arranged by the general practice upon which one relies. It is also possible that similar favourable reports would be obtained if clients were given the same amount of time by an untrained, warm and caring befriender or by a self-help group who could also offer practical assistance on a longer-term basis.

Utilisation of medical services

Studies have investigated utilisation of medical services and used this as a measure of outcome (assuming clients have improved if they visit the doctor less or stop taking psychotropic drugs). A number of studies have indeed shown a reduction in visits made to the doctor (Marsh & Barr, 1975; Waydenfeld & Waydenfeld, 1980) after counselling, in contrast to the period immediately before. Studies have also found a reduction in the number of psychotropic and other drugs prescribed (Cohen, 1977; Meacher, 1977; Waydenfeld & Waydenfeld, 1980) or a reduction in referrals to psychiatrists after a counselling attachment had been instigated (Illman, 1983; Corney, 1986). Again, these results have to be interpreted with caution, since it is likely that the client will be referred at a time of crisis when attendance is also likely to be high. Visits to the doctor may have decreased over time without the intervention of a counsellor.

Other studies have attempted to find out whether counselling is cost effective by comparing the cost of employing a counsellor with the money saved by a reduction in clients' use of medical and other services. Careful consideration needs to be given, however, on whether we should try to argue the case for attaching counsellors in general practice only in terms of cost effectiveness. A successful attachment of a counsellor may result in more time being spent in discussing cases with other members of the primary health care

---

Subjective accounts
  Patient satisfaction questionnaires
  Team discussion

Changes in utilisation of services
  Consultation rates
  Prescriptions for psychotropic drugs
  Referrals to other mental health professionals

Outcome measures
  Anxiety and depression rating scales

Box 8.3 *Evaluating the impact of counselling.*

team. It may also result in the primary health care professionals spending more time in their consultations with patients as they start to adopt a more patient-centred approach. While this change in approach may have far-reaching consequences in terms of comprehensive care and may eventually reduce medical costs, these effects may be extremely difficult to trace and cost accurately. Studies need to address the efficacy of counselling in terms of client outcome as well as cost effectiveness (Box 8.3).

Clinical trials of counselling

Although all clinical trials are difficult to undertake, they are even more problematic if the treatment under consideration is counselling. Most clinical trials evaluating counselling are flawed in a number of ways and many would argue that it was too early for us to proceed with this medical and scientific form of evaluation. It must be remembered that we are at an early stage in refining our techniques of evaluation. For example, many consider that the outcome measures used are crude and inappropriate to assess changes brought about by counselling.

Difficulties encountered include: defining who is the client group, deciding what constitutes improvement and how to measure it, deciding when to carry out follow-up assessments, how to assess the treatment given, what to use for control groups (for example, deciding on what constitutes a placebo), how to assess the quality of the counsellor's skills, how to assess client motivation and the quality of the relationship developed between client and counsellor (Corney, 1992a).

Ideally, any study should also evaluate the other effects of having a counsellor based in the practice in addition to improvements in the patients counselled. For example, a counsellor may increase the sensitivity of other team members to psychological problems and help them feel more confident in managing some of these problems (Corney, 1992b).

This chapter will not include the results of individual clinical trials undertaken in general practice which have been reported elsewhere (Corney, 1992a). In general, the results are mixed, although more recent studies have yielded results more in favour of counselling. However, we are not in a position to generalise from the results of these studies for the reasons outlined above. We are far from knowing the answers and any assumption that we do know is unwise.

There is, however, limited support from the result of a meta-analysis of 11 British studies of specialist mental health treatment in general practice. This meta-analysis was undertaken by Balestrieri and colleagues (1988). In each study the outcome of treatment by a specialist mental health professional located in general practice was compared with the outcome of the usual treatment by general practitioners. The main finding was that treatment by mental health professionals was about 10% more successful than that usually given by general practitioners. Counselling, behaviour therapy, and general psychiatry proved to be similar in their overall effect. The influence of counselling seemed to be greatest on social functioning, whereas behaviour therapy seemed mainly to reduce contacts with the psychiatric services.

The effectiveness of the counselling skills of other members of the primary health care team must also be evaluated. Some studies have already been conducted (although these are beset with the same problems as the above) and the results are encouraging. A controlled trial suggested that health visitors given training in non-directive counselling can bring about an improved outcome in women diagnosed with postnatal depression (Holden, Sagovsky & Cox, 1989) (see Chapter 4).

In another study by Catalan and colleagues (1984), brief counselling by general practitioners was found to be as effective as drug therapy. In this study, patients were randomly assigned to receive either a prescription for anxiolytics or brief counselling by their general practitioners. Improvements at one and seven months were similar in both groups. The authors suggested that such counselling need not be intensive or specially skilled and concluded that anxiety may often be reduced to tolerable levels by means of explanation, exploration of feelings, reassurance and encouragement.

Kiely & McPherson (1986) compared the use of self-help packages for 'stress' administered by the general practitioner compared with routine treatment. Patients were included in the study if they had psychological problems that were potentially stress related. The authors found greater improvement at 3 months in those receiving the package, and this group also visited the general practitioner less often for psychological problems.

The results of these three studies indicate the importance of developing the counselling skills of all primary care team members rather than just relying on employing a counsellor.

Evaluation of counselling within the practice

It may be particularly worthwhile if the primary health care team carries out its own evaluation of counselling within the practice. This can aid decisions on the best way to use the counsellor's time. Counsellors are limited in the number of clients that they can see each week, and it may be important that each referral is considered carefully. Other options should also be considered. An evaluation may address whether the consultative role of the counsellor (giving other team members support or advice regarding their patients) is as valuable as the counsellor seeing clients directly. Alternatively, an evaluation might explore whether running a group for clients (for example, a support group for those wishing to withdraw from tranquillisers) is more cost effective than seeing patients individually. Assessments may also yield information on the types of patients who seem to benefit most from seeing a counsellor as well as those who find it difficult to accept this type of help.

In planning an evaluation of counselling in general practice, the following areas should be considered by general practitioners and counsellors:

(a) an assessment of the counsellor's roles;
(b) the characteristics of patients referred to the counsellor;
(c) the characteristics of patients who fail to attend or drop out of treatment;
(d) the type of 'treatment' offered to clients and the number of sessions given;
(e) the counsellor's views on the effectiveness of the treatment with specific clients and in this setting;
(f) the views of other professionals on the effectiveness of the counsellor with specific patients;
(g) the views of clients on effectiveness referred to the counsellor;
(h) whether the provision of counselling alters the workload of other professionals;
(i) an assessment of attitudes of other professionals and clients towards counselling in general.

Development of good practice guidelines

It may be of value for a counsellor not only to deal with individual cases but to consider how the service offered by the primary health care team could be changed to meet more effectively the psychological needs of all the patients in the primary care setting. If a counsellor is not employed, another designated interested individual could be selected.

Protocols could be written and developed on which patients (and when) should be referred on for more experienced counselling help. The counsellor could also make sure that information on agencies is made available, such as self-help groups or befrienders (Chapter 3) who could help and support the client. Arranging for these groups to give talks on their work to the practice may facilitate a number of developments.

The way the primary health care team manages acute and chronic physical illness could also be considered. Discussions could include: how to develop the skills of the team in giving information about illnesses and make sure that this information is assimilated by patients, how to break bad news, prepare patients for distressing life events, or help patients make complex decisions about their treatment. The team could consider how best to support patients and their relatives in setting up self-help and carers' groups. The mass of psychological problems seen in primary care indicates the need to train and develop the skills of all workers in this setting and to organise the service so that the best use of these skills can be made.

References

Anderson, S. A. & Hasler, J. C. (1979). Counselling in general practice. *Journal of the Royal College of General Practitioners*, **29**, 352–6.

Balestrieri, M., Williams, P. & Wilkinson, G. (1988). Specialist mental health treatment in general practice: a meta-analysis. *Psychological Medicine*, **18**, 711–17.

Byrne, P. & Long, B. (1976). *Doctors Talking to Patients*. London: HMSO.

Catalan, J., Gath, D., Edmonds, G. & Ennis, J. (1984). The effects of non-prescribing of anxiolytics in general practice. I: Controlled evaluation of psychiatric and social outcome. *British Journal of Psychiatry*, **144**, 603–10.

Chester, R. (1971). Health and marriage breakdown: experience of a sample of divorced women. *British Journal of Preventive and Social Medicine*, **25**, 231–5

Cohen, J.S.H. (1977). Marital counselling in general practice. *Proceedings of the Royal Society of Medicine*, **70**, 495–6.

Corney, R. (1986). Marriage guidance counselling in general practice. *Journal of the Royal College of General Practitioners*, **36**, 424–6.

Corney, R. (1990). A survey of professional help sought by patients for psychosocial problems. *British Journal of General Practice*, **40**, 365–8.

Corney, R. (1992*a*). Studies of the effectiveness of counselling in general practice. In *Counselling in General Practice*. Corney, R. and Jenkins, R., eds. London: Routledge.

Corney, R. (1992*b*). Evaluating counsellor placements. In *Counselling in General Practice*. Corney, R. and Jenkins R., eds. London: Routledge.

Corney, R. & Jenkins, R. (1992). *Counselling in General Practice*. London: Routledge.

Cummings, N. (1990). The impact of psychological intervention on health care utilization and costs: the Hawaii Medicaid Project. (Unpublished manuscript)

DiMatteo, M. (1985). Physician–patient communication: promoting a positive health care setting. In *Prevention in Health Psychology*. Rosen, J. and Solomon, L., eds. Hanover New Hampshire: University Press of New England.

Di Matteo, M. & DiNicola, D. (1982). *Achieving Patient Compliance*. New York: Pergamon.

Goldberg, D. & Huxley, P. (1992). *Common Mental Disorders*. London: Routledge.

Harris C. M. (1987). Let's do away with counselling. *Medical Annual*. pp. 105–111. Bristol: Wright.

Herink, R. (1980). *The Psychotherapy Handbook; The A-Z Guide to More Than 250 Therapies in Use Today*. New York: Meridian Books.

Holden, J., Sagovsky, R. & Cox, J. (1989). Counselling in a general practice setting: controlled study of health visitor intervention in treatment of postnatal depression. *British Medical Journal*, **298**, 223–36.

Howe, D. (1993). *On Being a Client*. London: Sage Publications.

Illman, J. (1983). Is psychiatric referral good value for money? *British Medical Association News Review*, **9**, 41–2.

Irving J. & Heath V. (1989). *Counselling in General Practice: A Guide for General Practitioners*. Rugby: British Association for Counselling. Revised edition.

Kelleher, D. (1989). The general practitioner as counsellor: an examination of counselling by general practitioners. *Counselling Psychology Review*, British Psychological Society, **4**, 7–13.

Kiely, B.G. & McPherson, I.G. (1986). Stress self-help packages in primary care: a controlled trial evaluation. *Journal of the Royal College of General Practitioners*, **36**, 307–9.

Korsch, B., Gozzi, E. & Francis, V. (1968). Gaps in doctor–patient communication: 1 Doctor–patient interaction and patient satisfaction. *Journal of Paediatrics*, **42**, 855–71.

Ley, P. (1988). *Communicating with Patients*. London: Croom Helm.

McCleod, J. (1992). The general practitioner's role. In *Counselling in General Practice*. Sheldon, M., ed. London: RCGP Enterprises.

Marsh, G. & Barr, J. (1975). Marriage guidance counselling in a group practice. *Journal of the Royal College of General Practitioners,* **25**, 73–5.

Mayou, R., Foster, A. & Williamson, B. (1978). Psychosocial adjustment in patients one year after myocardial infarction. *Journal of Psychosomatic Research,* **22**, 447–53.

Meacher, M. (1977). *A Pilot Counselling Scheme with General Practitioner: Summary Report*. London: Mental Health Foundation. Unpublished.

Mitchell, R. (1981). *Someone to Turn to*. Aberdeen: Aberdeen University Press.

Murray, J. (1992). Prevention and the identification of high risk groups. *International Review of Psychiatry,* **4**, 281–6.

Nichols, K. (1984). *Psychological Care in Physical Illness*. London: Croom Helm.

Noon, J. (1992). Counselling general practitioners: the scope and limitations of the medical role in counselling. *Journal of the Royal Society of Medicine,* **85**, 126–8.

Querido, A. (1959). Forecast and follow up – an investigation into the clinical, social and mental factors determining the results of hospital treatment. *British Journal of Preventative and Social Medicine,* **13**, 33–49.

Rowland, N. (1992). What is counselling? In *Counselling in General Practice*. Corney, R. and Jenkins, R., eds. London: Routledge.

Rowland, N., Irving, J. & Maynard, A. (1989). Can general practitioners counsel? *Journal of the Royal College of General Practitioners,* **39**, 118–20.

Sutton C. (1987). The evaluation of counselling; a goal attainment approach. *Counselling,* **60**, 14–20.

Truax, C.B. & Carkhuff, R.R. (1976). *Towards Effective Counselling and Psychotherapy Training and Practice*, Chicago: Aldine.

Tuckett, D., Boulton, M., Olson, C. & Williams, A. (1986). *Meetings Between Experts: An Approach to Sharing Ideas in Medical Consultations*. London: Tavistock Publications.

Tyndall N. (1985). The work and impact of the National Marriage Guidance Council. In: *Marital Therapy in Britain,* Vol 1. Dryden, W., ed. London: Harper and Row.

Waydenfeld, D. & Waydenfeld, S.W. (1980). Counselling in general practice. *Journal of the Royal College of General Practitioners,* **30**, 671–7.

Part two

Early detection in primary care

[9] Secondary prevention of childhood mental health problems

Peter Hill and Quentin Spender

Introduction

Secondary prevention of child mental health problems is the prompt recognition and treatment of the early stages of emotional and behavioural problems in children and adolescents. It should prevent their escalation and the development of chronicity or secondary complications. Psychological problems are not uncommon in childhood: at any one time about one in six children will show excessive or inappropriate emotional responses or behaviours which are associated with substantial personal distress or impair ordinary psychosocial development and functioning (Hill, 1996). The term psychiatric disorder is used to cover the problems of this appreciable minority of children and teenagers (here termed children for short) and is often preferred as a term to mental illness which is retained to describe more severe or entrenched problems of apparently endogenous origin. Many children with problems of emotions, behaviour or relationships (childhood psychiatric disorder) have developed them in relation to adversity, and they can quite often be regarded as problems in adaptation or adjustment; hence the older term 'maladjusted'. More boys than girls are affected, hence our use of male pronouns. Most are brought to the notice of health services by their mothers.

Because children are not the instigators of their own referral, clinical problems of children's emotions, behaviour and relationships present to doctors only when they have become a source of concern to parents or teacher. This means they are often well established, even ingrained, when first seen. In a primary health care setting, the front line professional for young children is most likely to be the health visitor. It is therefore important that her attitudes to, and information about, these clinical problems establish her as enthusiastic and competent in their detection and, where appropriate, their treatment. We have used the otherwise rather clumsy term 'healthcare professional' in the knowledge that the doctor may not be the first person to assess and treat a mental health problem in a child.

Detection of psychological problems in childhood

In UK studies, 2–5% of children seen in primary care settings are presented by their parents with mental health problems as the main complaint. Hyperactivity, anxiety or behavioural problems are the principal concerns (Garralda, 1994). About 25% of all children seen, in other words ten times as many, will not have a primary psychiatric disorder but have physical problems which are seen by their doctor to be complicated by psychological issues (Bailey, Graham & Boniface, 1978). Interview studies of children, brought to general practitioners for whatever reason, show that about a quarter will have a psychiatric disorder (Garralda & Bailey, 1986b). In other words, detection of psychiatric disorder is about one-tenth of what it could be even though practitioners' sensitivity to contributory psychological issues in physical symptoms is high.

With this in mind, the primary care clinician needs to have a weather eye open for psychological trouble. The children most likely to suffer or display it are those with the characteristics listed in Box 9.1.

Clearly, the ability of a primary care clinician to detect early signs of psychiatric disorder is a prerequisite for early intervention or referral and the evidence is that this ability could be developed. There are at least two ways in which the matter might be approached:

1. screening questionnaires;
2. the clinician assesses mental health routinely in all children seen for whatever reason.

Chronic physical illness

Low intelligence

Damaged brain

Parental psychiatric disorder

Family disruption

Angry, bitter family relationships

Rejection by parents

Rejection by peers

Box 9.1 *Factors increasing vulnerability to psychiatric disorder.*

Questionnaires

Asking questions about mental health issues regardless of the problem leading to a consultation is educational and good practice but is time consuming. Accordingly, there have been experiments with questionnaires, particularly in American primary care paediatrics. Compared with active questioning, a little time is saved if the questionnaire yields negative results, but a positive result still needs clinical enquiry for confirmation.

This follows from the derivation of most questionnaires from epidemiological research in which they have been used to screen the general population. As a result they are sensitive with a high false-positive case identification rate. This results in the clinician having to assess a number of children who obtain high questionnaire scores but will not prove to have a psychiatric disorder. Cultural specificity of questionnaire items is a further problem, especially with problems arising in very young children.

Some well-known questionnaires are simply too bulky for parents or teenagers to complete. With this in mind, Jellinek, Murphy and Burns (1986) compiled a 34-item checklist, each item being marked on a 3-point scale by a parent. When used for 6–12-year-old children, it compared reasonably with the more cumbersome but familiar research tool, the Child Behaviour Checklist in identifying probable cases. Unfortunately, the authors did not validate it against clinical evaluation. Selecting a cut-off score of 28, they identified 12% of paediatric outpatients, of which 18% were false-positives. On the face of it this is worthwhile. But the face validity of the questionnaire is tenuous since its structure means that what counts is a large number of items scoring positive. A few items relevant to a particular diagnosis will only generate a small score because of the limited severity scale. In other words, a generally disturbed child with numerous mild behaviour and emotional symptoms would score much higher than a severely anxious one. It is possible that children with relatively specific disorders which are amenable to treatment are those most likely to be missed.

Mild cases, when treated, often do no better than controls either because the spontaneous clear up rate is high or because the non-specific measures which serve as a control are actually effective in their own right. On the other hand, severe or chronic cases do badly simply because they are chronic and severe. Treatment success is most likely to result from targeting moderate problems (Nicol, Stretch & Fundudis, 1993).

With this in mind, it is worth considering the use of questionnaires for detecting specific disorders rather than the presence of overall disturbance. Within an adolescent population seen in primary care services, fair sensitivity is obtained. About one-quarter of teenagers will score 16 or above on the Children's Depression

Inventory and about one-third of these will have clinical depression (Scott-Smith *et al.*, 1990; Wortman *et al.*, 1986). Probably only a small percentage will be false-negatives (Schubiner & Robin, 1990). In view of the very low rate of detection of adolescent depression by professionals, there may be a case for its use, but it is not known whether substituting a simple verbal question or two posed by a general practitioner or school doctor would be better. Simply asking: Do things get you down? Have you been out with your friends recently? Can you enjoy things? with further questions for clarification would be a straightforward procedure.

Questionnaires are not always good at differentiating between grades of severity but the judgement of an individual clinician can. Nor can a parent- or self-completed questionnaire substitute for clinical judgement when a diagnosis is required, though there has been an unwelcome tendency to rely on questionnaire data in the diagnosis of hyperactivity syndromes. In one study examining just this, parent-completed Conners' questionnaire scores contained 70% error variance when compared with clinician judgement (Taylor, E., personal communication).

The occasional use of questionnaires by secondary care services for parents and children is in order to provide a vocabulary for discussion or monitor progress, not to detect early disorder.

The overall conclusion is that questionnaires are a crude device when used for general screening for mental health problems. They are better suited to screening for specific conditions such as depression, but it is not clear that they are more efficient than brief direct enquiry.

Assessment for mental health problems

Nicol *et al.* (1993, p.218), in rejecting the value of questionnaire screening, take the view that 'a more helpful approach might be to alert general practitioners and health visitors to the fact that effective intervention is possible for preschool children with behaviour problems'. Yet the clinician still has to spot the problem.

Hall, Hill and Elliman (1994) have suggested a framework for child mental health surveillance which emphasises risk factors and is reproduced here (Box 9.2). It can be combined with knowledge of the risk factors which are present (Box 9.1). Many of these children will be presented by a parent who complains of a physical problem. Unfortunately, the type of physical problem initially presented by the parent is of little use in identifying psychiatrically disordered children (Garralda & Bailey, 1986*a*, *b*). The presence of psychiatric disorder in a child is most likely to be indicated by extremes of energy – too much or too little – (Garralda, 1994) or excessive anxiety, misery, irritability or difficulties in relationships, especially with parents. If the child's emotional responses are outwith the normal range and are an impairment to his ordinary

1. Are the parents competent?

2. What is their attitude towards the child?

3. What are the quality of the child's attachments?

4. What is the overall quality of the relationship between child and parent?

5. What is the child's temperament and how does it square with the parent's attitudes?

6. Are the parents mentally healthy?

7. What is the child's capacity to learn?

8. Is the child's language development satisfactory?

9. Is the child learning appropriate ways of coping with challenges posed by development?

10. Can the child form and maintain friendships?

Box 9.2 *Child mental health surveillance: ten questions.*

functioning or if the child is suffering, there is a clinical problem. The clinician can therefore ask the parent directly how the child's emotional state is and how he gets on with others at home and school. Teenagers can be asked directly.

However, it is not always easy to insert such questions into the semisocial conversation that many doctors use with teenagers who consult them about physical problems. Experience with deaf teenagers has shown that a doctor's overeagerness to engage an adolescent in a clinical interview can lead the teenager asked about their experience of life to provide socially appropriate responses along 'very well thank you' lines (Hindley, Hill & Bond, 1993). A concerned tone of voice may be a prerequisite for enquiring about psychological difficulties. Even so, a number of adolescents find it easier to brush off such questioning by providing answers which they believe will cause them or their parents the least trouble.

With this latter point in mind, it is wise to endeavour to interview adolescents on their own without a parent being present. Some doctors find it awkward to ask a parent to leave, particularly when it is the parent who has brought the child to all previous consultations. Simply saying 'You're old enough for me to see you on your own', while asking the mother to wait in the waiting room for a minute may suffice.

Assessment

Although it is possible to place a child's mental health problems in a diagnostic framework such as that provided by the International Classification of Diseases (ICD-10), this is a less important exercise than formulating the problem. A convenient way of doing this is to consider elements in the child, family and general situation which predispose the child to develop the problem, might have precipitated it and which are perpetuating it (the three Ps of causation). Thus the child might be vulnerable to developing a disorder because of a chronic physical condition, low intelligence or the presence of discordant relationships within the family. These will predispose him to developing a psychiatric disorder but may require a precipitant such as parental divorce, bullying at school or academic failure to initiate problematic behaviour or emotional response. Although some such responses will subside with time as the child copes positively and adaptively with the precipitant, others will persist because the response becomes self-perpetuating due to secondary gain. The child may become anxious following his father's departure from the family home and cling to mother because of fear that she may also leave. This clinging makes attendance at school impossible and so provides an answer to any problems that child may be having with other children at school. In this instance, avoidance of contact with peers becomes the main motivation for a problem of school non-attendance based on anxiety. The perpetuating mechanism is often different from the precipitating event.

Working out the contribution of such factors need not be complex and can be achieved by drawing up a simple table (Box 9.3). It avoids being drawn into a hasty and often mistaken attribution of causation to a precipitating event, and thus an expectation that things will sort themselves out in the long run. They often do not. For instance, a number of studies of children in the general population demonstrate the persistence of psychiatric problems over years. For instance, about half of adolescents with psychiatric

Factors	Individual	Family	Social
Predisposing			
Precipitating			
Perpetuating			

Box 9.3 *A model for fomulating a psychological problem.*

disorder have had their condition since childhood. This is also true for some behaviour patterns which are insufficiently extensive to be regarded as disorders. Aggressive behaviour, for example, shows remarkable persistence over time unless a way is found of stopping it. Some of this persistence reflects an underlying deficit: the aggressive child may lack the skill of negotiating interpersonal conflict. An impulsive child lacks the capacity to postpone gratification. That is why the problem persists; it is not that the child chooses to be aggressive or impulsive, rather that no other option is available to him unless the underlying deficit is corrected.

In order to gather enough information to construct a formulation, it is necessary to obtain a description of the child's problem from a parent. Interviewing both parents is not always easy to arrange but worthwhile since the adversities confronting young children often have their roots and reverberations within general family relationships. Ask for descriptions of actual instances of the problem, especially if its manifestation is episodic such as a tantrum. This may allow you to establish its ABC: the *A*ntecedents before the tantrum; the *B*ehaviour itself during a tantrum, its frequency and severity; and the immediate *C*onsequences of the tantrum such as the parent giving in to the child's angry demand. Over the age of about six, interviewing the child allows an extra dimension to be included. For instance, a common precipitant for a tantrum is a put-down or other stinging remark by a parent, but the parent is not the person who is going to tell you that.

For problems with other children, observations by playgroup, nursery or school staff are crucial and can be obtained by telephone or requested by letter. Remember that children's behaviour is quite often different at home and at school, or different with one parent compared with another. The cause of the problem is often in the interaction between the child and his personal environment, not entirely inherent in him.

A sequence of actions
A child is presented with an emotional, behavioural or relationship problem. A healthcare professional may or may not know how to deal with it. If not, or if uncertain, the following steps (see Fig. 9.1) provide a logical framework. They take the form of self-directed questions.

Is this problem normal for a child of this age?
There are no easy answers and no reference book in which population norms and tolerated deviations from these are registered. General knowledge and experience provide the best guide. Parents can be asked if the child's friends or relatives have behaved similarly. A specialist can be asked to comment without a referral being made. If the problem is associated with impairment of the child's

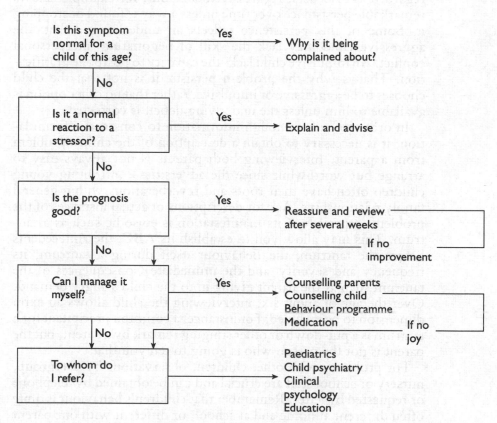

Fig. 9.1 *An approach to children's psychological problems.*

ability to function at home, at school or in play with other children, then some intervention is likely to be necessary. Similarly, if the child is suffering, the problem cannot be easily dismissed. Some unhappiness is inevitable in certain situations: parental death, painful or irritating physical conditions, parental divorce, for instance. Yet even then, it is appropriate to ensure that the child is receiving sufficient support in the form of affection, explanation and encouragement.

If the child's behaviour is thought to be normal, the next question is why his mother is concerned. She may be ignorant of what is normal, particularly if she is a first-time parent. Alternatively, she may have been misinformed that a behaviour is a sign of future trouble or an emotional response, such as a toddler's clinging is under the child's voluntary control. The behaviour may strike a sensitive chord in her own or her husband's past and provoke her concern even though normal. Or she may be parading the child's problem so that she can slip in a 'While I'm here, doctor . . .'. Only when all these have been considered is it appropriate even to consider terms such as 'overprotective' or 'neurotic' to describe unwarranted parental anxiety.

Is it a reaction to a time-limited event which will subside?

Children have, by definition, an immature range of coping reactions to adverse events. Many of these will elicit help or protection from parents. If upset, ill or in pain they tend to cling to their parents, particularly their mother, since the attachment relationship is a source of emotional security. This is often termed regression and is most evident in children aged six and under. Events themselves which include a separation from mother, such as first being left at playgroup, will also produce clinging. Anticipatory anxiety about a move of house or school examinations can be quite intense and present in masked form as hypochondriasis or demanding behaviour. In older children, nightmares following an accident are common and usually subside within a few weeks.

Some adversities reveal themselves as processes rather than events. One of the commonest is parental divorce. Some children are relieved by a divorce which brings an end to parental rowing, but more are disturbed and distressed by the warfare which continues between their parents, whose relationship with each other deteriorates during the legal process and the subsequent sharing of finances and care arrangements. The prognosis for the child becomes the prognosis for the relationship between the parents and a child who is caught up in the continuing dispute suffers even more (Buchanan, Maccoby & Dornbusch, 1992). It is important, when considering prognosis, to be sure that an apparent event is time limited and not part of a continuing adversity.

Does it have a good prognosis?

If it does, reassurance will suffice. A reaction to an event as mentioned above will clear up if the child is provided with emotional support and no perpetuating factors develop. A few conditions like simple tics and blue breath-holding attacks are very likely to clear up on their own. On the other hand, reactions to continuing adversity (such as chronic discord in family relationships) and some specific problems such as aggressive behaviour are very persistent, and reassurance is inappropriate. Some vulnerability factors such as poor relationships with other children ('can't make and keep friends of his own age') or low intelligence are indicators of a probable poor prognosis for a variety of emotional and behavioural problems.

When reassuring, make sure that you know what the parent and the child are concerned about. Stating that the recurrent abdominal pain is not appendicitis is of little help if one of them is sure it is cancer and also convinced that you have missed it, as happened with Auntie Jane. Reassure the right person. Cover yourself by making a forward appointment for review which can be cancelled by them if no longer necessary.

Can I treat it myself?

A large number of emotional, behaviour and relationship problems can and should be treated in primary care. For a few conditions there are studies which demonstrate this and the cure rates for enuresis and sleep problems which can be achieved in clinic settings use techniques which can readily be employed in primary care.

The sorts of approach which are likely to prove useful are the provision of sensible information and advice, counselling older children (11 and over), counselling parents, simple behaviour programmes such as star charts and the occasional use of medication.

To whom do I refer?

There are a number of professionals with something to offer. Within the National Health Service, the largest number of children's mental health problems are encountered by paediatricians, particularly school doctors and other community paediatricians. The quality of assessment and treatment offered will vary enormously between localities but a competent psychologically aware paediatrician is like gold dust. The specialist services in child and adolescent psychiatry and clinical child psychology are chronically underfunded with long waiting lists and are often slow to respond to referrals. This matters less with entrenched and complex problems when complex assessment procedures and multifaceted team approaches prove their worth, but obtaining a quick response to problems in their early phase is difficult unless repeatedly requested, and when purchaser power may force a change in the pattern of service delivery. Educational and social service provisions for children with mental health needs have been cut during the last decade and are now increasingly reserved for 'statutory' instances such as child abuse or children with a 'statement' of special educational needs (see Chapter 15). Some voluntary services are superbly sympathetic, particularly when dealing with oppressed young mothers or difficult teenagers, but their efficacy is largely untested. The simplest recommendation is to know your patch and discover who is worthwhile. For the early stages of emotional and behavioural problems, no single discipline or agency stands out as the obvious one to refer to.

In the present climate of diminishing funding for patient care it is probable that most agencies will need to apply some form of allocating priorities to referrals. In a sense this has always been done for obvious emergencies and urgencies. In some child mental health services now there is a requirement in purchaser contracts for all referrals to be 'prioritised'. As a rough rule of thumb, the more information in the referral letter, the higher the priority allocated. Sparse letters simply do not contain what is needed for a service to judge whether the child needs seeing quickly. It is perfectly reasonable to make the case that a recent onset of a clinical problem is grounds for an early appointment.

Problems with the current structure of services

Mental health services for children and adolescents have evolved in closer partnership with education and social services than any other area of medicine. The contribution of psychiatric social workers in particular was huge, and it was generally intended that they should outnumber psychiatrists by a substantial ratio. In most parts of the UK, social services still fund the social workers in child psychiatry services and historically this would have accounted for most of the funding for such services. Until relatively recently, child guidance clinics were frequently housed in buildings owned by the education authorities so many child and adolescent psychiatrists practised in community settings away from other medical colleagues. Some were employed by Local Authorities rather than by the National Health Service. The end result was a service somewhat isolated from medicine and indeed from adult psychiatry, which operated for much of its time as a primary health care resource, seeing self-referrals and referrals made by non-medical professionals such as teachers, educational psychologists, education welfare officers and social workers. In many clinics, referrals by general practitioners were in a minority. Treatments were predominantly social and psychotherapeutic, protracted and involved several staff working as a team.

In recent years, a number of changes have occurred. Educational psychologists have effectively withdrawn from child guidance clinics. Psychiatric social workers have been increasingly replaced by less trained social workers or been redirected to child protection work elsewhere in social services. Education authorities have wanted their premises for other purposes. Child psychiatrists have adopted rigorous training standards and become both more biological and more eclectic. Increasing awareness of children's mental health problems and possibly some social changes have led to a higher rate of referral.

With this in mind, it is not surprising that new forms of child mental health service are currently being explored. A theme is emerging of a tiered service with primary care as one level (Department of Health, 1995; Williams & Richardson/Health Advisory Service, 1995; Royal College of Psychiatrists, 1994). There is an expectation that cases will be seen at different levels according to their complexity and severity. The important issue for secondary prevention is the existence of a level of provision containing mental health professionals operating solo, not as team members. This should, if adequately provided, facilitate a speedy response to children whose problem is in its early stages of development.

Some people have suggested that it may be necessary to facilitate the transition from primary care to the next level of care. Historically this has been poorly done, perhaps for some of the reasons above. A suggestion (Hall & Hill, 1994) that a new form of professional – a child mental health worker – might be created to work in both general practice and child psychiatric services taking cases with them from one level to another in order to work with a mental heath professional or team proved unpopular because of the number of different professions and agencies already claiming a stake in the field. It is possible that the problem might be alleviated by special training for health visitors and there have been various attempts to develop this concept and evaluate their contribution (Stevenson, 1990; Nicol et al., 1993). To date, results have been rather disappointing. For instance, Nicol et al.'s (1993) study examined the impact on pre-school children's mental health of intensive health visiting, family therapy and mother and toddler groups. Although a number of clinical problems were helped in the medium term, in the longer term social adversity wiped out nearly all treatment gains. Furthermore, there is the problem of reach. Many parents experiencing the most severe problems with their children refused outside help (Nicol et al., 1987).

Early active management of selected problems

Child and adolescent psychiatry and psychology are low technology specialties. It is reasonable to attempt to import their contributions into a primary care setting. The drawback is that the techniques are time consuming. Even so, there are a number of manoeuvres which can be carried out and these are referred to here in a section organised by clinical problem. This presumes that reassurance and common-sense measures deriving from a formulation have been considered.

Studies of the management of children's psychological problems and personal experience suggest that two interventions which are overused in primary care settings are inappropriate reassurance and sedative medication (Adams, 1991; Bailey et al., 1978). Both have their place but there is a need to make sure that the child's problem is being dealt with; not just the parents' concerns or the doctor's uncertainty.

The detail of management plans cannot be covered here but as far as young children are concerned, the relevant sections in Hall, Hill and Elliman (1994) provide detail.

Excessive tantrums in young children

Ensure that remedial causes of frustration have been addressed and poor parental communication dealt with. The child deserves clear instructions as to what behaviour is required in terms he can understand. Tantrums themselves are met with 'structured ignoring' (time-out) in which the parent removes themselves, will not respond or removes the child from the company of others for one minute per year of age, keeping a record and looking for gradual change rather than immediate contrition.

Aggressive behaviour

This needs stopping as soon as possible in view of its tendency to persist over time. It may result from an ignorance of what else can be done to solve a dispute or may be a result of anger or resentment. In some families it is a reflection of parental aggressive behaviour. Parents should be urged to attempt to prohibit the behaviour and where feasible apply time-out. The latter is best if coupled with an incentive programme to build pro-social behaviours such as turn-taking or sharing.

Non-compliance in young children

Parents need to be sure that their instructions are sufficiently clear for their child to understand and that they are positive rather than a nagging, error-triggered whine whereby the child is told repeatedly to stop virtually everything they do instead of being told what is expected.

Once this is achieved, a simple star chart whereby the child earns stars for doing a specified action is often effective. The acid test is that the child should be able to tell you what they have to do to get a star. Star charts (or beads on a string, ticks on a calendar, etc.) can be used with children aged between 3 and 10 years for about three weeks before they lose their appeal. It is not necessary to couple stars with tangible rewards, praise is usually sufficient.

Sleep problems

Difficulties settling to sleep in the evening can be addressed by measures which allow the child to learn how to settle themselves to sleep alone. Since most children wake during the night, but those who cannot settle themselves back to sleep will cry, a large proportion of so-called night-wakers can also be managed by attending to how they are settled to sleep in the evening.

Meal refusal

Children who refuse to eat what is put in front of them but are thriving are obtaining food from somewhere. The first step is to demonstrate to the parent by means of a growth chart that there is no physical cause for concern. Secondly, and often with the help of a food diary, it is important to ensure that there is no calorie intake between meals. Once this is achieved, attention can then be turned to the meal process itself and issues such as a maximum time for the meal, the food offered and the style of parent–child interaction when feeding (praise for eating, ignoring for spitting out, etc.) be tackled.

Excessive clinging

Clinging to an attachment figure is normal in toddlers and will return when the child is tired, ill, fearful or in pain. If rejected, it will intensify. A common cause for its persistence is an anxious child and a common cause for the latter is that the parent has made threats to abandon the child. These may have been overheard in a marital row or used openly as a disciplinary measure. The child needs reassuring that he is secure and will not be abandoned. Learning through experience complements verbal reassurance, and the parents should persevere with brief separations, building the duration of these so that the child has a repeated experience of parents returning after separations. Simply instructing the parent to keep calm when dealing with the child may suffice (though is difficult to implement).

Enuresis

Unless enuresis is a consequence of infection, its first-line management is a star chart which can be expected to be effective in about one-third of cases. Those who do not respond will nearly always learn continence with the aid of an enuresis alarm. This takes a few weeks to work but offers a much higher rate of cure than medication. Desmopressin is an effective short-term measure but has a high relapse rate on discontinuation and is no substitute for an alarm unless the latter is impossible to administer. Imipramine will stop wetting in many cases but virtually all relapse when it is discontinued. It has no advantages over desmopressin and, in view of the danger of accidental overdose to the child and siblings, it should no longer be used outside a specialist clinic (and only exceptionally within one).

Faecal soiling

Most children who soil are constipated with a loaded colon which can be palpated abdominally or faeces found on rectal examination. They can be managed by emptying the rectum with an oral laxative, thereafter arranging for the child to be rewarded, by means of a star chart for defaecating in an appropriate receptacle. The chart may need to be maintained for a month or so and stars may therefore need to be backed up with a tangible reward.

Phobic anxiety

Irrational fears are common in children and need only be treated if they represent a handicap to the child's ordinary activities. The key principle is one of graded exposure to the feared object or situation, something to be carried out supportively by the parents (who not uncommonly share the same fear). Fear of school is not uncommonly a complex anxiety which can be rational. If not, it should be managed by arranging the earliest return to school possible with parents, teachers and educational welfare officers acting in concert. A common breeding ground for school phobia is protracted convalescence or repeated sick notes for trivial complaints and appropriate caution is required when medical sanction for avoiding school is requested.

Hyperactivity

Many parental complaints that their child is hyperactive are really complaints about disobedience, boisterousness or excitability. Hyperactivity means inattentive restlessness with fidgeting and squirming so that tasks ar never completed. It is quite a common phenomenon and 5–10% of primary school-age children will show this as a pattern with an onset in early childhood. Some parents use the old American term attention deficit disorder as an explanantion for all sorts of impatient, difficult behaviour. The modern term, hyperkinetic disorder, refers to the existence of inattentive restlessness across several types of situation to the extent where it becomes handicapping. In such a sense, it affects 1–2% of children, mainly boys.

Hyperactivity as a phenomenon is a vulnerability state for the development of antisocial behaviour, academic failure, peer rejection and low self-esteem. It is worth treating actively and parents should promote solitary self-occupation by the selective use of praise, insist on the completion of tasks, and boosting self-esteem by avoiding too much criticism while remarking positively on the child's achievements. Methylphenidate and allied stimulants are potent promoters of focused, settled attention but are best initiated by specialists in view of their side-effects, particularly on growth (see Chapter 15). Dietary restriction with the identification and elimination of foods which produce irritability and disrupted attention are effective in some children but not powerfully so. The simple diets which aim to exclude all additives are ineffective and potentially harmful. Any dietary intervention should be reviewed and supervised by a paediatric dietician.

Oppositional behaviour

Grumpy, argumentative or abusive behaviour can arise at any age in childhood and adolescence. In children aged under five years it can be managed along the lines detailed above for tantrums or aggressive behaviour. In older children, one can reasonably presume resentment and an interview with the child on his own or a family interview may shed some light. Advising parents to focus on praise for positive behaviour helps, but not all will feel able to put this into practice without support. Truculent or rebarbative adolescents can sometimes be helped by a reciprocal contract set up between them and their parents (you will need to see both parents), treating the matter along the lines of a marital dispute. Each side is urged to state their demands of the other and these demands are put into an exchange which can be reviewed weekly while the doctor holds the ring in each interview and insists on fair play.

Stealing from home

Incorrigible stealing from home is usually a sign that the child is experiencing rejection in the home or from the peer group. Although parental supervision is, across the board, the best way of minimising thieving, an interview with the child can reveal unhappiness which may be remediable. Parents need to keep valuables locked away and not leave then around to 'test' the child.

Obsessive–compulsive disorder

Children commonly create rituals as part of games but compulsive rituals which are experienced as compelling and distressing by the child should be taken seriously. Typically a child or adolescent with obsessions is cagey about revealing them, fearing ridicule because of their apparent nonsensical nature. Open discussion in a family interview may be sufficient. Failing this, some teenagers respond promptly to clomipramine 25–50 mg daily as a starting dose.

Misery

Children who are chronically unhappy are usually responding to circumstances rather than suffering a primary depressive illness. However, depression becomes a substantial mental health problem in adolescence, especially among girls and should be actively enquired about. If detected, situational adversity at home and school should be asked about and the parents advised to tackle it directly if it is present. If it cannot be remedied, the child will need support from parents or a counsellor or both but it must be a counsellor conversant with children's needs and skilled in working with them. Antidepressants are often thought to be effective in primary depressive disorders in adolescents but it is wise to prescribe one that is fairly safe in overdose such as lofepramine. Teenagers usually require an adult dose. Selective serotonin reuptake inhibitors are also safe in overdose but can produce excited reactions in some children and young teenagers so that they require expert handling.

Anorexia nervosa

Anorexic attitudes towards food are more numerous than anorexia nervosa itself. Self restrictive dietary practices and the belief that one mouthful more than a self-imposed maximum will result in visible fattening can progress to anorexia nervosa in those girls who are predisposed. In the early stages it is probably wise to advise parents to monitor eating and weight, even though they may be reluctant to do so. Once calorie restriction has resulted in a weight of below about 48 kg it is very difficult to reverse the mental and physical changes which ensue (see Chapter 12) and it is sensible to avoid the weight falling below 50 kg or to the point where amenorrhoea supervenes. Parents can be encouraged to use their authority to insist on adequate weight gain and maintenance. In general terms, the psychological problems which are associated with anorexia nervosa maintain rather than initiate self-starvation.

Coda

There are rich possibilities in the field of secondary prevention of mental health problems in children and adolescents. This can prove to be rewarding clinical work, given a modicum of knowledge and good sense. It is also likely to be more welcome to parents than simply making a referral to a secondary centre or service with a long waiting list with the consequence that the problem is even more ingrained by the time it is dealt with.

References

Adams, S. (1991). Prescribing of psychotropic drugs to children and adolescents. *British Medical Journal*, **302**, 217.

Bailey, V., Graham, P. & Boniface, D. (1978). How much child psychiatry does a general practitioner do? *Journal of the Royal College of General Practitioners*, **28**, 621–6.

Buchanan, C.M., Maccoby, E.E. & Dornbusch, S.M. (1992). Caught between parents: adolescents' experience in divorced homes. *Child Development*, **62**, 1008–29.

Department of Health (1995). *Child Mental Health*. London: HMSO.

Garralda, E. (1994). Primary care psychiatry. In *Child and Adolescent Psychiatry*. Rutter, M., Taylor, E. and Hersov, L., eds. 3rd ed. Oxford: Blackwell Scientific Publications.

Garralda, M.E. & Bailey, D. (1986a). Psychological deviance in children attending general practice. *Psychological Medicine*, **16**, 423–9.

Garralda, M.E. & Bailey, D. (1986b). Children with psychiatric disorders in primary care. *Journal of Child Psychology and Psychiatry*, **27**, 611–24.

Garralda, M.E. & Bailey, D. (1989). Psychiatric disorders in general paediatric referrals. *Archives of Disease in Childhood*, **64**, 1727–33.

Hall, D. & Hill P. (1994). Community Child Health Services. In *Health Care Needs Assessment*. Stevens, A. and Raftery, J., eds. Oxford: NHSME Radcliffe Medical Press.

Hall, D., Hill, P. & Elliman, D. (1994). *The Child Surveillance Handbook*. 2nd ed. Oxford: Radcliffe Medical Press.

Hill, P. (1996). Child and adolescent psychiatry. In *Essentials of Psychiatry*. Murray, R., Hill, P. and McGuffin, P., eds. Cambridge: Cambridge University Press (In press).

Hindley, P., Hill, P. & Bond, D. (1993). Interviewing deaf children, the interviewer effect. *Journal of Child Psychology and Psychiatry*, **34**, 1461–67.

Jellinek, M.S., Murphy, J.M. & Burns, B.J. (1986). Brief psychosocial screening in outpatient pediatric practice. *Journal of Pediatrics*, **109**, 371–8.

Nicol, A.R., Stretch, D.D., Fundudis, T., Smith, I., & Davison, I. (1987). The nature of mother and toddler problems, I: Development of a multicriterion screen. *Journal of Child Psychology and Psychiatry*, **28**, 739–54.

Nicol, R., Stretch, D. & Fundudis, T. (1993). *Preschool Children in Troubled Families*. Chichester: John Wiley & Sons.

Royal College of Psychiatrists (1994). *Purchasing Psychiatric Care*. London: Royal College of Psychiatrists.

Schubiner, H. & Robin, A. (1990). Screening adolescents for depression and parent–teenager conflict in an ambulatory medical setting: a preliminary investigation. *Pediatrics*, **85**, 813–18.

Scott-Smith, M., Mitchell, J., McCauley, E.A. & Calderon, R. (1990). Screening for anxiety and depression in an adolescent clinic. *Pediatrics*, **85**, 262–6.

Stevenson, J. (ed.) (1990). *Health Visitor Based Services for Pre-school Children with Behaviour Problems*. Occasional papers No.2. London:Association for Child Psychology & Psychiatry.

Williams, R. & Richardson, G. (1995). *Together We Stand*. London: Health Advisory Service.

Wortman, R.N., Donovan, D.S., Woodburn *et al.*, (1986). Depression and its relationship to somatic complaints in adolescent patients. *Journal of Adolescent Health Care*, **7**, 295.

[10] The secondary prevention of depression

André Tylee

The recognition of depression in general practice

Whilst general practitioners recognise much of the psychiatric morbidity suffered by their patients, a review found that overall around half goes unrecognised (Goldberg & Huxley, 1980). In major depression specifically, around a half of those identified by psychiatric research interviews go unrecognised by general practitioners, whether the patients are attending with a new episode of illness (Bridges & Goldberg, 1987) or for any reason (Skuse & Williams, 1984; Freeling *et al.*, 1985). Although another 10% are subsequently recognised and 50% of those unrecognised will remit, the remaining 20% may remain unrecognised even after six months and may develop a chronic depression (Freeling *et al.*, 1985).

General practitioners have a difficult and highly skilled task when faced with several presenting problems first to make a decision about the likelihood of a patient having a physical disorder, and if so whether it is mild or potentially life threatening, whilst simultaneously considering the possibility of emotional disorder also. With depression, this task is also made difficult by the frequency in general practice of presentations with somatic symptoms and of depression related to physical disorders.

Reasons why depression is missed

Two broad reasons why depression is missed in general practice settings are:

First, that patients whose depression is correctly recognised differ systematically in their personal characteristics (i.e. demographic, psychiatric or physical characteristics) or in what they mention to their general practitioners from those patients whose depression is missed (Box 10.1).

Secondly, that depression is missed because the general practitioners who are good at recognising depression differ

---

Increasing recognition
   female sex
   middle-aged
   unemployed
   bereaved or separated
   looks depressed
   white

Decreasing recognition
   adolescent or young adult
   elderly
   students
   physically ill
   presents with physical complaints
   unwilling to consider psychological problem
   presents psychological cues late in the interview, or not at all

---

Box 10.1 *Patient characteristics affecting the detection of depression.*

systematically in their personal characteristics or in their consulting behaviour from general practitioners who are poor at recognising depression (Box 10.3).

Patient characteristics

Freeling and colleagues (1985) found no demographic differences between their patients whose depression was recognised and those whose depression went unrecognised. Patients aged over 65 may be perceived by general practitioners as differing from younger ones in so far as depression is concerned. In one study (MacDonald, 1986) 27.7% of attenders aged 65 and over scored positively on the depression scale (Gurland & Wilder, 1984) and only 2.5% of these were rated by their general practitioner as having no depression at all. However, there was little relationship in this study between the opinion regarding depression recorded by a general practitioner and any action taken. Elderly patients from deprived areas may be seen as more likely to experience depressive illness (Copeland, 1987), whereas the incidence of depressive illness in those aged 65 and over does not correlate positively with the degree of social deprivation.

Marks and colleagues (1979) identified patient characteristics associated with whether the psychiatric diagnosis was made. Female patients are more likely to be perceived as psychiatrically disturbed than males and this was confirmed for patients attending male doctors but not for those attending female ones, among whom there was a higher prevalence of disturbance (Marks *et al.*, 1979). Male patients are more likely than females to have their psychiatric health rated accurately by their doctor (Marks *et al.*, 1979); general practitioners were most accurate with middle-aged patients and least accurate with patients aged 15–24. Widowed patients were more likely to be perceived by their doctors as psychiatrically disturbed, although this finding was not confirmed by the screening instrument. The unemployed were least likely to have their psychiatric illness go unrecognised. Students were most likely to have their psychiatric illness missed. Those who had stayed in education until 23 years and over were more likely to have their psychiatric illness missed than were those completing education younger.

Patient presentation

Most of the contacts between general practitioners and their patients are initiated by the patient. Differences in patients' help-seeking behaviour will affect the process, content and probably the outcome of the consultation. A poll (Mori Poll, 1992) commissioned for the launch in 1992 of the Defeat Depression Campaign organised by the Royal College of Psychiatry in association with the Royal College of General Practitioners asked people to identify someone to whom they would go if they suspected that they themselves might be depressed. Of respondents, 60% identified the general practitioner. Large numbers of the same respondents, however, felt that depression carried a stigma and that general practitioners might consider that a patient presenting with depression was lacking in 'backbone'. Many of the respondents also thought that they needed to be listened to but that their general practitioner would not have much time. They did not want to be prescribed antidepressant pills because they (mistakenly) thought that they are addictive.

Bucholz and Robin (1987) found that females rather than males are more likely to discuss their symptoms when they have several symptoms and patients who discuss their symptoms are more likely to have experienced hopelessness, cognitive difficulties, appetite and loss of weight than were non-discussers. Other factors associated with having discussed depressive symptoms with a doctor were being aged over 36, experiencing worse physical health, and having used specialist mental health facilities previously. Being both female and recently separated or widowed predicted discussion (Bucholz & Robin, 1987) as did having symptoms of panic and phobic disorders, whilst patients who abused drugs or were drug dependent were less likely to have discussed depressive symptoms (Bucholz & Dinwiddie, 1989).

The symptom of hopelessness was reported as discriminating

patients with psychiatric illness from those with only physical illness (Blacker & Clare, 1988).

A key task for the general practitioner is to distinguish between psychiatric and non-psychiatric disorder and then between forms of psychiatric disorder. It would be helpful to general practitioners to know which symptoms are particularly valuable in pointing to depression. Williams and Skuse (1988) found that depressive thoughts were commonly reported by attenders to a South London practice and that their occurrence correlated more with the psychiatrist's diagnosis of depression than the general practitioner's. Blacker and Clare (1988) used discriminant analysis to show that two symptoms may be particularly valuable in pointing to depression; depression of mood which is persistent and pervasive and loss of motivation, interest and drive. Other pointers are fatigue, insomnia, low self-opinion, loss of concentration and hopelessness.

Freeling and colleagues (1985) compared patients whose depression had been recognised with those whose depression had been missed without controlling for the accuracy or bias of the doctors involved and found that their two groups hardly differed in their psychiatric characteristics. There was, however, considerable overlap between the groups on all three scales so that some patients whose depression went unrecognised were rated by the research psychiatrist as more severely depressed than some patients whose major depression was recognised. The unrecognised group showed less overt evidence of depression, as they looked less depressed, and they were less likely to attribute their illness to depression. The unrecognised depressives were more likely to have had their depressive illness for more than a year and more likely to have concurrent physical illness contributing to their depression.

In another study, patients whose depression went unrecognised were more likely to be somatising their distress (Bridges & Goldberg, 1987). Somatisation is manifested by patients who seek help for the somatic manifestations of their psychiatric disturbance as opposed to seeking help for a co-existing physical illness (Bridges & Goldberg, 1985). By their definition, a patient who somatises:

(a) does not mention psychological symptoms;
(b) attributes the manifestations to a physical problem when they consult their general practitioner;
(c) does report symptoms to a researcher which justify a psychiatric diagnosis;
(d) has somatic symptoms assessed by the researcher as likely to revert to their original level or to disappear with psychiatric treatment.

Of patients with new inceptions of illness, 33% had psychiatric diagnoses according to the American Diagnostic and Statistical Manual (DSM-III-R) criteria (Box 10.2) and 13% had Adjustment

Duration of at least two weeks
    One of either:
        depressed mood
    or
        markedly diminished interest or pleasure in normal activities
    Plus four of:
        significant weight loss or gain
        insomnia or hypersomnia
        agitation or retardation
        fatigue or loss of energy
        feelings of worthlessness or excessive guilt
        reduced ability to concentrate or make decisions
        thoughts of death or suicidal thoughts or actions

Box 10.2 *Diagnostic criteria for major depression. (American Psychiatric Association, 1987.)*

Disorders. Of new inceptions, 10% had a psychiatric disorder alone. Pure somatisation was the presentation for 32% of all DSM-III-R psychiatric illness. Somatisation accounted for a half of all undetected psychiatric disorder and nearly half of the remaining unrecognised group had a physical illness. A patient classified by these criteria as a somatiser is often aware of symptoms contributing to a psychiatric diagnosis even if unwilling to accept it in principle and difficult to convince of their need for psychiatric treatment (Wright, 1990). It would seem then that somatisation, for some of these patients at least, is the result of an unspoken contract with their doctor and thus may be related to the concept of a first-contact doctor prematurely 'organising' his patient's malaise into a mutually preferred disease (Browne & Freeling, 1976). These more covert aspects of diagnosis can only be examined by careful study of the process and content of consultations. It is worth noting that Marks in his 1979 study comments that, whilst his ability to identify depression (identification index) *was* higher than those of general practitioners, when he relied on the information obtained by witnessing their consultations his ability to rate severity congruently with patients was *not*. Another study found that psychiatrists assessing patients in a general practice setting had difficulty judging whether the patients had a discrete psychiatric diagnosis when physical illness was present (Mann, Jenkins & Belsey, 1981).

Davenport and colleagues (1987) suggest that patients who are more disturbed are more likely to give cues (verbal, vocal, and postural) in their consultations, but some doctors seem able to suppress the expression of verbal and vocal cues by their patients although not of postural ones.

Ormel and colleagues (1990a,b) found that patients who presented with a psychological or social reason for their encounter with their doctor were more likely to be recognised as were those whose present symptoms were of more recent origin and that patients with more than one psychiatric diagnosis, and those with severe illness were more likely to be recognised than less ill patients. They also found that patients who in the previous year had received a psychiatric diagnosis from their general practitioner were more likely to be recognised at re-presentation than those presenting for the first time, but they are also more likely to be diagnosed as psychiatrically ill when they were not.

Tylee and colleagues (1993) used the same psychiatric interview as Freeling and colleagues (1985) but controlled for the doctor characteristics and found fewer differences between recognised and unrecognised patients. They (1993) did find that female patients seen by general practitioners who had physical illness were up to five times less likely to have a concurrent major depression recognised than female attenders who had no physical illness.

It is essential to determine what are the behaviours and underlying attitudinal characteristics which foster or impair patients' willingness and ability to communicate with their doctor about their depression. It seems likely that there is positive feedback between good consulting habits, the willingness of the patient to volunteer psychiatric symptoms and improvement in the patient's mental health (Ormel et al., 1990a,b).

General practitioner characteristics

Schulberg and McClelland (1987) postulated that a doctor's failure to assess depression might arise from any combination of the following:

1. a lack of knowledge regarding depressive symptoms and their management;
2. a failure to consider the diagnosis of depression despite the availability of relevant cues because of a preoccupation with possible organic pathology;
3. a failure to elicit affective, cognitive, and/or somatic symptoms relevant to the diagnosis of depression;
4. an under-rating of depression's severity or treatability after considering this diagnosis relative to the competing medical ones;
5. an awareness of the presence of depression, but a failure to diagnose it because psychiatric illness is not properly treated in primary care practice.

These and several other reasons will be discussed in terms of the role of the general practitioner, the structure of general practice, the process of decision making in general practice and the knowledge, skills and attitudes of the general practitioner.

The role of the general practitioner

A general practitioner needs to be alert to non-verbal or verbal patient cues of depression which is particularly pertinent if patients wait to share psychosocial concerns until late in the consultation (Burack & Carpenter, 1983) and if problems mentioned later in the consultation are just as important as problems mentioned early (Beckman & Frankel, 1984). Once a cue has been identified by the general practitioner, assessment is necessary to establish as soon as is feasible the probability of the patient suffering from a depressive illness. This entails not only exploring the sufferer's experience but also excluding, or identifying and treating, any of a range of physical conditions which can be linked or not to the depression. Once a depressive illness is recognised, the general practitioner may choose to acknowledge it to the patient in a manner which conveys some hope and explain that depression is a syndrome rather than a single symptom or normal mood which might be treated by the sufferer 'pulling him or herself together'. Then management can be decided upon in collaboration with the patient after explaining the probabilities, problems, benefits and risks of the different methods available. General practitioners sometimes postpone some of these steps to a later interview. Although general practitioners average ten minutes or less per consultation, they have the advantage of being able to arrange frequent, even daily, contact. General practitioners will make mistakes in recognising depression if they do not require the same number of symptoms to be present as do psychiatrists or if they accept as relevant only a more limited repertoire of symptoms. Such differences in criteria would produce both false-positive and false-negative diagnoses when general practitioners are assessed against research 'gold standards' which themselves have been validated against the clinical work of specialist psychiatrists. Often, one symptom repeatedly mentioned by the patient can carry the same weight to a general practitioner as the mention of several different symptoms once each. These differences in diagnostic approaches could easily arise from the tendency for general practitioners to make diagnoses over a series of relatively short patient contacts and would be associated with the structure of UK general practice.

The structure of general practice

British general practice has many large group practices with several partners sharing lists with each other, plus vocational trainees and medical students. The work of these practices is increasingly proactive, seeking to provide preventive care and to modify lifestyles. This work may in many practices result in depressed patients making their first contact with, for example, a practice nurse. Balint's (1957) notion of a 'collusion of anonymity' can now easily occur with a patient seeing different primary health care team members within a group practice. Some patients play on the lack of intimacy. A general practitioner covering for an absent partner may be less likely to be 'cued' into underlying depression by recognising an inconsistency in the patient's behaviour (Freeling, 1983) or to have the pre-existing relationship necessary for a patient to open with a statement about mood. Alternatively, however, depression can be missed by the doctor who regularly sees a patient whilst a new doctor may recognise it by the incongruity of affect which is produced (Freeling, 1983). If patients are not instantly familiar to their doctors, perhaps more emphasis is needed in training on the skills necessary to recognise depression.

The process of general practice

History taking, physical examination, investigation, diagnosis and treatment are not always present in general practitioner consultations, and general practitioners often make management decisions first and formulate a diagnostic label that fits (Howie, 1972). Because patients present an undifferentiated mix of physical, psychological, and social symptoms and the early symptoms of serious disease may be impossible to distinguish immediately from those of self-limiting ones, general practitioners have adopted a problem-solving approach based on likely probabilities (Crombie, 1963; Royal College of General Practitioners, 1972). General practitioners need to estimate the degree of threat of a condition and the effectiveness and availability of interventions. A model of the process general practitioners thought they used to identify depressed patients and decide upon their management was derived by two groups of general practitioners (Burton & Freeling, 1982) who decided that they were first 'cued' to consider depressive illness and that they then applied a checklist of symptoms. If depressive illness seemed likely, they assessed recent life events, and 'depressive tendencies' which include past or family history of depressive illness, or an adverse upbringing. Management decisions are based on this information. When the general practitioners applied their model to an audit of their care of depressive illness, their most commonly used cue proved to be a volunteering by the patient of a single symptom of depression (82%), second was the patient saying 'I feel depressed' (52%), third was the ill-defined cue that the doctor 'felt' the patient was depressed (53%), and fourth was the recurrent presentation of symptoms without identifiable organic cause (44%). Only rarely did a single cue trigger the process of seeking supporting evidence. This group of general practitioners as in most other studies showed great variability in their rates of diagnosis: one of them reported nearly a half of all cases audited.

In another study by Jenkins and colleagues (1985), 27 experienced general practitioners with an interest in psychological medicine differed widely in their response to videotaped consultations and vignettes over whether cases were primarily psychological and over categorisation of the psychological disorder. Agreement between the general practitioners was higher for the predicted outcome for the patient than on categorisation and also on the presence or absence of most psychological, physical, personality and social features. It does not seem surprising that experienced and interested general practitioners should show some agreement about outcome. The problems about categorisation are certain to impair any possible agreements about suitability of interventions. Also, a comparison of decision-making by trainee general practitioners with that by trainee psychiatrists (Wilkinson, 1988) showed a low level of agreement overall between groups and within groups. There was low agreement about the magnitude of psychosocial stressors, prognosis, and the diagnosis of depression and high agreement about the use of psychotropic drugs and good agreement about the use of counselling. Differences in interpretation between general practitioners and psychiatrists may make it a little difficult to use case discussion as a teaching method unless emphasis is placed on exploring the differences between general practitioners rather than eliminating differences between them and psychiatrists.

General practitioners vary in their willingness to attach a definite psychiatric diagnosis even in patients categorised as having psychiatric illness (Ormel et al., 1990a, b). Goldberg and Huxley (1980) have pointed out that there are two qualities, 'bias' and 'accuracy', which may account for systematic differences between general practitioners. A doctor with a high bias will tend to allocate many of his patients to a psychiatric diagnosis but may do so with a low degree of accuracy, i.e. with little relationship to the number of psychiatric symptoms experienced by his patients. Accuracy can be measured in one of two ways, *agreement* with a gold standard diagnostic schedule such as DSM-III, or *congruence* of ratings for severity with the patient's score on a screening instrument for psychological distress such as the General Health Questionnaire (GHQ). There have been a number of studies seeking to determine systematic differences between general practitioners who are good, and those who are poor at recognising psychiatric or depressive illness and not all utilise the distinctions drawn by Goldberg and Huxley (1980). Differences postulated between general practitioners could be classified under the rubrics 'knowledge', 'skills', and 'attitudes'.

General practitioners' knowledge

'Age and experience' might be seen as a surrogate for a general practitioner's knowledge. This dimension includes years in practice, age, and higher qualifications and did not show strong associations with accuracy (Marks *et al.*, 1979). Relevant academic ability has been shown to have associations with accuracy: academically more able doctors who possessed an appropriate concept of minor psychiatric illness as seen in general practice were more likely to rate their patients' degree of emotional distress congruently. They were also more likely to possess and use more directive interview approaches.

General practitioners' skills

The verbal and non-verbal behaviours of the doctor did not predict accurate identification in the study by Marks *et al.* (1979). Some general practitioners are more accurate than others in recognising depression (Marks *et al.*, 1979; Goldberg & Huxley, 1980; Millar & Goldberg 1991; Goldberg & Huxley, 1992; Goldberg *et al.*, 1993). Those who are better able to identify depression tend to make more eye contact with the patient, to be less likely to interrupt the patient or show signs of being in a hurry, and tend to be 'good listeners'. They are also more likely to ask direct questions with a psychological and social content. These behaviours are likely to encourage the patient to reveal depressive cues. Some behaviours of the doctor will make it more difficult to detect depression, because they will have the effect of inhibiting a distressed patient. These behaviours include asking many 'closed' questions (that is to say, questions that can readily be answered with a simple 'yes' or 'no') and asking many questions derived from medical theory rather than from what the patient has just said (Box 10.3).

Davenport and colleagues (1987) concluded that the reason why some doctors are better able than others to detect psychiatric illness is that they are more likely to allow patients to express verbal cues about lowered mood as well as somehow permitting 'vocal' (paraverbal) cues such as sighing. This giving of permission is probably related to, and may account in part for, the wide variation among general practitioners in their ability to detect psychiatric disorders (Shepherd *et al.*, 1966) which has been attributed to the personal bias of individual doctors towards or away from such problems (Marks *et al.*, 1979).

Awareness of the link between personal idiosyncrasy and general practitioner variability led to a series of efforts to improve general practitioners' performance with patients who have emotional disorder or psychiatric illness (Box 10.4). In the 1950s and 1960s these efforts lay largely in the field of what has come to be called Balint training. The training consisted of the discussion, in small groups comprising peers, of case reports made by the responsible doctor. The emphasis was on acquiring an understanding of the patient rather than agreeing a diagnosis and relied especially on the nature of the relationship and transaction between doctor and patient.

Increasing recognition
knowledge
about the symptoms of depression
about the treatments available
attitudes
showing interest and concern
asking about the home, work and family
sensitivity to verbal and non-verbal cues
skills in interviewing
giving more eye contact
listening, not interrupting
asking open-ended questions initially
asking about feelings
making empathic comments

Decreasing recognition
conservative personality types
a tendency to prescribe hypnotics

Box 10.3 *Doctor characteristics affecting the detection of depression.*

Education about the causes and effects of depression
medical students
vocational trainees
established general practitioners
other primary health care professionals
the public (The 'Defeat Depression Campaign')

Balint training

Increasing the continuity of care
personal lists
more/longer follow-up appointments

Training in interview skills (video feedback)

Screening questionnaires

Box 10.4 *Ways of improving the detection of depression.*

Successful training was reported to produce a 'small but significant change in the doctor's personality' (Balint *et al.*, 1965). For many doctors such a successful outcome might take five years of meeting once weekly for two hours for three 13-week terms a year. Originally all groups were led by psychoanalysts; later, leadership spread to general practitioners who had themselves experienced the training and for whom a 'group of groups' was often provided. The fact of continuing responsibility of the doctor for the patient was seen originally as very important; nevertheless the technique has been adopted for vocational trainees with considerable success. None of these interventions had been studied to see if patient outcome can be improved also.

The recognition of depression in general practice has been shown to be improved by training general practitioners in interview skills using video feedback (Gask *et al.*, 1987). There may also be value in organising consultations so as to achieve continuity of contact between the patient and the same general practitioner, in follow-up appointments to provide additional time or repeated contacts over a period. Screening using questionnaires or computer administered interviews has also been shown to improve recognition, particularly in high risk groups, but needs to be supplemented by the appropriate interview skills (Hoeper *et al.*, 1979). Many of the issues in improvement of recognition are educational, requiring the education of medical students, vocational trainees, general practitioners, and also public education of the general public to reduce stigma and encourage self recognition, acknowledgement to the doctor and recognition by families. Attempts have been made to replace the need for a general practitioner to have a high degree of sensitivity to cues of emotional disturbance by providing them with the results of screening questionnaires applied in the waiting room. Providing American family doctors with scores from the 28-item GHQ (Goldberg & Hillier, 1979) produced no increase in the recognition of mental disorder (Hoeper *et al.*, 1984) although one general practitioner with a known interest in psychiatry found the results of the 60-item GHQ helpful (Johnstone & Goldberg, 1976) and another study found that providing feedback made a significant difference to the doctors' recognition (Magruder-Habib, Zung & Feussner, 1990). It has been suggested that rather than replacing the emotional antennae of the general practitioner with a printout of a screening test it would be sensible to replace the general practitioner with a specially trained worker for some groups known to be at high risk. Interviewing behaviours have been taught to, and shown to increase the accuracy of, American family practice trainees in recognising psychiatric disorders although those who performed poorly at onset seemed also to need teaching about approaches to management (Goldberg, Steele & Smith, 1980*a*; Goldberg *et al.*, 1980*b*).

The technique of problem-based interviewing developed at McMaster University (Lesser, 1985) has successfully been taught to general practitioner trainees (Gask *et al.*, 1988) and to a self-selected group of established general practitioners (Gask *et al.*, 1987). The latter improved their skills in psychiatry which were already good (Gask *et al.*, 1987). There must be a suspicion that, as hypothesised above, the improvement in performance is related in part to the group work and not only to the technique learnt. However, it has been demonstrated that communication skills training of general practitioners has increased patient satisfaction (Evans *et al.*, 1987) and also that interviewing skills taught to undergraduates persist into professional life (Maguire, Fairbairn & Fletcher, 1986) so that the acquisition of appropriate techniques is in itself likely to be of lasting value. An international consensus view is that communication skills can be taught and that the subsequent benefits to medical practice are demonstrable, feasible on a routine basis and enduring (Simpson *et al.*, 1991). It still remains that good recognisers of depression are better than poor recognisers at a whole range of consulting activities which follow after diagnosis (Millar and Goldberg, 1991) as well.

General practitioners' attitudes
General practitioners vary in their preferred length of consultations and are not always able to consult at their preferred speed. It has been demonstrated (Howie *et al.*, 1991) that general practitioners can be classified as faster (average of 6.99 minutes or less per patient), intermediate and slower (9.0 minutes or more per patient), that patient satisfaction was greater with longer consultations, and that relevant psychosocial health problems were more likely to be dealt with in longer consultations, whatever the predilection of the general practitioner as regards length of consultation. On the other hand, Marks *et al.* (1979) found doctors whose consultations lasted longer to be no better at detecting psychiatric illness.

'Interest and concern' is a dimension which involves high empathy (Truax & Carkhuff, 1967), being interested in psychiatry, and asking questions about family and problems at home. It is associated with correctly recognising psychiatric disorder and with rating it congruently (Marks *et al.*, 1979). In the same study, a dimension, 'conservatism', was identified which 'is associated with lack of congruence in rating psychiatric disorder'. It embraces a measure of resistance to change on a social attitude inventory (Wilson, 1975), along with extraversion, use of hypnotics, and a tendency to make contentless statements during consultations. A third dimension, 'psychiatric focus' by the doctor, was found to be associated with bias but not with accuracy. In contrast, in another study, 'psychological orientation' (Cockburn, Reid & Sanson-Fischer, 1987) was significantly correlated with broader indicators of good quality of care provided in a consultation (Howie *et al.*, 1991).

Recognition improves patient outcome

There is general agreement that an improvement in the recognition of major depression by general practitioners is desirable (Rutz *et al.*, 1989; Regier *et al.*, 1988; Secretary of State, 1992; Priest 1991).

Some general practitioners' failure to recognise depressive illness may result from their belief that a patient will not benefit from a mental health intervention. Depressed patients about whose outcome their doctors were optimistic and who were therefore not prescribed antidepressants fared significantly worse than those who were treated (Zung *et al.*, 1985).

Freeling and colleagues found that patients with unrecognized major depressive disorder did slightly worse over three months (personal communication) than the recognised patients who were prescribed inadequate dosages of antidepressant drugs and rarely had a second contact within the three months with anyone in the practice. This finding confirmed those of Johnson (1973). Given the frequency with which depressive illness goes unrecognized, it seems important to determine whether such failure is disadvantageous. Weissman and colleagues (1981) suggest from the USA that there are some patients who, once missed, stay that way for a long time, although another study has described how depressives are eventually recognised (Widmer & Cadoret, 1978). We need more studies of natural history to inform us about the link between depression being missed and whether this adversely affects patient outcome.

Ormel and colleagues (1990a, b) looked at the effect of general practitioner recognition on management and patient outcome, and whether such effects are confounded by the severity of the condition, duration of condition, concurrent morbidity, reason for encounter and diagnostic category. Nearly 2000 attenders to 25 general practitioners underwent a standard two-stage psychiatric interview that included a disability scale. They describe three types of 'caseness' for psychiatric disorder: a 'case' defined by the general practitioner, a 'case' defined by the screening instrument and finally a 'case' defined by the detailed psychiatric interview. These three techniques obtained different prevalences for psychiatric disorder: the general practitioners declared a prevalence of 26%, the screening instrument 46% and the psychiatric interview 15%. When they simply considered those patients with new psychiatric morbidity the rates were 14%, 38% and 10%, respectively. The general practitioners missed half of the cases identified on the psychiatric interview and depression was more readily recognised than anxiety disorder. The detection rate by the general practitioner increased in proportion to the severity of the illness. General practitioners tended to provide diagnoses that were less specific than the psychiatric instrument in the patients that they recognised. Patients recognised as having a psychiatric disorder by the general practitioner were more likely to receive mental health intervention. These patients also fared better in terms of psychopathology and social functioning than the non-recognised group. Initial severity, psychological reasons for encounter, recent onset, diagnostic category and psychiatric co-morbidity were all related to better recognition and outcome.

If general practitioners do not know the range of depressive symptoms to ask about, they will be unable to make an accurate diagnosis. Similarly, if a doctor does not know, or believe, or value the effectiveness of certain kinds of management, then he/she may eschew diagnoses which would lead to those managements. Whilst deficiencies in knowledge can be rectified relatively easily, changing beliefs and values is likely to be more difficult, particularly if they have not been elicited. If a doctor is preoccupied with possible organic pathology, this may be due to lack of confidence in his ability to diagnose and manage organic pathology and correcting that lack may be too onerous a task. The lack of confidence could originate in cognitive deficit, in mind set, or in personality. Lack of confidence should be determinable. A failure to elicit appropriate information could stem from any of the above but a specific and isolated lack of communication skill is possible and then correctable.

An under-rating of comparative severity suggests that the doctor is applying a Cartesian dichotomy between mind and body normally held to be inappropriate and ineffective in modern medical care (Engel, 1977). It seems unlikely that there is widespread in primary care a mind set which construes psychiatric illness as lying outside the ambit either of doctors in general or of general practitioners in particular. It seems reasonable to suggest, first, that being a good recogniser of depressive illness is simply a subset of a much wider set of being a good general practitioner and that this is itself related to particular types of decision-taking and problem-solving and may be associated with attitudes towards personal risk-taking.

Research needs to determine the extent to which recognition of depression is a subset of a much wider range of competence in general practice, and the extent to which recognition is a product of mind set and personality. Global ratings do not allow for the stage in the consultation at which recognition may have occurred. There remain those problems which arise from the responsibility to provide whole-person care in general practice to people who have, simultaneously, physical symptoms and affective disorder. Concern about physical illness is not only reasonable but desirable. On the other hand, it is not appropriate for all patients to be fully investigated for organic disorder before the psychosocial aspects of their problems are tackled. This is reported as happening frequently in the USA (Katon 1984; Rodin & Voshart, 1986).

The complexity of the problems faced by general practitioners is highlighted by the fact that many of these missed and somatising depressives had a physical disorder also. The co-existence of different disorders in a single patient is the very fabric of a generalist discipline and general practitioners are familiar with the problems of treating for acute and new illness patients with the care of whose chronic disorders they are already involved (Stott & Davis, 1979). For the general practitioner, the main conclusion is the importance of familiarity with a relatively direct interview for the main specific symptoms of depression, (Box 10.2) and of being willing to ask these questions.

Conclusion

Depression is a common condition and is eminently treatable if recognised. A combined approach that encourages patients to discuss it more readily, and general practitioners to be more willing and able to manage it with the help of the primary health care team, seems at present to be the most pragmatic approach to prevention in the absence of clear evidence for the possibility of primary prevention.

References

American Psychiatric Association (1987). *Diagnostic and Statistical Manual of Mental Disorders*. 3rd ed. revised. Washington DC: APA.

Balint, M. (1957). *The Doctor, the Patient, and the Illness*. London: Pitman Medical.

Balint, M., Balint E., Gosling R. & Hildebrand P.A. (1965). *A Study of Doctors*. London: Pitman Medical.

Beckman, H.B. & Frankel R.M. (1984). The effect of physician behaviour on the collection of data. *Annals of Internal Medicine* **101**, 692–6.

Blacker, C.V.R. & Clare A.W. (1988). The prevalence and treatment of depression in general practice. *Psychopharmacology*, **95**, S14–17.

Bridges, K. & Goldberg, D. (1985). Somatic presentation of DSM-III in psychiatric disorders in primary care. *Journal of Psychosomatic Research*, **29**, 563–9.

Bridges, K. & Goldberg, D. (1987). Somatic presentation of depressive illness in primary care. In *The Presentation of Depression: Current Approaches*. Freeling, P., Downey, L.J. and Malkin, J.C., eds. London: Royal College of General Practitioners.

Browne, K. & Freeling, P. (1976). *The Doctor–Patient Relationship*. London: Churchill Livingstone.

Bucholz, K.K. & Dinwiddie, S.H. (1989). Influence of non-depressive symptoms on whether patients tell a doctor about depression. *American Journal of Psychiatry*, **146** (5), 640–4.

Bucholz, K.K. & Robin, L.N. (1987). Who talks to a doctor about existing depressive illness? *Journal of Affective Disorders*, **12**, 241–50.

Burack, R.C. & Carpenter, R.R. (1983). The predictive value of the presenting complaint. *Journal of Family Practice*, **16**, 749–54.

Burton, R.H. & Freeling, P. (1982). How general practitioners manage depressive illness: developing a method of audit. *Journal of the Royal College of General Practitioners*, **32**, 558–61.

Cockburn, J., Reid, A.L. & Sanson-Fisher, W. (1987). The process and content of general practice consultations that involve prescription of antibiotic agents. *Medical Journal of Australia*, **147**, 321–4.

Copeland, J.R.M. (1987). Prevalence of depressive illness in the elderly community in the presentation of depression: In *Current Approaches*. Freeling, P., Downey, L.J. and Malkin, J.C., eds. Exeter: Royal College of General Practitioners.

Crombie, D.L. (1963). Diagnostic methods. *Journal of the Royal College of General Practitioners*. **6**, 579–89.

Crombie, D. (1974). *Changes in patterns of recorded morbidity*. In *Benefits and Risks in Medical Care*. Taylor, D., ed. London: Office of Health Economics.

Davenport, S., Goldberg, D. & Millar T. (1987). How psychiatric disorders are missed during medical consultations. *Lancet*, **ii**, 439–40.

Engel, G.L. (1977). The need for a new model: a challenge for biomedicine. *Science*, **196**, 129–36.

Evans, J., Kiellerup, F.D., Stanley, R.O., Burrows, G.D. & Sweet, B. (1987). A communication skills programme for increasing patients' satisfaction with general practice consultations. *British Journal of Medical Psychology*, **60**, 373–8.

Freeling, P. (1983). *A Workbook for Trainees in General Practice*. Bristol: Wright PSG.

Freeling P. (1985). Health outcomes in primary care: an approach to the problem. *Family Practice*, **23**, 177–81.

Freeling, P., Rao, B.M., Paykel, E.S., Sireling, L.I. & Burton, R.H. (1985). Unrecognised depression in general practice. *British Medical Journal*, **290**, 1880–3.

Gask, L., McGrath, G., Goldberg, D.P. & Millar, T. (1987). Improving the psychiatric skills of established general practitioners: evaluation of group teaching. *Medical Education*, **21**, 362–8.

Gask, L., Goldberg, D., Lesser, A.L. & Millar, T. (1988). Improving the psychiatric skills of the general practice trainee: an evaluation of a group training course. *Medical Education*, 22, 132–8.

Goldberg, D.P. & Hillier, V.F. (1979). A scaled version of the General Health Questionnaire. *Psychological Medicine*, 9, 139–45.

Goldberg, D.P. & Huxley, P. (1980). *Mental Illness in the Community. The Pathway to Psychiatric Care*. London: Tavistock.

Goldberg, D.P. & Huxley, P. (1992). *Common Mental Disorders – A Biosocial Model*. London: Routledge.

Goldberg, D.P., Steele, J.J. & Smith, C. (1980a). Teaching psychiatric interviewing skills to family doctors. *Acta Psychiatrica Scandinavica*, 62, 41–7.

Goldberg, D.P., Steele, J.J., Smith, C. & Spivey, L. (1980b). Training family doctors to recognise psychiatric illness with increased accuracy. *Lancet*, ii, 521–3.

Goldberg, D.P., Jenkins, L., Millar, T. & Faragher, E.B. (1993). The ability of trainee general practitioners to identify psychological distress among their patients. *Psychological Medicine*, 23, 185–93.

Gurland, B.J. & Wilder, D.E. (1984). The CARE revisited: development of an efficient systematic clinical assessment. *Journal of Gerontology*, 39, 120–37.

Hoeper, E.W., Nycz, P.D., Cleary, P.D., Regier, D.A. & Goldberg I.D. (1979). Estimated prevalence of RDC mental disorder in primary mental care. *International Journal of Mental Health*, 8, 6–15.

Hoeper, E.W., Kessler, L.G., Burke, J.D. & Pierce, W. (1984). The usefulness of screening for mental illness. *Lancet*, i, 33–5.

Howie, J.G.R. (1972). Diagnosis – the Achilles heel. *Journal of the Royal College of General Practitioners*, 22, 310–15.

Howie, J.G.R., Porter, A.M.D., Heaney. D.J. & Hopton, J.L. (1991). Long to short consultation ratio: a proxy measure of quality of care for general practice. *British Journal of General Practice*, 41, 48–54.

Jenkins, R. & Clare A. (1985). Women and mental illness. *British Medical Journal*, 291, 1521–2.

Jenkins, R., Smeeton, N., Marinker, M. & Shepherd, M. (1985). A study of the classification of mental ill health in general practice. *Psychological Medicine*, 15, 403–9.

Johnson, D.A.W. (1973). Treatment of depression in general practice. *British Medical Journal*, 2, 1061–4.

Johnstone, A. & Goldberg, D. (1976). Psychiatric screening in general practice: a controlled trial. *Lancet*, i, 605–8.

Katon, W. (1984). Depression: relationship to somatisation and chronic illness. *Journal of Clinical Psychiatry*, 45, 4–11.

Lesser, A.L. (1985). Problem-based interviewing in general practice: a model. *Medical Education*, 19, 209–304.

MacDonald, A.J.D. (1986). Do general practitioners 'miss' depression in elderly patients? *British Medical Journal*, **292**, 1365–7.

Magruder-Habib, Zung, W.K. & Feussner, J.R. (1990). Improving physicians' recognition and treatment of depression in general medical care. Results from a randomised clinical trial. *Medical Care*, **28**, 239–50.

Maguire, G., Fairbairn, S. & Fletcher C. (1986). Benefit of feedback training in interviewing as students persist. *British Medical Journal*, **1**, 268–70.

Mann, A.H., Jenkins, R. & Belsey, E. (1981). The twelve month outcome of patients with neurotic illness in general practice. *Psychological Medicine*, **11**, 535–50.

Marks, J.N., Goldberg, D. & Hillier, V.F. (1979). Determinants of the ability of general practitioners to detect psychiatric illness. *Psychological Medicine*, **9**, 337–53.

Millar, T. & Goldberg, D.P. (1991). Link between the ability to detect and manage emotional disorders: a study of general practitioner trainees. *British Journal of General Practice*, **41**, 357–9.

Mori Poll. (1992). *Defeat Depression Campaign*. London.

Ormel, J., Koeter, H., van den Brink, W. & van de Willige G. (1990*a*). The extent of non-recognition of mental health problems in primary care and its effect on management and outcome. In *The Public Health Impact of Mental Disorder*. Goldberg, D. and Tantam, D., eds. Basle: Hogrefe-Huber. pp. 154–164.

Ormel, J., Van den Brink, W., Koeter, M.W.J., Giel, R., Vandermeer, K., & Van de Willige G. *et al.* (1990*b*). Recognition, management and outcome of psychological disorders in primary care: a naturalistic follow-up study. *Psychological Medicine*, **20**, 909–23.

Priest, R.G. (1991). A new initiative on depression (editorial). *British Journal of General Practice*, **41**, 487.

Regier, D., Boyd, J., Burke, J., Rae, D., Myers, J. & Kramer M. *et al.*, (1988). One month prevalence of mental disorders in the United States. *Archives of General Psychiatry*, **45**, 977–85.

Rodin, G. & Voshart K. (1986). Depression in the medically ill: an overview. *American Journal of Psychiatry*, **143**, 696–705.

Royal College of General Practitioners. (1972). *The Future General Practitioner. Learning and Teaching*. London: British Medical Journal Publishing.

Rutz, W., Walinder, J., Eberhard, G., Holmberg, G., von Knorring, A-L., & von Knorring, L. *et al.* (1989). An educational programme on depressive disorders for general practitioners on Gotland: background and evaluation. *Acta Psychiatrica Scandinavica*, **79**, 19–26.

Rutz, W., von Knorring, L. & Walinder J. (1992). Long term effects of an educational program for general practitioners given by the Swedish Committee for the Prevention and Treatment of Depression. *Acta Psychiatrica Scandinavica*, **85**, 83–8.

Schulberg, H.C. & McCelland, M. (1987). A conceptual model for educating primary care providers in the diagnosis and treatment of depression. *General Hospital Psychiatry*, **9**, 1–10.

Secretary of State (1992). *Health of the Nation*. London: HMSO.

Shepherd, M., Cooper, M., Brown, A.C. & Kalton G. (1966). *Psychiatric Illness in General Practice*. Oxford: Oxford University Press.

Simpson, M., Buckman, R., Stewart, M., Maguire, P., Lipkin, N., Novack, D. & Till J. (1991). Doctor–patient communication: The Toronto Consensus Statement. *British Medical Journal*, **303**, 1385–7.

Skuse, D. & Williams, P. (1984). Screening for psychiatric disorder in general practice. *Psychological Medicine*, **14**, 365–77.

Stott, N.C.H. & Davis, R.H. (1979). The exceptional potential of each primary care consultation. *Journal of Royal College of General Practitioners*, **29**, 201–5.

Truax C.B., & Carcuff, R.R. (1967). *Toward effective counselling and psychotherapy. Training and Practice*. Chicago: Aldine Atherton.

Tylee, A.T., Freeling, P. & Kerry, S. (1993). Why do general practitioners recognise major depression in one woman patient yet miss in it another? *British Journal of General Practice*, **43**, 327–30.

Weissman, M.M., Myers, J.K. & Thompson, W.D. (1981). Depression and its treatment in a US urban community 1975–76. *Archives of General Psychiatry*, **38**, 417–21.

Widmer, R.B. & Cadoret, R.J. (1978). Depression in primary care: changes in pattern of patient visits and complaints during a developing depression. *Journal of Family Practice*, **7**, 293–302.

Wilkinson, G. (1988). A comparison of psychiatric decision-making by trainee general practitioners and trainee psychiatrists using a simulated consultation model. *Psychological Medicine*, **18**, 167–77.

Williams, P. & Skuse, D. (1988). Depressive thoughts in general practice attenders. *Psychological Medicine*, **18**, 167–77.

Wilson, G.D. (1975). *Manual for the Wilson Patterson Attitude Inventory* (WPAI). London: NFER.

Wright, A.F. (1990). A study of the presentation of somatic symptoms in general practice by patients with psychiatric disturbance. *British Journal of General Practice*, **40**, 459–63.

Zung, W.W.K., Zung, E.M., Moore, J. & Scott, J. (1985). Decision making in the treatment of depression by family medicine physicians. *Comprehensive Therapy*, **11**, 19–23.

[11] The prevention of anxiety disorders

Helen Kennerley

Introduction

This chapter describes the types of anxiety disorders seen in primary care settings, the risk factors associated with those disorders, and possibilities for early intervention to avoid their progression.

Anxiety problems in the community

Anxiety and related difficulties are very common in primary care. Every general practitioner encounters patients with irrational fears; health visitors may be familiar with new mothers who have developed agoraphobia; and the community nurse will certainly come into contact with anxious relatives of ill patients.

Around one in six adults consulting general practitioners are 'generally anxious' (Lader, 1992). Others present with specific phobias, discrete panic disorder or obsessional–compulsive disorder, so the prevalence of anxiety disorders in primary care settings is at least 15%. Minor affective disorders, that is anxiety and mild depression or both, account for a large proportion of consultations in general practice (Goldberg & Huxley, 1980). Anxiety is more common even than depression and is usually managed in primary care, rather than being referred on for specialist attention (McPherson, 1987).

Primary care workers are well placed to help

The primary health care team is in contact with the majority of the individuals who need help in coping with anxiety. Furthermore, studies show that primary care professionals can be highly successful in helping the anxious to overcome problems using psychological methods. Catalan *et al.* (1984) found that general practitioners can successfully use problem-solving techniques rather than prescribe anxiolytic medication, while Marks (1985) established that trained practice nurses could work well as behaviour therapists in a primary care setting.

There are other good reasons for anxiety to be tackled at the primary care level. General practitioners see more than two-thirds of their patients in a year and more than 90% every five years (Gray & Fowler, 1983) and thus are ideally placed to identify at-risk groups and to spot the early signs of anxiety disorders opportunistically. Where early identification is possible, the prognosis is improved. The stigma of attending specialist mental health services can be avoided if the patient is treated in primary care. People with psychological problems prefer to see their family doctor, rather than a mental health worker (Barker *et al.*, 1990). The familiar faces of members of the primary health care team can be a comfort to those going through a stressful time – indeed, general practitioners are the most trusted of health workers and their advice carries most weight (McCron & Budd, 1979). In addition, their knowledge of a person's background can contribute to a better understanding of the problems and to a more effective intervention.

Finally, there are greater opportunities for health education in primary care than in specialist clinics, and it is this which is fundamental to the prevention of anxiety-related problems.

Types of anxiety-related problems
Anxiety is, of course, a normal and expected response to stress and common to us all. The anxiety response triggers physical, psychological and behavioural changes which prepare an individual for coping with stressors, and which remit once danger has passed. On most occasions the response is reasonable or even vital.

Normal responses to stress
The signs and symptoms of normal anxiety will be familiar. Essentially, the person is preparing for 'fight or flight' and there are appropriate mental and bodily changes. The physical indicators include muscular tension, hyperventilation, increased blood pressure and digestive changes, all of which increase a person's readiness for action. The psychological changes precipitated by anxiety include cognitive and emotional shifts which, again, facilitate coping under stress. Thinking becomes more focused, there can be a improvement in concentration and problem-solving, and a range of affective responses including increased irritability, on the one hand, or even a sense of well-being on the other. The behavioural sequelae of anxiety are usually forms of escape or vigilance: jumping out of the way of a bus or being particularly determined to hold onto the steering wheel of a car during a skid, for example.

Problem anxiety
Anxiety neuroses, on the other hand, are defined as 'various combinations of physical and mental manifestations of anxiety, not

attributable to real danger and occurring either in attacks or as a persistent state' (Gelder, Gath & Mayou, 1989). This overestimation of danger tends to be accompanied by an underestimation of personal coping resources or of the likelihood of being rescued from a frightening situation.

The natural bodily changes, if sustained for prolonged periods, can give rise to a range of psychosomatic problems such as general aches and fatigue, tension headaches, loss of appetite, weight loss, chest pains, irritable bowel syndrome, skin problems, and respiratory difficulties. Patients often come to the attention of primary health care professionals with such complaints. The mood changes linked with extended periods of anxiety can include oversensitivity, lability and demoralisation, while the cognitive changes often involve exaggerated perceptions of threat, rumination over problems, impaired memory and poor concentration. The most common problem behaviour is avoidance in some form.

The precipitants of anxiety-related problems might be external or internal. For example, a man with a snake phobia would experience distress on seeing a real snake or a picture of a snake. He would have the same response if he believed that he had seen a snake or that he was likely to come into contact with a snake.

Whether the stimulus is real or perceived, the common theme in anxiety problems is the cycle which maintains the response after it has been triggered. Maintaining cycles may be physical, psychological, behavioural or systemic.

Physical maintaining cycles
The physical experience of anxiety can be alarming and can lead to greater levels of tension and worry. For example, muscle tension can turn into marked pain or spasm, or increased respiration can become hyperventilation with subsequent alkalosis. Even though a person recognises that the muscular pain and difficulties in breathing are simply anxiety symptoms, the experience can be so aversive as to trigger a fear of the symptoms of anxiety: a fear of fear. Anticipation of this discomfort can then cause anxiety in turn, even in the absence of a continuing external source of stress and so anxiety can become long term.

The physical symptoms associated with anxiety, such as shaking, sweating, nausea and faltering voice, can impair a person's performance, particularly in public or social settings. An awareness of this can easily undermine the confidence of an anxious person, increasing performance worries and exacerbating the physical symptoms in turn.

Psychological maintaining cycles
Cognitive distortions are magnified as fear levels increase. This exacerbates anxiety and causes further distortion. The most

common of the cognitive distortions are catastrophising, dichotomising, exaggerating, over-generalising and ignoring the positive (Beck, Emery & Greenberg, 1985) (see Chapter 17).

When *catastrophising*, the anxious person anticipates disaster as the only outcome, for example, assuming that dizziness indicates a stroke, or expecting that minor surgery will result in death.

Dichotomising means seeing only black and white categories and not experiencing more moderate responses: 'I will always feel this bad,' rather than, 'I feel bad at the moment but I could get better with help,' or 'Everyone always picks on me,' rather than 'Sometimes I am criticised and sometimes this is unjustified.'

Exaggerating refers to the process of magnifying the negative or frightening aspects of one's experiences and is often coupled with *over-generalising* and then jumping to erroneous conclusions. An example of this would be a man who feared redundancy and who subsequently began to note and exaggerate only his mistakes and errors. As thinking errors tend to co-exist, a single mistake could trigger: 'I'll never be able to complete this task (dichotomising) and the manager will see me as incompetent (jumping to conclusions) and I'll lose my job (catastrophising).'

Ignoring the positive is a process of mentally filtering out positive and reassuring facts and events, not noticing compliments, not acknowledging achievements, not recognising one's strengths.

Scanning is another cognitive process which perpetuates problem anxiety. Scanning or searching for phobic stimuli increases the likelihood of experiencing fright, either because a person is more likely to see, feel or hear the feared object, or because that person is experiencing false positives which alarm. For example, mistaking fluff on the carpet for a spider, presuming a benign swelling is a malignancy.

Finally, the mood changes that are sometimes associated with stress can themselves in turn further impair the patient's ability to cope with stress. Thus the experience of chronic anxiety can be increasingly demoralising, promoting a hopelessness which undermines coping, while irritability or lability of mood can handicap someone in their performance or social functioning and thus feed into further anxieties about failure.

Behavioural maintaining cycles

One of the natural reactions to perceived danger is to flee from, or avoid, the threatening situation. This immediately reduces anxiety, but such behaviour may serve to maintain the problem because a person never stays around long enough to learn to cope. Avoidance and escape can take overt or covert forms. Overt avoidance and escape is demonstrated by the person who never enters a frightening shopping mall or who walks in only to race out again. Covert avoidance or escape might involve entering the shopping mall but only if accompanied by a friend or leaning on a shopping trolley for support. The anxious person never learns that it is possible for them to face their fear without support and so the original fears persist or worsen.

Another common behaviour which exacerbates anxiety is the use of stimulants in response to stress: lighting up a cigarette, making a coffee, comfort-eating a chocolate bar, turning to alcohol – which becomes a stimulant as it is metabolised.

Systemic maintaining cycles

Not all maintaining factors are internal; sometimes problems are perpetuated by the direct or indirect actions of others. For example, an anxiety disorder might not remit because of background stress caused by ongoing difficult work situations or domestic problems or long-term unemployment. Difficulties and loss of confidence might be maintained because a wife responds to her husband's pleas for reassurance about his health or because a neighbour fetches an agora-phobic friend's shopping: both collude in maintaining an anxiety-related problem. General practitioners should consider whether they may exacerbate agoraphobia by agreeing to regular home visits rather than insisting the person comes down to the surgery.

The management of anxiety-related problems requires an under-standing of the development of these cycles and the application of strategies to break them.

Presentation of anxiety-related problems

Different categories of anxiety neurosis are characterised by dif-ferent presentations, although certain features are common to them

---

Phobias
  Simple phobias, e.g. of dogs or heights
  Social phobia
  Agoraphobia

Panic disorder – often co-exists with agoraphobia

Generalised anxiety disorder

Obsessive–compulsive disorder (rare)

Somatisation and hypochondriasis

Burn out

Post-traumatic stress disorder

Box 11.1 *Types of anxiety disorders.*

all. The types which are likely to be seen in general practice are: phobias, panic disorder, generalised anxiety disorder (GAD), obsessive–compulsive disorder (OCD), somatic problems and hypochondriasis, 'executive' stress or 'burn out', and post-traumatic stress disorder (PTSD) (Box 11.1).

Phobias

Mild fears are common but become a problem when the fear response is inappropriately intense or when it leads to avoidance of certain situations or objects. The main categories of phobia are: simple, social and agoraphobia. Simple phobias are discrete fears of specific stimuli such as dogs or heights while social phobia is the fear and avoidance of situations where one might be exposed to the evaluation of others – public speaking, for example. Agoraphobia is the fear of leaving a place of safety because of an expectation that something terrible will happen, and is often associated with panic attacks.

Phobias tend to be maintained by the sufferer's consistent over-estimation of the risk of danger coupled with avoidance, which then prevents testing of the validity of the fear and subsequent desensitisation to the phobic stimulus.

Panic

Panic describes intense feelings of apprehension or impending disaster. The onset of a panic attack is rapid and physical symptoms are very marked, especially if the individual hyperventilates. There are many possible triggers for a panic attack: chest pain mis-construed as a heart attack or dizziness misinterpreted as an impending stroke, for example. The condition is frequently main-tained by such catastrophic misinterpretation of common bodily sensations, and by hyperventilation and avoidance. Panic can occur in combination with other anxiety disorders.

Generalised anxiety disorder (GAD)

Generalised anxiety disorder refers to persistent, pervasive feelings of anxiety which give rise to chronic bodily, psychological and behavioural symptoms. The patient will often describe GAD as 'constant' and occurring 'out of the blue'. However, it is generally thought to be underpinned by chronic worry or the misinterpreta-tion of a wide range of situations as threatening (Beck *et al.*, 1985). These collections of fears need to be teased out in treatment and each tackled individually.

Obsessive–compulsive disorder (OCD)

This involves a subjective compulsion to carry out acts or to dwell on intrusive cognitions – repetitive images or thoughts which are abhorrent to the sufferer and difficult to dismiss. The triggers for such cognitions tend to be perceived dangerous or contaminating situations, thoughts or actions. This then sets off the compulsion to 'neutralise' the thought, either by perseverating on a positive cognition or by carrying out a ritualistic behaviour such as touching objects in a certain way or repeated checking. Coping with OCD is most often in the form of avoidance, e.g. washing to avoid contamination, or not reading newspapers to avoid the word 'death'.

Somatic problems and hypochondriasis

This type of presentation of anxiety is very commonly seen in general practice and might be dealt with as a physical problem initially. Indeed, psychosomatic problems are by definition physical, and stressful life events can both cause and maintain these conditions (Alexander, 1950). Classically, psychosomatic presentations include insomnia, irritable bowel syndrome, headaches, hypertension, asthma, psychogenic difficulty in swallowing, vomiting, and diarrhoea.

Hypochondriasis specifically describes an anxiety-related problem where there is distress in response to perceived symptoms, often associated with hypersensitivity to normal bodily sensations or a preoccupation with the fear of catching a serious disease. Hypochondriacal worries tend to be resistant to reassurance yet maintained by reassurance seeking and it is important that the practitioner tries to help the patient to acknowledge and desensitise themselves to the health fears rather than simply repeating that there is nothing physically wrong with them.

Burn out

This term describes a reaction to chronic stress, which is particularly common among caring professionals (Freudenberger, 1974). The stress can be 'positive', such as overwork, pressured deadlines, or impossible targets, or 'negative' such as job boredom, lack of autonomy, or frustration. Symptoms are similar to the other anxiety disorders but tend to be more marked because the stress is ignored or dismissed until it has reached a debilitating level. It may be ignored through habit or because stress is construed as 'excitement' or because an individual's drive over-rides their awareness of stress.

Post-traumatic stress disorder (PTSD)

This may follow unusually traumatic events such as road traffic accidents, rapes, witnessing a major disaster, or being involved in military combat. The main features, which are usually accompanied by symptoms of anxiety, are recurrent intrusive flashbacks or dreams of the event; emotional numbing or hyper-alertness; guilt; or memory impairment. PTSD often remits without active intervention, although it can run a chronic course. Barlow (1988) suggests that the latter happens when the person experiencing the trauma has a biological vulnerability to anxiety, a lack of a sense of control in a dangerous situation and subsequent avoidance of anything likely to stimulate memories of the traumatic event. Avoidance can take the form of behavioural avoidance of situations or persons who trigger distress, or cognitive avoidance of the recall of events. In treating PTSD in rape victims, Foa *et al.* (1991) established that exposure and desensitisation to traumatic memories was a more effective treatment than counselling or stress inoculation training.

Risk factors

Risk factors for the development of anxiety-related problems may be characterological, (personality type) familial, cognitive, behavioural or social (Box 11.2).

Personality type

The significance of personality type remains controversial, though many would agree with Snaith's (1981) opinion: 'It is probable that some degree of abnormality of a specific personality trait underlies the liability to develop a phobic neurosis . . .'.

In the early 1960s, Friedman and Rosenman identified a 'Type A' personality which seemed to confer an increased risk of heart disease, raised blood pressure and other stress-related problems.

Personality type (can be assessed by questionnaire)
Eysenck's 'neuroticism'
Friedman and Rosenman's 'Type A'
Spielberger's 'trait anxiety'

Family history
Genetic or acquired?

Life events
Involving threat rather than loss

Cognitive style

Maladaptive coping behaviours
e.g. Substance misuse

Lack of social support

Box 11.2 *Risk factors for the development of anxiety disorders.*

Such individuals were said to be identifiable through competitive behaviour, ambition and a tendency to ignore stress symptoms.

In his theory of personality, Eysenck (1967) defined the opposing constructs of neuroticism and stability based on learning theory. Those classified as neurotic showed more intense autonomic nervous activity and slow rates of habituation to stimuli and were therefore more likely to experience anxiety and less able to desensitise to aversive stimuli.

Although a cognitive theorist, Spielberger (1985) considered anxiety as a *trait*, predisposing an individual to anxiety problems, when it is a chronic condition. This he distinguishes from *state* anxiety, a transitory emotional state triggered by a stressor. 'Type A' personality, Eysenck's 'neuroticism' and Spielberger's 'trait anxiety' are each measurable, using questionnaires devised by the authors. Such psychometric data could provide primary health care teams with useful markers of their patients' vulnerability to develop anxiety disorder.

Family history

The presence of innate fears in infancy, such as those of strangers, heights, novelty, or separation, suggests that some fears are genetic and therefore the possibility that fears can be passed on in families (Marks, 1987).

There is evidence of a familial pattern in anxiety disorders from studies, such as that of Crowe *et al*. (1983), who studied the relatives of patients with panic disorder, and Torgersen (1983) who stated that, although genetic factors were not evident for GAD, they did seem to influence the development of other anxiety disorders, especially panic and agoraphobia. However, clustering of disorders within families could also be accounted for by imitation and learning: a mother can communicate her health anxieties to her young daughter; a father's frequent warning that dogs bite might predispose his son to developing a dog phobia.

Thus an awareness of family history and problems can alert the primary care worker to vulnerability in an individual.

Stressful life events

These have been implicated in the onset of affective disorders (Finlay-Jones & Brown, 1981; Brown, 1993) (see Chapter 3). Whereas events involving loss are associated with the development of depression and those involving hope with its remission, events involving threat seem to be linked with the onset of anxiety disorders and events promoting security with the amelioration of anxiety.

It is not only life events in the present which increase the risk of developing anxiety related problems. A person is more likely to be distressed in response to a life event if that event matches a traumatic event in childhood (Brown, Bifulco & Harris, 1987). For example, a boy involved in a serious road traffic accident would react more severely to witnessing a car crash later in life than a person who had not experienced a similar early trauma. Young (1994), amongst other cognitive theorists, suggested that early experience determines our beliefs (schemata) about our self and our world. His model predicts the development of schemata involving threat and a sense of uncontrollability in response to childhood experiences of danger and insecurity. These schemata then negatively bias perceptions so that a person is more likely to interpret events as dangerous and the self as vulnerable.

Cognitive style

It has been established that perceptions are state congruent, that is that interpretation of current events and recall of past events accords with a person's current mood state (Bower, 1981). Thus, the person in crisis perceives and remembers with a strong sense of threat which can be powerful in exacerbating anxiety. In these states of heightened anxiety, individuals are more likely to be subject to the thinking biases and cognitive distortions outlined earlier in this chapter and these, in turn, will fuel an anxiogenic style of thinking. When this happens, anxiety can become self-perpetuating.

Skills deficits

Although Barker et al. (1990) discovered that the majority of the general population have good coping strategies for managing psychological problems, a proportion turn to unhelpful means such as substance misuse, leading to even greater problems. In the absence of knowledge of helpful coping techniques, individuals may employ maladaptive strategies and will run the risk of worsening a problem which could have been arrested.

Social support

According to Brown and Harris's 1979 model of the social origins of depression, vulnerability to depression increases with reduced levels of social support (Chapter 3). This is particularly marked if a person has no confidant(e), and even worse if that person suffers the loss of a confidant(e). Carroll et al. (1985) established that this is also the case with PTSD – the greater the available social support, the more buffered is the victim of trauma. Barlow (1988) suggests that this finding is likely to be the case for all anxiety disorders.

A person's vulnerability is often determined by a combination of factors rather than a single variable. For example, an obsessive disorder might emerge in a person with a psychological predisposition combined with serious life events and in the absence of a confidant. This highlights the importance of having knowledge of a person's background. Primary health care professionals are often better informed about patients than other health professionals and thus may be in a better position to recognise those at risk.

Non-pharmacological prevention in general practice

There are good reasons for adopting a psychological, rather than a pharmacological approach to managing anxiety disorders. Anxiolytic drugs such as benzodiazepines have proved no more effective than psychological management of anxiety disorders (Catalan & Gath, 1985) and they are subject to problems of side-effects and dependency (see Chapter 13). Drugs can also provide a means of subtle avoidance for the user who can then become psychologically if not physically dependent on medication.

Psychological methods of prevention will be addressed at the primary, secondary and tertiary levels. At any level, it is necessary that the patient understands the function of anxiety, the development of problem anxiety, its triggers and maintaining factors.

Primary prevention

This is directed towards the person 'at risk' and requires the adoption of an educational, rather than a therapeutic role. The primary health care professional has more contact with an individual than any other health professional and is in a unique position to practise primary prevention when a patient suffers stressful life events such as bereavement, job loss, or threat of redundancy (Chapter 3). Identification of the vulnerable could be facilitated by the future development of record systems and computers, as described by Gray and Fowler (1983), to store relevant information for reference and to alert primary health care professionals to act pre-emptively.

Most people are well able to help themselves and prefer informal to formal help (Barker et al., 1990), thus, there are good reasons to anticipate individuals responding well to primary prevention. Barker and co-workers surveyed help-seeking and coping patterns in a UK sample and found that individuals experiencing psychological problems mostly turn to adaptive, rather than maladaptive coping strategies. The most commonly used were keeping busy, problem-solving and 'trying not to worry', while the least popular methods of coping were using pills, alcohol or smoking. Individuals were most likely to turn to a partner or close relative for support, followed by a friend and then the family doctor.

Interventions at the level of primary prevention could take the form of booklets and guides in the surgery, drop-in clinics, educational videos, and so on. A short list of useful texts for patients is given in the Appendix.

Secondary prevention

This depends upon the detection of the problem in its early stages when action can arrest or reverse the process. Again the primary health care team is in a good position to identify those who would benefit from early intervention and to help patients understand the development and maintenance of their problems before maladaptive responses become fixed.

Guided self-help

Marks (1991) showed that persons with anxiety disorders can benefit from self-administered behavioural treatments involving gradually increasing exposure to feared objects or situations. So successful did he regard such self-help that he concluded that 'Therapist-accompanied exposure is now known to be largely redundant.' His intervention requires a therapist to assess the problem, to help the patient draw up a hierarchy of feared situations and then to guide and supervise progress, while the client carries out systematic exposure alone.

Sorby, Reavley & Huber (1991) validated an intervention in a primary care setting, which involved even less professional input. The study focused on panic and GAD patients who received a self-help booklet on the management of anxiety symptoms as a supplement to the general practitioner's usual treatment and advice. Results of the study indicated that this did indeed enhance anxiety management without the general practitioner having to spend more time with the patient.

Management strategies

A range of coping strategies can help modify the physical, the psychological and the behavioural symptoms associated with problem anxiety (Box 11.3). These are described in detail in texts such as France and Robson (1986) and Kennerley (1995) and only a few can be summarised in this chapter. The techniques listed below are particularly suitable for the primary care setting and all are skills which need to be practised regularly to be effective.

Management of physical symptoms

Two useful techniques for managing unpleasant bodily sensations associated with anxiety are controlled breathing and relaxation.

Controlled breathing

The procedure for teaching controlled breathing is described fully by Clark, Salkovskis and Chalkley (1985). In their article, they advise first explaining the link between hyperventilation and the unpleasant symptoms of anxiety or panic, followed by training in slow, regular breathing. The suggested rate of breathing is 8–12

Controlled breathing exercises

Relaxation training

Distraction techniques
physical exercise
re-focusing
mental exercises

Problem-solving

Exposure therapy
graded exposure
unaccompanied (guided self-help) or accompanied

Box 11.3 *Management strategies in secondary prevention of anxiety disorders.*

breaths per minute and this should be nasal and diaphragmatic. Diaphragmatic breathing is taught by getting the patient to place a hand on their chest and a hand on their abdomen and instructing them to breathe more deeply so that their lower hand moves up and down more than their upper hand. In a 'provocation test' the patient practises hyperventilating whilst supervised by the therapist, to encourage recognition of its role in the development of symptoms. The patient is then instructed to introduce controlled breathing and to recognise how the symptoms abate.

Relaxation training

There is a wide range of relaxation exercises available and it is important that patients try a few to find out which works best for them. Descriptions of various exercises can be found in Charlesworth and Nathan (1982) and Kennerley (1995). One of the simplest and most adaptable to general practice, is the 'relaxation response' (Benson, 1975) which requires a patient to use a soothing or relaxing image or word.

The patient sits in a comfortable position, allows the body to become as relaxed as possible and then focuses on inhaling slowly. On the outbreath, the patient brings to mind a soothing image or word and then repeats the cycle, always breathing slowly and using the diaphragm. This need only be maintained for a few minutes, but practised at intervals throughout the day this brief exercise can diminish physical tension and help the patient develop a skill which can be applied as needed in an anxiety-provoking situation.

Management of psychological symptoms

The alarming worries and distressing images which can exacerbate and maintain anxiety disorders can be modified through distraction and problem-solving.

Distraction is based on the fact that none of us can concentrate on two things at once: if one attends to something neutral or positive, one cannot also focus on worries and alarming thoughts. There are three categories of distraction: physical exercise, re-focusing, and mental exercise. It is important that patients try to learn distraction techniques from each of these categories so that they can adapt to different settings.

A repertoire of physical distractions could include activities such as playing squash, or taking the dog for a walk as well as more subtle forms such as tidying a handbag or re-organising a filofax. The re-focusing technique requires a person to attend to their surroundings. For example, counting tins on supermarket shelves, reading leaflets in a waiting room, describing in detail a visible piece of artwork. Mental exercises involve the self-generation of distractors such as carrying out mental arithmetic, reciting poetry or holding a soothing image in mind. Different strategies will suit different circumstances, and the most compelling distractors will be those which are of interest to the user.

Problem-solving

Catalan and colleagues (1984) established that general practitioners could help their anxious patients by teaching them a simple problem-solving technique which proved as effective as anxiolytic drug treatment. Problem-solving offers a structure for breaking out of cycles of unproductive worry. Each aspect of a problem is defined and subjected to the six steps set out in Box 11.4. This is best done as a written exercise, taking one aspect of a problem at time.

---

1. Define the worry. Who does it involve? Under what circumstances?

2. Brainstorm possible solutions without censure and using other people's suggestions if needed.

3. Choose and rank the most helpful solutions.

4. Take the first solution and plan how to implement it in detail.

5. Try it out.

6. Evaluate the outcome. If the solution did not work, return to Step 4.

Box 11.4 *The steps in problem-solving.*

Management of behavioural consequences

The most common problem behaviour associated with anxiety is avoidance and this responds readily to graded exposure. The keys to successful exposure are: grading, planning, and practice. The patient first defines the problem situation. What is avoided? When? Under what circumstances? This gives the target which is then worked towards in a series of safe steps.

The first step must be a challenge to the patient but must also seem achievable. At this point one would incorporate factors to ease distress (such as having a friend present) and the circumstances of this step would be well planned with a prepared contingency plan to adopt in case of initial failure. Once the first step is accomplished, it is rehearsed until it is manageable with ease and then the process is repeated for step two and so on until the target is reached.

Relapse prevention

The long-term management of anxiety problems depends on a patient being able to predict future problems and plan how to cope with them (Marlatt & Gordon, 1985). A relapse prevention plan incorporates a list of potential problem situations and early warning signs of distress coupled with specific management plans. For example, a man worried that his phobia of flying might be re-kindled when he next had to fly on business could draw up a plan including the use of controlled breathing and relaxation to calm him before the flight, carrying a novel and worry beads to provide distraction during the flight, and allowing himself the option of going by train as a contingency plan.

A combination of these management strategies will often be necessary to the patient and teaching them could be carried out individually or in groups.

Tertiary prevention

This is the management of an established anxiety disorder and might be best carried out in primary care, using the above tech-niques, or by referral to a specialist for behavioural, cognitive or dynamic psychotherapy, especially when the problem is chronic and has not responded to self-help instruction or brief intervention. Although the focus of treatment is then handed over to another professional, the general practitioner or other practice worker will still be in contact with the patient or the family and can continue to be involved in supportive work and relapse prevention.

Assessing the efficacy of interventions

To evaluate the usefulness of interventions to manage anxiety, ideally data should be collected at the start of intervention and then progress monitored and followed up after intervention has ceased. This could include behavioural observations, simple self-ratings or standardised symptom questionnaires. Such prospective assessments of change and progress are likely to be more accurate than retrospective recall of change. Two frequently used and well-validated questionnaires which the primary care worker would find useful are the Beck Anxiety Inventory (Beck *et al.*, 1988) and the Spielberger State-Trait Anxiety Inventory (Spielberger *et al.*, 1983). A comprehensive review of assessment strategies can be found in Hersen and Bellack (1981).

Conclusion

There is now good evidence that primary health care professionals can successfully intervene to prevent the progression of their patients' anxiety problems. It should be possible to avoid the development of chronic intractable anxiety states in many cases, and long-term dependence on anxiolytic drugs should become a thing of the past. General practitioners and practice nurses might consider seeking training in problem-solving techniques and exposure therapy. The possession of such skills might prevent much misery, avoid the need for more difficult remedial treatments later in the progression of a disorder, and add to the job satisfaction of the primary health care team.

Appendix

Useful texts for patients
Benson, H. (1975). *The Relaxation Response*. Fount paperbacks.
Butler, G. (1985). *Managing Anxiety.* Oxford: Oxuniprint.
Butler, G. (1992). *Managing Social Anxiety.* Oxford: Oxuniprint.
Charlesworth, E. A. & Nathan, R. G. (1982). *Stress Management.* Corgi books.
Fennel, M. & Butler, G. (1985). *Controlling Anxiety.* Oxford: Oxuniprint.
Hambly, K. (1983). *Overcoming Tension*. London: Sheldon Press.
Kennerley, H. (1996). *Worries, Fears and Anxieties: A Guide to Recovery* London: Robinson Health.
Mills, J.W. (1982). *Coping with stress*. New York: Wiley Press.

References

Alexander, F. (1950). *Psychosomatic Medicine, Its Principles and Application*. Norton. New York.
Barker, C., Pistrang, N., Shapiro, D.A. & Shaw, I. (1990). Coping and help-seeking in the UK. adult population. *British Journal of Clinical Psychology*, **29**, 271–86.

* Available from The Department of Clinical Psychology, Warneford Hospital, Oxford OX3 7JX.

Barlow, D. H. (1988). *Anxiety and its Disorders*. New York: Guilford Press.

Beck, A. T., Emery, G. & Greenberg, R.L. (1985). *Anxiety Disorders and Phobias*. New York: Basic Books Inc.

Beck, A.T., Epstein, N., Brown, G. & Steer, R.A. (1988). An inventory for measuring clinical anxiety: psychometric properties. *Journal of Consulting and Clinical Psychology*, **56**, 893–7.

Benson, H. (1975). *The Relaxation Response*. Fount Paperbacks.

Bower, G.H. (1981). Mood and memory. *American Psychologist*, **36**, 129–48

Brown, G.W. (1993). Life events and affective disorder: replications and limitations. *Psychosomatic Medicine*, **55**, 248–59.

Brown, G.W. & Harris, T.O. (1978). *Social Origins of Depression: A Study of Psychiatric Disorder in Women*. London: Tavistock Publications.

Brown, G.W., Bifulco, A. & Harris, T.O. (1987). Life events, vulnerability and the onset of depression: some refinements. *British Journal of Psychiatry*, **150**, 30–42.

Carroll, E.M., Rueger, D.B., Foy, D.W. & Donahoe, C.P. (1985). Vietnam combat veterans with post traumatic stress disorder: analysis of marital and cohabiting adjustment. *Journal of Abnormal Psychology*, **94**, 329–37.

Catalan, J. & Gath, D. (1985). Benzodiazepines in general practice: a time for decision. *British Medical Journal*, **290**, 375–6.

Catalan, J., Gath, D., Edmonds, G. & Ennis, J. (1984). The effects of non-prescribing of anxiolytics in general practice. *British Journal of Psychiatry*, **144**, 593–602.

Charlesworth, E.A. & Nathan, R.G. (1982). *Stress Management*. Corgi books.

Clark, D. M., Salkovskis, P.M. & Chalkley, A. J. (1985). Respiratory control as a treatment for panic attacks. *Journal of Behaviour Therapy and Experimental Psychiatry*, **16**, 23–30.

Crowe, R.R., Noyes, R., Pauls, D.L. & Slymen, D.J. (1983). A family study of panic disorder. *Archives of General Psychiatry*, **40**, 1065–69.

Eysenck, H.J. ed. (1967). *The Biological Basis of Personality*. Springfield, IL: Charles C. Thomas.

Finlay-Jones, R. & Brown, G.W. (1981). Types of stressful life event and the onset of anxiety and depressive disorders. *Psychological Medicine*, **11**, 803–15.

Foa, E.B., Olasov Rothbaum, B., Riggs, D.S. & Murdock, T. B. (1991). Treatment of post traumatic stress disorder in rape victims: a comparison between cognitive–behavioural procedures and counselling *Journal of Consulting and Clinical Psychology*, **59**, 715–23.

France, R. & Robson, M. (1986). *Behaviour Therapy in Primary Care: A Practical Guide*. Croom Helm.

Freudenberger, H.J. (1974). Staff burn out. *Journal of Social Issues*, **30**, 159–65.

Gelder, M.G., Gath, D.H. & Mayou, R. (1989) *The Oxford Textbook of Psychiatry*. Oxford: Oxford University Press.

Goldberg, D. & Huxley, P. (1980). *Mental Illness in the Community: The Pathway to Psychiatric Care*. London: Tavistock Publications.

Gray, M. & Fowler, G. (1983). *Preventative Medicine in General Practice*. Oxford: Oxford Medical Publications, Oxford University Press.

Hersen, M. & Bellack, A.S. (1981). *Behavioral Assessment: A Practical Handbook*. New York: Pergamon Press.

Kennerley, H. (1995). *Managing Anxiety: A Training Manual*, Oxford: Oxford Medical Publications, Oxford University Press.

Lader, M.H. (1992). Guidelines for the management of patients with generalized anxiety. *Bulletin of the Royal College of Psychiatry*, **16**, 560–5.

McCron, R. & Budd, J. (1979). Communication and health education: a preliminary study. Unpublished document prepared for the Health Education Council, University of Leicester Centre for Mass Communication Research, October 1979, Chapter 8.

McPherson, I. G. (1987). Clinical psychology in primary healthcare. In *Reconstructing Psychological Practice*. McPherson, I.G. and Sutton, A. eds. London: Croom Helm.

Marks, I.M. (1985). A controlled trial of psychiatric nurse therapists in primary care. *British Medical Journal*, **290**, 1181–84.

Marks, I.M. (1987). *Fears, Phobias and Rituals: Panic Anxiety and their Disorders*. Oxford: Oxford University Press.

Marks, I.M. (1991). Self-administered behavioural treatment *Behavioural Psychotherapy*, **19**, 42–6.

Marlatt, G.A. & Gordon, J.R., eds. (1985). *Relapse Prevention*. New York: Guilford.

Rossenman, R.H. Friedman, M. & Straus, R. (1964). A predictive study of CHD. *Journal of the American Medical Association*, **195**, 86–92.

Snaith, P. (1981). *Clinical Neuroses*, Oxford: Oxford University Press.

Sorby, N.G.D., Reavley, W. & Huber, J.W. (1991). Self-help programme for anxiety in general practice: controlled trial of an anxiety management booklet. *British Journal of General Practice*, **41**, 417–20.

Spielberger, C. D. (1985). Anxiety, cognition and affect: a state-trait perspective. In *Anxiety and the Anxiety Disorders*. Tuma, A. H. and Maser, J. D., eds. Hillsdale, NJ: Erlbaum.

Spielberger, C.D., Gorsuch, R.L., Lushene, R., Vagg, P.R. & Jacobs, G.A. (1983). *Manual for the State-Trait Anxiety Inventory*. Palo Alto CA: Consulting Psychologists Press Inc.

Torgersen, S. (1983). Genetic factors in anxiety disorders. *Archives of General Psychiatry*, **40**, 1085–9.

Young, J.E. (1994). *Cognitive Therapy for Personality Disorders: A Schema-focused Approach*. Sarasota: F.L. Professional Resource Exchange, Inc.

[12] The prevention of eating disorders

Frances Raphael

Introduction

Prevalence of eating disorders

The reported prevalence of eating disorders has risen exponentially over the last 30 years and continues to rise. Some have questioned whether this is due to a true change in incidence or merely a reflection of greater public and professional awareness of the disorders. It may also be that the total sum of neurotic disorder within a given population is constant, but the type of problem presented varies with time, ethnicity and gender.

Changing patterns of neurosis

Regarding women and neurosis generally, hysterical symptoms are not the everyday occurrence they once were. One view is that the recognition of eating disorders parallels their evolution. Vomiting was not part of the original descriptions of anorexia nervosa. As the condition evolved, vomiting may have made the condition more visible. Restrictive anorexia nervosa was the standard form in the 1960s, the bulimic variant was recognised in the 1970s, before normal weight bulimia nervosa firmly established itself as a separate entity in the 1980s (Box 12.1). Although they are still in the minority, the number of women with the multi-impulsive form of bulimia nervosa is increasing through the 1990s.

It is most likely that a combination of explanations is relevant. As methods of epidemiological research have improved a consensus has been reached that the prevalence of disorder among women according to the strict American Diagnostic and Statistical Manual (DSM-III-R) diagnostic criteria is between 1% and 2% for bulimia nervosa (Fairburn & Beglin, 1990) and between 0.02% and 0.04% (Rooney et al., 1995; Hoek, 1991) for anorexia nervosa. Box 12.1 gives DSM-IV diagnostic criteria.

Above and beyond those who meet diagnostic criteria for complete syndromes, large numbers of women have some or other

Anorexia nervosa

Refusal to maintain body weight above 85% of that expected

Intense fear of gaining weight, though underweight

Disturbed experience of body weight or shape, or undue influence of shape on self-image

Amenorrhea in women, for three months

(May include bingeing and purging too)

Bulimia nervosa

Recurrent episodes of binge eating, far beyond normally accepted amounts of food (at least twice a week for three months)

Inappropriate compensatory behaviour to prevent weight gain, such as vomiting, and use of laxatives, diuretics and appetite suppressants

Self-image unduly influenced by body shape

(May be purging or non-purging types)

Box 12.1 *Diagnostic criteria for eating disorders (DSM-IV). (American Psychiatric Association, 1994.)*

symptoms of eating disorders. A large cross-sectional population survey by Bushnell *et al.* (1990) reported that 22.5% of women engaged in recurrent binge-eating at some stage in their lives, which supports similar earlier findings.

Children and adolescents

There are numerous reports of eating disorders, both anorexia nervosa and bulimia nervosa, being recognised in children and adolescents but reliable prevalence data in this age group are not yet available. Even if children do not have adult type eating disorders, it is clear that concerns regarding body image and dieting are prominent at an earlier age than was previously recognised (Childress *et al.*, 1993). This raises the possibility of preventing progression to more severe states.

Obesity

Neither DSM-IV (APA, 1994) nor the World Health Organisation's (1992) International Classification of Diseases (ICD-10) recognise obesity as an eating disorder. They prefer obesity to be considered a physical disorder unless there is particular evidence that psychological factors are of importance in its aetiology. This denies the extent to which obesity is a major, everyday problem in western society. According to a recent nationwide survey, 45% of male informants and 36% of female informants could be classified as overweight (OPCS, 1994). There are often psychological consequences to obesity but the origins of obesity are undoubtedly multifactorial and not always psychological. The prevention of obesity is beyond the scope of this chapter which will be restricted to anorexia nervosa and bulimia nervosa.

The consequences of eating disorders

The costs to the community of eating disorders, including absenteeism from work, social security benefits and health service costs, are difficult to quantify. The physical, psychological and social morbidity of the disorders is extensive. The physical consequences are summarised in Box 12.2. There is significant overlap between the eating disorders but physical complications of starvation and refeeding are most likely in anorexia nervosa whereas complications arising from purging are likely to occur in both anorexia nervosa and bulimia nervosa. Physical complications are more likely in children and prepubertal starvation can delay menarche and permanently minimise breast development.

Risk factors

The understanding of the aetiology of eating disorders is far from complete but some risk factors have been identified (Box 12.3).

Demographic characteristics

Both anorexia nervosa and bulimia nervosa occur overwhelmingly in women. The ratio of women to men is 9 : 1 for anorexia nervosa. The literature on bulimia nervosa in men is scanty but records from a specialist eating disorder clinic show that, among more than 500 cases, where over 75% had bulimia nervosa, only 9 cases (less than 2%) were men (Hubert Lacey, personal communication). This figure may even be inflated by referral bias, in that men are more often referred to specialist clinics because of their rarity. Closer examination of men apparently suffering from bulimia nervosa sometimes reveals that they are, in fact, suffering from the bulimic variant of anorexia nervosa.

Anorexia nervosa is associated predominantly with middle or upper social class backgrounds (Garner & Garfinkel, 1982) whereas bulimia nervosa arises equally in all social classes (Lacey, 1991). Bulimic women are less likely to be black or Asian, or to be married (Lacey & Dolan, 1988). Although the average ages of development of anorexia nervosa and bulimia nervosa are similar, the ages at which individuals tend to present differ. On average, women with bulimia nervosa present at around 25 years of age, while those with anorexia present at around 16 years.

Body system	Starvation	Purging	Re-feeding
Cardio-vascular	Bradycardia Hypotension	Cardiac arrhythmias Cardiac failure ECG abnormalities Sudden death	Cardiac failure
Gastro-intestinal	Delayed gastric emptying (sensation of bloating)	Erosion of dental enamel Enlarged salivary glands Severe vomiting Oesophageal ulcers Altered bowel habit Malabsorption Fatty liver	Acute dilatation of the stomach Stomach rupture Duodenal dilatation Acute pancreatitis
Nervous		Epileptic seizures Tetany	
Renal	Reduced glomerular filtration Poor concentrating capacity Pitting oedema	Electrolyte abnormalities Hyperphosphataemia Hypomagnesaemia Refractory hypocalcaemia Renal calculi	Hypophosphataemia Peripheral oedema
Blood	Mild anaemia Thrombcytopenia Pancytopenia		
Skeletal	Short stature Retarded bony maturation Osteoporosis Pathological fractures	Muscle weakness	
Endocrine	Menstrual abnormalities Ovarian changes Increased cortisol Increased growth hormone Diabetes insipidus Reduced thyroxine		
Metabolic	Lowered metabolic rate Poor temperature regulation		
Other	Poor skin and hair Lanugo	Calluses on backs of hands	

Box 12.2 *Physical consequences of eating disorders.*

Demographic characteristics
  Female sex
  Middle and upper class
  Younger age group
  Less common in ethnic minorities
  Less likely to be married

Occupation
  Models
  Dancers
  Actresses
  Athletes

Introverted perfectionist personality type

A history of strict dieting

Positive family history

Emotional problems in the family

Box 12.3 *Risk factors for eating disorders.*

Personality

There is no universal personality type that characterises sufferers of anorexia nervosa but they are often described as introverted, compliant and perfectionist. Women with bulimia nervosa tend to be more extroverted. Some normal-weight bulimic women display impulsive behaviours and may have features of the 'borderline' personality disorder (Box 12.4) (Lacey & Evans, 1986).

Drug abuse

Alcohol abuse

Deliberate self-harm:
  Repeated overdosing
  Self-cutting
  Self-burning

Stealing

Sexual disinhibition

Box 12.4 *Behaviours encountered in the minority of bulimic women who have a multi-impulsive or borderline personality disorder.*

Social and cultural influences

Women working in professions which require a certain body weight such as dancers, models, actresses and athletes are more at risk of developing an eating disorder (Garner *et al.*, 1980; Joseph, Wood & Goldberg, 1982). However, the increased pressure that all women face in society through recent and continuing emphasis on thinness in the fashion world and the media should not be underestimated.

Latterly, the fashionable body shape has reached new heights of impossibility by asking women to be excessively thin but at the same time to have breasts. It is noteworthy that although slimness in women is widely considered an attractive feature by women, there is no evidence that men in general share this opinion (Garner *et al.*, 1980).

Women are pulled in all directions. They are required to be sexual beings. At the same time they have been encouraged to deny the sexual basis of their natural shape of full breasts and hips by responding to pressure to be thin and tubular rather than curvaceous. In parallel to this, they must progress and achieve in the work environment while managing the responsibilities of motherhood.

There have been tremendous changes in western society over the last century. Women's roles have changed and multiplied. Greater sexual freedom has been encouraged and fuelled by the easy availability of contraception, in particular the development of the oral contraceptive pill which is a direct way for women to have control over their bodies. These changes have produced a dilemma for women about whether to suppress or promote their sexuality. Because of the links between body shape and sexuality some women seem to have translated this dilemma into a confusion over weight and eating, and then to manifesting eating disorders.

Dieting

Dieting is, of course, commonplace in the western world. Nielsen's 1978 study showed that 45% of all households in America contained someone who dieted in that year. Such dieting has spread to quite young children and adolescents (Crowther, Post & Zaynor, 1985; Killen *et al.*, 1986). While the majority of teenage dieters eventually give up their restraint, however, very strict dieting is widely accepted as a risk factor for the subsequent development of either eating disorder.

Binge-eating, whether in anorexia nervosa or bulimia nervosa, always follows an extended period of severe dieting (Gandour, 1984). The inability to maintain a low carbohydrate diet leads to craving and binge-eating and then to purging and further restriction and thus the destructive 'binge–purge cycle' (Lacey, Coker & Birtchnell, 1986).

Genetic predisposition

Anorexia nervosa can run in families. Twin studies, and the increased incidence of affective disorders in the families of women with either anorexia nervosa or bulimia, support the hypothesis of a genetic component (Garner & Garfinkel, 1982; Gershon *et al.*, 1984) but the precise mechanism remains unclear.

A few researchers have emphasised the familial links with affective disorders and the response of some sufferers to antidepressants. They have argued that disordered eating, particularly bulimia nervosa, is a variant of depression (Swift, Andrews & Barklage, 1986), but most workers in the field regard eating disorders as distinct entities.

Family dynamics

Studies of the families of anorexic women have pointed to problems such as alcohol dependence in parents, excessive preoccupation with feeding and physical fitness, and a tendency to respond to stress by avoidance and denial. These families have also been described as rigid, overprotective, and involving the patient in parental conflict. A number of studies have concluded that there is generally more psychopathology in the families of normal weight bulimic women and of bulimic anorectic women than there is in the families of those with abstaining anorexia.

Bulimic women often report poor relationships with their parents. The parents have often sought professional help for their own emotional problems. The most common diagnosis for mothers of women with bulimia nervosa is depression whilst that for fathers is alcohol abuse. For example, a bulimic daughter may describe that prior to her illness, during her adolescent years, she was being used as an 'unofficial therapist' by her mother who was lonely and estranged from her husband.

In recent years much attention has been paid to possible links between childhood sexual abuse and psychological morbidity in later life. Research in this area is fraught with difficulties because of varying definitions of sexual abuse and degrees of severity as well as confounding factors of poor parenting generally. The general consensus is that sexual abuse produces psychological morbidity in some individuals but that it may present in a variety of ways including depression, alcohol and drug abuse. It is no surprise that, when women with eating disorders are questioned, a proportion disclose previous sexual abuse. There is little evidence that this association is any stronger than in any other psychiatric disorder. The exception to this is women who have multi-impulsive bulimia nervosa. In this case there is a higher than expected association with childhood sexual abuse either within the family or by others.

Preventing eating disorders

Primary prevention

Any preventive intervention should ideally meet certain standards. The advantages of prevention should be clear in terms of reducing the costs of caring for the morbidity and disability produced by the disorder. The other half of the equation is the cost of the prevention strategy itself. Prevention also needs to be acceptable and appropriate, both politically and morally. Some elements of the primary prevention of eating disorders may not be readily accepted. It is easy to see the benefit of a preventive vaccination programme but suggesting that someone's beliefs about or attitudes to their body or behaviour are wrong leads into the potentially much more contentious area of the social control of deviant behaviour.

With this in mind, it should also be clear who should carry out the prevention, as it is important to distinguish between medical and societal roles. Most of these issues have not as yet been resolved. However, there are a number of ways in which primary care professionals could be involved in primary prevention.

The media

The work of Garner and Garfinkel et al. (1980) illustrates the pressure women face, using data about Playboy centrefolds and Miss America Pageant contestants over a 20-year period. They showed a significant trend toward a thinner, more tubular standard shape in the context of increasing population weight norms. They also noted a coincident increase in the number of diet related articles in popular women's magazines.

Currently, in western society women believe themselves to be more attractive to men if they are slender (Furnham & Radley, 1989; Freeman, 1987; Franz & Herzog, 1987). Despite changes in the representation of women in all popular media, however, there is no evidence to support the notion that any particular body shape or size is more appealing to men in general than any other (Smith, Waldorf & Trembath, 1990).

Some, including Vandereycken and Meermann (1984) contend that primary prevention of eating disorders is impossible because of the difficulty of changing such widely and firmly held beliefs in society. They emphasise the improbability of industry forfeiting large profits from slimming aids for altruistic reasons. Others, however, are more optimistic, pointing out that if views have changed in one direction in a relatively short period it ought to be possible to influence them in the reverse direction too (Yager, 1985).

There has been an increase in the number of articles in women's magazines and on television highlighting the incidence of eating disorders, the distress involved and how to seek help. Public awareness is slowly being raised. However, concern has been expressed that such programmes may actually encourage eating disorders (Garner, 1985; Chiodo & Latimer, 1983; Fairburn & Cooper, 1982). There is some evidence that bulimic patients learn their unhealthy weight control methods from magazines or television programmes. Withholding knowledge is unlikely to be effective, however, and attempts to do so may be self-defeating.

To counteract these concerns, it is important that health professionals take any opportunities they have to collaborate actively with journalists and public figures in the field of eating disorders, not just to warn about the perils of weight manipulation but to present more positive images of women and more constructive role models than those which focus entirely on weight and shape. Film and fashion industries may be hard to penetrate, but women's magazines are more accessible as an easy, cost-effective way of reaching large numbers of women.

Primary prevention also involves education of those at risk of eating disorders so they are better able to interpret media messages. This can take place in a number of ways.

Educating parents in primary care

Opportunities for educating parents about normal eating patterns may arise in child health surveillance sessions, at the pre-school stage. One major risk for the development of an eating disorder is childhood obesity. This should be tackled whenever possible. There is some evidence that breast-feeding has advantages over bottle-feeding in terms of preventing obesity in childhood and later life. Except for the extremely obese child, it is wiser not to suggest weight loss but to look at how to slow down the weight gain so as to make use of their growth to return to normal limits of weight-for-height. Appropriate levels of exercise should be encouraged.

Taking the focus off food, removing the arguments and battles around meal times, as well as direct advice and intervention over intake are likely to be helpful. Helping parents to find alternative ways to reward their children and to find other representations of love than food are important. General practitioners and health visitors might encourage parents to examine their own eating patterns and attitudes to weight and shape to help them become better role models for their children in the development of normal eating routines. Parents can be encouraged to be sensitive towards the emotional difficulties their children face, especially at vulnerable periods such as early adolescence.

Schools

Primary care professionals could contribute to local parent–teacher meetings addressing aspects of child health and behaviour, including information about eating disorders. A general practitioner might be able to build on personal links with the local school doctors and nurses. High school and college education programmes have been established in other countries to target young adolescents (Shisslak, Crago & Neal, 1990; Moreno & Thelen, 1993; Killen *et al.*, 1993). Students have shown an increase in knowledge after such programmes and even changes in attitudes, but unfortunately this may not equate to changes in behaviour and a reduction in eating disorders.

Some, including Crisp (1986) and Noordenbos (1994), consider that focusing specifically on eating disorders in such programmes may be too specific. Adolescents may be seen as ill-equipped to deal with emotional conflict and the greater stresses of life today. Tackling self-esteem, self-confidence, assertiveness and problem-solving skills generally may promote development of better coping strategies in all areas of life, not just eating.

Slimming clubs

In the community it is important to remember organisations such as *Weight Watchers*, other diet organisations, and health and fitness centres. These are now major industries. Some organisations are becoming more aware of the risks of excessive dieting or exercise. Supervisors can disseminate more appropriate approaches to weight loss and recognise when individuals are driving themselves too far. The primary health care team should be aware of such possibilities in any of their patients who are attending slimming clubs.

The research evidence, especially from the schools studies above, suggests that labour intensive educational programmes directed at the whole community do not work very well. It might be better to target high-risk groups, for example families at risk of eating disorders and people in certain occupations (Box 12.5). Members of the primary health care team are often well placed to offer education to such groups.

Secondary prevention

Chronicity of illness is usually associated with a poor outcome, while early acceptance of treatment is more hopeful prognostically. Established anorexia nervosa is easier to recognise than bulimia. Milder levels of either disorder can be very difficult to identify because the symptoms and signs are very subtle. Functioning at work is often not adversely affected in eating-disordered women who are frequently high achievers and perfectionists. Social functioning may be affected earlier. High levels of denial and secrecy due to a sense of personal shame also add to the difficulties of recognition.

Families with emotional problems

History of eating disorder in the family

Previous history of weight disorder

Obese patients

Seriously underweight patients

Those with frequent dieting or weight fluctuation

Occupational risk groups
   Athletes, gymnasts
   Dancers
   Models, actresses

Girls' boarding schools

Box 12.5 *Risk groups for targeted education.*

Opportunistic screening and education

The general practitioner has frequent opportunities to educate young women about eating disorders and to look for eating disorders among surgery attenders. Appointments for family planning and cervical smears may be used to ask questions about possible eating disorder. Consultations for children, particularly in child health surveillance sessions, often give an opportunity to gauge how relaxed a mother is about her own eating, weight and shape.

Particular attention should be paid to young women who attend surgery repeatedly for non-specific problems including abdominal pain, menstrual problems or gynaecological symptoms. Where weight loss is not directly obvious, suitable introductory questions could include:

- How much exercise do you do?
- Are you happy with your weight?
- Do you diet?
- Do you feel in control of your eating?
- Do you ever find you can't stop eating when you want to?
- Do you ever fast for whole days at a time?

It may then be possible to ask more direct questions about binge-eating, vomiting, laxative use and menstrual abnormalities. Particular attention should be paid to those in the occupational risk groups mentioned above. Given the established associations with drug and alcohol abuse and with any form of repeated deliberate self-harm, eating must be assessed in such presentations. Although the majority of sufferers are women, men from similar high-risk groups can develop eating disorders too.

If there is the possibility of an eating disorder, it is essential to look for any of the aetiological factors described. Bearing in mind (but not necessarily declaring) the possibility that food is being used by the individual in an attempt to cope with emotions or conflict, it is good practice to try to explore any emotional difficulties in the individual or family. This may take patience and several visits because even if they are aware of an eating problem, they may be quite unaware of its roots.

Suggested strategies for the prevention of eating disorders in primary care are summarised in Box 12.6.

Educate patients individually in surgery
  Young women
  High-risk occupations

Make surgery staff more aware of the problem

Health education talks aimed at
  Parents
  School children

Tackle childhood obesity

Opportunistic screening
  Smear appointments
  Family planning checks
  Child health surveillance checks
  New registration checks for young women patients
  High-risk occupations

Question requests for prescriptions of
  Laxatives
  Diuretics
  Appetite suppressants

Give information about self-help organisations:
  In waiting room
  To individuals

Use purchaser role to improve treatment services

Box 12.6 *Preventive strategies in primary care.*

Intervention in primary care

Having recognised the presence of an eating disorder and engaged the patient, treatment must be offered in line with available re sources. Helping the patient to recognise her problem and the need for help are essential to engage her in the process of treatment. Entering treatment as early as possible is a strong indicator for good outcome. Individuals with uncomplicated bulimia nervosa and milder cases of anorexia nervosa can be treated in primary care either by a general practitioner or a trained counsellor.

Efforts at this stage may prevent the patient progressing to a more entrenched position which is then harder to tackle and which carries greater risks of physical, social and psychological complications. Exposing or witnessing a crisis, however, may be the only way an individual can be helped to recognise the extent of their difficulties.

Availability of specialist treatment

Greater education and awareness of eating disorders and early recognition are wasted if treatment is not then available. A recent survey by a working group of the Royal College of Psychiatrists has highlighted the lack of treatment services nationally. A survey undertaken in 1991 identified only 21 units in the United Kingdom which could be classed as specialist units for the treatment of eating disorders. Of these, only 11 had inpatient facilities. In the context of the high prevalence of eating disorders, the report suggested that supra-regional specialist units alone are inadequate. Every region should ideally provide treatment with both inpatient and outpatient facilities for patients living within that region. Primary care professionals need to be aware of the facilities in their own region. Where there are no district or even regional services the general practitioner, in collaboration with voluntary bodies, has an important role to play in influencing purchasing authorities to ensure the availability of specialist help.

It is not the remit of this chapter to detail the specific steps of the various treatment approaches for eating disorders. Different treatments are available, depending on the level of pathology but the reader should look elsewhere (e.g. Crisp and McClelland, 1994; Freeman, 1991) for further information on treatment.

Self-help groups

One national network in the United Kingdom, the Eating Disorders Association, is particularly useful for sufferers, families and involved health professionals (see Appendix). However, they ought to be considered as complementary rather than as an alternative to treatment from the statutory health services. The primary health care team should be aware that some self-help groups can lead to competitive dieting, which has implications for the training of the leaders of such groups.

Conclusion

Primary health care professionals, particularly health visitors and general practitioners, are well placed to play a significant role in the prevention of eating disorders. Psychiatrists often do not see patients until their problem has become well established and difficult to treat. Established anorexia nervosa in particular carries a significant risk of death at a young age. Members of the primary health care team need to be aware of the risk factors for eating disorders, the early clues, and strategies for intervention if they are to prevent what can be extremely serious illnesses in their young women patients.

Appendix

Eating Disorders Association, Sackville Place, 44 Magdalen Street, Norwich, Norfolk NR3 1JU, UK.

References

American Psychiatric Association (APA) (1994). *Diagnostic and Statistical Manual of Mental Disorders*. 4th edn. Washington DC: APA.

Bushnell, J.A., Wells, J.E., Hornblow, A.R., Oakley-Browne, M.A. and Joyce, P. (1990). Prevalence of three bulima syndromes in the general population. *Psychological Medicine*, **20**, 671–680.

Childress, A.C., Brewerton, T.D., Hodges, E.L. & Jarrell, M.P. (1993). The Kid's Eating Disorder Survey (KEDS): a study of middle school students. *Journal of the American Academy of Child and Adolescent Psychiatry*, **32**, 843–50.

Chiodo, J. & Latimer, P.R. (1983) Vomiting as a learned weight-control technique in bulimia. *Journal of Behavior Therapy and Experimental Psychiatry*, **14**, 131–35.

Crisp, A.H. (1986). The integration of 'self-help' and 'help' in the prevention of anorexia nervosa. *British Review of Anorexia Nervosa and Bulimia*, **1**, 27–39.

Crisp, A.H. & McClelland, L. (1994). *Anorexia Nervosa: The St George's Approach*. Department of Mental Health Sciences, St George's Hospital Medical School, London SW17 0RE, UK.

Crowther, J.H., Post, G. & Zaynor, L. (1985). The prevalence of bulimia and binge eating in adolescent girls. *International Journal of Eating Disorders*, **4**, 15–29.

Fairburn, C.G. & Beglin S.J. (1990). Studies of the epidemiology of bulimia nervosa. *American Journal of Psychiatry*, **147**, 401–8.

Fairburn, C. & Cooper, P. (1982). Self-induced vomiting and bulimia: an undetected problem. *British Medical Journal*, **284**, 1153–5.

Franz, S.L. & Herzog, M.E. (1987). Judging physical attractiveness: what body aspects do we use? *Personality and Social Psychology Bulletin*, **13**, 19–33.

Freeman, C.P. (1991). Recent advances in the treatment of bulimia nervosa. *Journal of Psychosomatic Research*, **35**, Suppl. 1.

Freeman, H.R. (1987). Structure and content of gender stereotypes: effects of somatic appearance and trait formation. *Psychology of Women Quarterly*, **11**, 59–68.

Furnham, A.F. & Radley, S. (1989). Sex differences in the perception of male and female body shapes. *Personality and Individual Differences*, **10**, 653–62.

Gandour, M.J. (1984). Bulimia: clinical description, assessment, etiology and treatment. *International Journal of Eating Disorders*, **3**, 3–38.

Garner, D.M. (1985). Iatrogenesis in anorexia nervosa and bulimia nervosa. *International Journal of Eating Disorders*, **4**, 701–26.

Garner, D.M., Garfinkel, P.E., Schwartz, D. & Thompson, M. (1980). Cultural expectations of thinness in women. *Psychological Reports*, **47**, 483–91.

Garner, D.M. & Garfinkel, P.E. (1982). *Anorexia nervosa: A Multidimensional Perspective*. New York: Brunner Mazel.

Gershon, E.S., Schreiber, J.L., Hamovit, J.R., Dibble, E.D., Kaye, W., Nurnburger, J.L., Anderson, A.E. & Elbert, M. (1984). Clinical findings in patients with anorexia nervosa and affective illness in their relatives. *American Journal of Psychiatry*, **141**, 1419–22.

Hoek, H.K. (1991). The incidence and prevalence of anorexia nervosa and bulimia nervosa in primary care. *Psychological Medicine*, **21**, 455–60.

Joseph, A., Wood, I.K. & Goldberg, S.C. (1982). Determining populations at risk for developing anorexia nervosa based on choice of college major. *Psychiatry Research*, **7**, 53–8.

Killen, J.D., Taylor, C.B., Telch, M.J., Saylor, K.E., Maron, D.J. & Robinson, T.N. (1986). Self-induced vomiting and laxative and diuretic use among teenagers: precursors of the binge–purge syndrome? *Journal of the American Medical Association*, **255**, 1447–9.

Killen, J.D., Taylor, C.B., Hammer, L.D., Litt, I., Wilson, D.M., Rich, Hayward, C., Simmonds, B., Kraemer, H. & Varady, A. (1993). An attempt to modify unhealthful eating attitudes and weight regulation practices of young adolescent girls. *International Journal of Eating Disorders*, **13**, 369–84.

King, M.B. (1989). Eating disorders in a general population: prevalence, characteristics and follow-up at 12–18 months. *Psychological Medicine,* Suppl 14.

Lacey, J.H., Coker, S. & Birtchnell, S.A. (1986). Bulimia: factors associated with its aetiology and maintenance. *International Journal of Eating Disorders,* **2**, 59–66.

Lacey, J.H. (1991). The treatment demand for bulimia: a catchment area report of referral rates and demography. *Psychiatric Bulletin* **16**, 203–5.

Lacey, J.H. & Evans, C.D.H. (1986). The impulsivist: a multi-impulsive personality disorder. *British Journal of Addiction,* **81**, 715–23.

Lacey, J.H. & Dolan, B. (1988). Bulimia in British blacks and Asians: a catchment area study. *British Journal of Psychiatry,* **52**, 73–9.

Moreno, A.B. & Thelan M.H. (1993). A preliminary prevention program for eating disorders in a junior high school population. *Journal of Youth and Adolescence,* **22**, 109–24.

Noordenbos, G. (1994). Problems and possibilities of the prevention of eating disorders. *European Eating Disorders Review,* **2**, 126–42.

Office of Population Censuses and Surveys (OPCS) (1994). *The Dietary and Nutritional Survey of British Adults.* London: HMSO.

Rooney, B., McClelland L., Crisp, A.H. & Sedgewick, P. (1995). The incidence and prevalence of anorexia nervosa in three suburban health districts in South West London, UK. *International Journal of Eating Disorders* (in press).

Shisslak, C.M., Crago, M. & Neal, M.E. (1990). Primary prevention of eating disorders. *American Journal of Health Promotion,* **5**, 100–6.

Smith, J.E., Waldorf, V.A. & Trembath, D.L. (1990). 'Single white male looking for thin very attractive . . .'. *Sex Roles,* **23**, 67–85.

Swift, W.J., Andrews, D. & Barklage, N.E. (1986). The relationship between affective disorder and eating disorder: a review of the literature. *American Journal of Psychiatry,* **143**, 290–9.

Vandereycken, W. & Meermann, R. (1984). Anorexia nervosa: is prevention possible? *International Journal of Psychiatry in Medicine,* **14**, 191–205.

World Health Organisation (1992). *International Statistical Classification of Diseases and Related Health Problems* (ICD-10). Geneva: WHO.

Yager, J. (1985). Afterword. In *Psychiatry Update: Annual Review,* Hales R. and Frances, A. eds., **4**, 481–502. Washington, DC: American Psychiatric Association.

[13] The prevention of alcohol and drug misuse

Hugh Williams and Hamid Ghodse

Introduction

Although the misuse of alcohol and of other substances have many features in common and often coexist in the same patient, for the convenience of the reader this chapter is divided into separate sections on alcohol and drug misuse respectively.

Alcohol related problems

Opportunities for prevention in primary health care

A report by the Royal College of General Practitioners (1986) suggested that any general practitioner will have on his list about 55 patients who are drinking at levels exposing them to a high risk of harm and a further 200 at levels with an intermediate risk of harm. General practitioners and other primary health care professionals are well placed to identify patterns of hazardous drinking early and to intervene in order to arrest progression and minimise damage.

In Britain, 70% of the practice population consult their general practitioner in any one year, offering obvious possibilities for opportunistic screening (Pollak, 1989). Other advantages of the primary care setting are the ease of accessibility, the long-term relationship which often exists between general practitioner and patient, the lack of labelling and stigma which may be associated with specialist alcohol services, and the opportunity for involvement of other members of the patient's family (Babor, Ritson & Hodgson, 1986).

Despite these advantages, many at-risk drinkers go unnoticed and research suggests that many general practitioners are reluctant to become involved with alcohol problems (Thom & Tellez, 1986). Reasons include a perceived difficulty in asking about drinking, reluctance to confront the patient, uncertainty regarding the diagnosis and a lack of adequate training. Many general practitioners express pessimism about the value of any intervention undertaken.

However there is now encouraging research evidence to suggest that harmful drinking can be reduced by intervention in primary care.

Levels of risk

The Royal Colleges of General Practitioners (1986), Psychiatrists (1986) and Physicians (1987) have produced useful and widely accepted guidelines relating the risk of damage to health to the average weekly consumption of alcohol (Box 13.1). These levels are convenient divisions of a continuum of increasing risk. The *Health of the Nation* document has set as a national target a reduction in the proportion of men drinking more than 21 units of alcohol per week from 28% in 1990 to 18% by the year 2005 and women drinking more than 14 units from 11% to 7% (Department of Health, 1991*b*).

A unit of alcohol (8 g of absolute alcohol), corresponds to a half-pint of ordinary strength beer or cider, a standard glass of wine, or a pub measure of spirits. Some strong beers or lagers can be two to three times the strength of ordinary strength beers.

Recent reports have suggested a possible protective effect of consuming one to three units of alcohol per day against coronary heart disease. This does not imply, however, that non-drinkers should be encouraged to drink, or that drinkers should increase the frequency of their drinking. Further controlled longitudinal studies are needed before such a pro-drinking policy could be adopted (Douds & Maxwell, 1994). At present such an attitude only serves to confuse the public.

Screening in general practice

Screening has been described as a preliminary diagnostic procedure directed at people who appear not to have a condition in order to identify those who probably have the condition (Babor *et al.*, 1992). Screening may help primary health care professionals to:

- identify problems before serious dependence has occurred;
- motivate patients to change their drinking behaviour.

	Men	Women
Low risk	less than 21	less than 14
Intermediate	21 to 50	15 to 35
High risk	greater than 50	greater than 35

Box 13.1 *Categories of risk – units of alcohol per week.*

Methods commonly employed for alcohol screening are interview or questionnaire techniques, laboratory investigations (biological markers), and recognition of clinical signs. A detailed review of screening procedures is provided by Babor *et al*. (1986).

Alcohol screening questionnaires

One of the best known and most widely used is the CAGE (Mayfield, McLeod & Hall, 1974). The CAGE consists of four questions, of which a positive reply to two suggests problem drinking:

- Have you ever felt you should Cut down on your drinking?
- Have people ever Annoyed you by criticising your drinking?
- Have you ever felt bad or Guilty about your drinking?
- Have you ever had a drink first thing in the morning to steady your nerves or to get rid of a hangover (Eye-opener)?

In a community sample, the CAGE identified approximately half the known problem drinkers (Saunders & Kershaw, 1980).

The Health Survey Questionnaire (HSQ) (Wallace & Haines, 1985) is a self-administered questionnaire which employs a quantity (of alcohol) times frequency (of drinking) scale to assess consumption and has been shown to be acceptable and effective in general practice (Cutler, Wallace & Haines, 1988). In general, screening questionnaires or interview techniques are quick, easy to administer, and reasonably accurate. However, they are subjective and clinicians may prefer to screen using biological markers.

Laboratory investigations

Gamma-gutamyl transferase (GGT) is a liver enzyme that is particularly sensitive to early liver involvement. Raised serum levels may occur after only a few weeks of heavy drinking and begin to return towards normal after a short period of abstinence. Increased enzyme activity does occur with other non-alcoholic liver conditions and with certain medications (e.g. barbiturates, anticonvulsants). Among hospitalised patients, increased levels of GGT have been reported in up to 60% of drinkers consuming over 50 units of alcohol per week (Lloyd, Chick & Crombie, 1982). A raised blood count mean corpuscular volume (MCV) is found in approximately one-third of heavy drinkers. Unfortunately, however, laboratory tests alone are not suitable for screening in general practice. Hoeksema & de Bock (1993) point out that the positive predictive value of GGT is only 25% in a general practice population with a 10% prevalence of drinking problems. Investigations can be useful, however, in confronting the patient with the effects of alcohol on their physical health, and serial estimations of GGT are useful in monitoring the patient's progress.

Clinical signs

Heavy drinking can have adverse effects on nearly every organ and system in the human body. The presence of certain clinical signs such as tremor, sweating and hepatomegaly, or a history of repeated trauma, have been used in screening for alcohol excess. However, as clinical signs often appear late they are of limited value in the early recognition of hazardous drinking.

Some screening procedures incorporate a combination of methods, in order to improve detection rates. The AUDIT (the Alcohol Use Disorders Identification Test) (Babor *et al.*, 1992) is a screening instrument developed by the World Health Organisation, designed specifically for use in primary care settings and tested in six countries. It consists of two parts: a ten-item questionnaire (the core AUDIT – Box 13.2) and a clinical screening instrument which includes a trauma history, clinical examination, and a GGT estimation. In a study of subjects attending primary health care facilities, 92% of hazardous drinkers had an AUDIT score of 8 or more. The false-positive rate was 6% (Saunders *et al.*, 1993). The AUDIT therefore appears to be particularly suitable for use in the primary care setting.

Assessment of alcohol consumption – where to start?

We suggest that all adult patients be asked about, and have their usual level of alcohol consumption recorded. If general practitioners feel uncomfortable about directly asking patients about their drinking habits, questions can be included in a more general enquiry about healthy life style including smoking, diet, exercise and leisure. This approach may also help the patient view alcohol consumption within a broader context of healthy living and health promotion.

A brief method of recording the patient's alcohol consumption is to ask:

- On how many days of the week do you normally drink?
- On a day when you drink how many drinks would you normally have?

By multiplying the two answers the patient's weekly consumption in units of alcohol is obtained and can be classified into low, intermediate or high risk categories.

For patients drinking at high risk (greater than 50 units per week for men and greater than 35 units for women) a more detailed assessment will need to be made. This involves a brief drinking history, a physical examination and laboratory investigations. In

Please circle the answer that is correct for you

1. **How often do you have a drink containing alcohol?**

   Never   Monthly or less   Two to 4 times a month   Two to three times a week   Four or more times a week

2. **How many drinks containing alcohol do you have on a typical day when you are drinking?**

   1 or 2   3 or 4   5 or 6   7 to 9   10 or more

3. **How often do you have six or more drinks on one occasion?**

   Never   Less than monthly   Monthly   Weekly   Daily or almost daily

4. **How often during the last year have you found that you were not able to stop drinking once you had started?**

   Never   Less than monthly   Monthly   Weekly   Daily or almost daily

5. **How often during the last year have you failed to do what was normally expected from you because of drinking?**

   Never   Less than monthly   Monthly   Weekly   Daily or almost daily

6. **How often during the last year have you needed a first drink in the morning to get yourself going after a heavy drinking session?**

   Never   Less than monthly   Monthly   Weekly   Daily or almost daily

7. **How often during the last year have you had a feeling of guilt or remorse after drinking?**

   Never   Less than monthly   Monthly   Weekly   Daily or almost daily

8. **How often during the last year have you been unable to remember what happened the night before because you had been drinking?**

   Never   Less than monthly   Monthly   Weekly   Daily or almost daily

9. **Have you or someone else been injured as a result of your drinking?**

   No   Yes, but not in the last year   Yes, during the last year

10. **Has a relative or friend, or a doctor or other health worker been concerned about your drinking or suggest you cut down?**

    No   Yes, but no in the last year   Yes, but during the last year

Procedure for scoring

Questions 1–8 are scored 0, 1, 2, 3 or 4.
Questions 9 and 10 are scored, 0, 2 or 4 only.
The response coding is as follows:

	0	1	2	3	4
Q. 1	Never	Monthly or less	Two to four times a month	Two to three times a week	Four or more times a week
Q. 2	1 or 2	3 or 4	5 or 6	7 to 9	10 or more
Q. 3–8	Never	Less than monthly	Monthly	Weekly	Daily or almost daily
Q. 9–10	No		Yes, but not in the last year		Yes, during the last year

The minimum score (for non-drinkers) is 0 and the maximum possible score is 40.
A score of 8 or more indicates a strong likelihood of hazardous or harmful alcohol consumption.

Source: Babor, T. F. *et al.* Audit, The Alcohol Use Disorders Identification Test; World Health Organisation (WHO) 1989.

Box 13.2 *The alcohol use disorders identification test (AUDIT).*

British general practice, where the average time per consultation is eight to nine minutes, it may be useful to carry out this assessment over a number of visits. The essential components are as follows:

- Start by enquiring about drinking during the past week, recording units of alcohol per day and the drinking pattern, whether daily or episodic binges.
- Identify events or situations that are particularly associated with heavy drinking.
- Ask about withdrawal symptoms (tremor, sweating, morning nausea, anorexia, irritability). More serious symptoms include convulsions or delirium tremens.
- Look for other evidence of alcohol dependency.
- Look for effects on physical and mental health, family life, work, finances and legal problems.
- Ask about periods of abstinence or times when the patient was able to reduce their drinking. How was this achieved and what triggers were associated with relapse?
- Check for alcohol on the breath, tremor, sweating, spider naevi and liver enlargement or tenderness.
- Order a full blood count, GGT and other liver function tests (aspartate transaminase (AST), alanine transaminase (ALT) and bilirubin).

Preventive interventions in primary care

Brief interventions which can be carried out effectively by primary care staff are now described. These are aimed at preventing alcohol problems and may not be suitable for patients who are already severely dependent or damaged by their drinking.

Low-risk category

For patients in the low-risk group, the majority of attenders, the risk of alcohol related harm is minimum. However, limits can never be absolute and there are exceptional circumstances. Patients consuming all their 'weekly allowance' of units on one or two separate occasions would not be regarded as low-risk drinkers. Similarly, driving with any amount of alcohol can be hazardous. Certain patients, by virtue of physical illness or mental illness, and those taking certain medications, may be particularly vulnerable to alcohol. Pregnant women should be advised to limit their intake to one to two units once or twice a week.

The consumption should be recorded in the patient's notes. This can be used as a baseline against which any future escalation can be compared.

Intermediate-risk category

Patients within this category are drinking at an increasingly hazardous level. For these patients Anderson, Wallace and Jones (1988) have suggested the following strategy:

- Ask the patient if they feel that their drinking is affecting their life.
- Fill in a drinking diary with the patient covering the previous week's drinking (Box 13.3).
- Point out where the patient's consumption lies compared to the general population (Box 13.4).
- Discuss the risks associated with continued drinking at this level and outline the benefits of reduction.
- Give firm advice to reduce drinking to safe limits.
- Supply appropriate educational material.
- Make a record of consumption in the notes and review in one to two months.

High-risk category

Patients who are regularly drinking at this level are highly likely to be damaging their health. Having completed a more detailed assessment as above the general practitioner should now discuss the findings, including the results of any investigations. This should be done in an open, supportive and non-judgemental manner. It is important that the patient has a clear and unambiguous understanding of their drinking and any harm it is causing if they are going to consider reducing their consumption. Attention should be drawn to the excessive level of consumption, in comparison with the rest of the population. Some patients genuinely underestimate their intake or consider their drinking to be normal because their friends drink corresponding amounts.

It is important at this point to find out whether the patient has contemplated changing his drinking behaviour or not. Some will need help in moving from indifference to thinking about change. Any alcohol-related problems the patient is experiencing should be highlighted and their relationship with alcohol explained. In a general practice study Pollak (1989) found that in every case of high-risk drinking alcohol was either responsible for, or associated with, the presenting problem. Frequently the patient may not have previously made the connection. Objective evidence of alcohol-related harm, for example, a raised GGT or other liver function test, reinforces the point.

A drinking diary

Day	How much?	When/where/who with?	What was the effect?	Units	Total
Monday					
Tuesday					
Wednesday					
Thursday					
Friday					
Saturday					
Sunday					
Total for the week					

Box 13.3 *A drinking diary.*

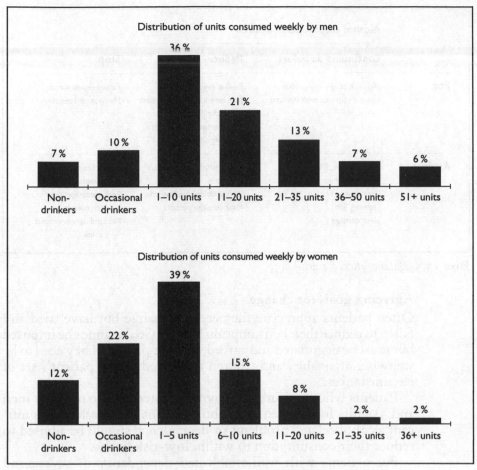

Box 13.4. *Units of alcohol consumed per week in Great Britain. Source: OPCS General Household Survey (1992).*

The nature and significance of any physical withdrawal symptoms experienced should be explained to the patient. Sometimes withdrawal symptoms will have been incorrectly attributed to other psychiatric conditions, for example, anxiety or depression. Drinking balance sheets (Box 13.5) which encourage the patient to weigh up the pros and cons of reducing consumption can be very useful at this stage in motivating the patient to change.

	Alcohol consumption desired		
	Continuing as before	**Reduce**	**Stop**
For	Help me forget my problems	Be like everybody else	Family wants me to
	Enjoy nights out with drinking friends	Not be a kill-joy at business lunches	My liver will recover
		Avoid embarrassment of being different	
Against	Wife says she'll leave me	Didn't work when I tried before	Could I cope with business lunch?
	Upsetting children	Wife wouldn't believe me	Feel uncomfortable with friends
	Lose driving licence	Liver damage persists	No confidence without a drink
	Lose my job		
	Liver damage		

Box 13.5 *Balance sheet for drinking.*

Agreeing goals for change

Often patients appreciate the need for change but have tried and failed to reduce their consumption before. Goals cannot be imposed but must be negotiated and agreed with the patient. They need to be stepwise, attainable, and tailored to the individual patient's set of circumstances.

Patients who are drinking heavily (greater than 50 units for men and 35 units for women) but who have not yet developed significant alcohol-related problems or dependency should be advised to reduce their consumption to within low-risk limits.

For patients with well-established dependency or severe and extensive alcohol related problems, total abstinence should be recommended. Not infrequently, however, these patients may be unwilling to consider abstinence and insist on the opportunity to reduce or 'control' their drinking. Rather than reaching a therapeutic impasse with the patient, it may be more beneficial in the long term to work at reduction only, and to repeat advice about abstinence at a future date, especially if the patient has been unable to achieve or maintain reduction.

A useful place to begin is to get the patient to take responsibility for monitoring their own drinking by keeping a drinking diary (Box 13.3) for a few weeks. The diary can help monitor the patient's progress and identify situations or triggers associated with heavy drinking, such as certain times of the day, social situations, particular company or anxious feelings. The patient can be helped to identify and possibly avoid these situations or to explore alternative methods of handling them (Marlatt & George, 1984). For example, a man who regularly finds he drinks excessively with work colleagues after a particularly tense day at work might be encouraged to return home directly or to find other ways of relieving tension, for instance through physical exercise. A helpful list of 'useful tips' designed to help patients reduce their consumption is given in Box 13.6. Involvement of the spouse or another family member is especially important. Some will have suffered as a result of the patient's excessive drinking and may need support in their own right (Ghodse, 1982). Others may encourage the patient in their attempt to reduce consumption, but note that often both members of a couple drink too much.

Follow-up and review

High-risk drinkers should be regularly followed up and have their progress monitored. A drinking diary or serial estimations of GGT as previously described can be used for this purpose. Success, however modest, should be praised and further progress encouraged. Failures or relapses should not be criticised nor viewed as a lack of motivation on the part of the patient but treated as a learning opportunity from which future strategies can be planned.

Common elements in brief interventions

In their review of brief interventions for alcohol problems Bien, Miller and Tonigan (1993), identified seven elements commonly included in brief interventions that have been shown to be effective. The first six, summarised by the acronym FRAMES, are as follows:

- *F*eedback of personal risk or impairment;
- emphasis on personal *R*esponsibility for change;
- clear *A*dvice to change;
- a *M*enu of alternative change options;
- therapeutic *E*mpathy as a counselling style;
- enhancement of *S*elf-efficacy.

Finally, the authors comment on the importance of follow-up for maintaining reduced consumption.

Detoxification

In most cases, alcohol detoxification can be achieved outside hospital under supervision by the general practitioner. We suggest:

- The patient should remain off work and at home.
- Family or friends should be involved to support and supervise.
- Regular visits (daily) should be made by the general practitioner or other member of the primary health care team.
- The patient should be advised to have a light healthy diet and encouraged to drink plenty of fluids (e.g. fruit juice).

Take smaller sips

Sip less often and take small sips. Count the number of sips it takes to finish a glass, and then try increasing the number for the next glass or so.

Occupy oneself

Do something else enjoyable while drinking that will help distract attention from the glass, and drink more slowly; for example, eating, listening to music, playing darts, talking and so on.

Change the drink

Changing the type of drink can help break old habits and reduce the amount drunk.

Drink for the taste

Drink more slowly and enjoy the flavour.

Imitate the slow drinker

Identify someone who drinks slowly and become a shadow, not picking up the glass until he does.

Put the glass down between sips

If the glass is held it will be drunk more often. Do something else with your hands instead of lifting the glass to the lips.

Dilute spirits

Top up spirits with non-alcoholic mixers.

Reduce amounts in rounds

Buy your own drinks or one round and then go solo; do not buy yourself a drink when it is your round; order non-alcoholic drinks every so often.

Drink and eat

Eat before drinking or whilst drinking; this slows down the absorption of alcohol and doing something else may also reduce the amount drunk.

Take days of rest

Abstain from alcohol at least one day per week, or preferably two, three or even four days per week. Take up other forms of entertainment or relaxation.

Start later

Start drinking later than usual: for example, go to the pub later.

Learn to refuse drinks

Rehearse ways of refusing drinks. For example, 'No thanks, I'm cutting down', or 'Not tonight, I've got a bad stomach.'

Source: Hazardous Drinking, Pollack, Smith & Wilson

The Medical Council on Alcoholism, 1990

Box 13.6 *Useful tips to reduce alcohol consumption.*

- All patients should receive oral supplements which include vitamin B1 (vitamin B compound tablets, strong). If there has been dietary neglect or if the patient is poorly nourished, intramuscular high-potency vitamin preparations should be given for five days.
- A long-acting benzodiazepine such as chlordiazepoxide should be given to ease withdrawal symptoms. The dosage will depend on the patient's size, sex, and degree of physical dependence but a typical regime for an average male would be chlordiazepoxide 25 mg four times a day reducing to zero over a week. Some general practitioners may prefer to use chlormethiazole. The British National Formulary should be consulted.

Referral

Patients with a history of severe withdrawal complications including convulsions or delirium tremens, those with serious medical or psychiatric conditions, or those with little in the way of social support are not suitable for home detoxification and should be referred to hospital.

Drug misuse and primary care

General practitioners are increasingly likely to come in contact with drug misusers as their number continues to rise. Glanz & Taylor (1986a) found that one in five general practitioners in England and Wales had contact with an opiate user in the previous four weeks. Two-thirds of these sought help with withdrawal or rehabilitation.

A report by the Advisory Council on the Misuse of Drugs (ACMD, 1993) states that general practitioners are the key to early and easy access to care for drug users and recommends increased involvement at a level of intervention appropriate for the practitioner and his practice.

Occasional drug users, those with a short history of use, patients using non-opiate drugs, and those with good social family support may be particularly suitable for interventions within the primary care setting (Richards, 1988; Cohen & Schamroth, 1989). Although primary care staff are often reluctant to become involved with drug addicts, a number of practitioners have reported successful and satisfying outcomes from treating these patients (Waller, 1993; Elander, Porter & Hodson, 1993).

Detecting drug misuse

Certain features of a patient's presentation (Box 13.7) may alert the practitioner to the possibility of substance misuse. A more pro-active approach to detection is possible, by incorporating questions

How the patient presents for help
    With a specific request for drugs of abuse.
    Outside normal GP surgery hours.
    As a temporary resident.

Symptoms and signs
    Puncture marks, scars and pigmentation over injection sites.
    Pupils markedly constricted or dilated.
    Unexplained constipation or diarrhoea.

Behaviour during consultation
    Unaccountably drowsy, elated or restless.
    Loss of former interest in appearance or work.

Social behaviour
    Family disruption.
    Frequent changes of GP.
    History of offences to obtain money.

Source: Drug Misuse and Dependence.
Guidelines on Clinical Management (DoH, 1991).

Box 13.7 *Features which suggest possible drug misuse.*

about the misuse of drugs into general screening questionnaires about lifestyle. This should include not only illicit substances such as heroin, cocaine, and amphetamines, but also legally prescribed drugs including opiate or opiate-related analgesics and benzodiazepines, as well as over-the-counter preparations such as cough mixtures and volatile substances.

Assessment of drug misuse

This involves a drug history, a mental state and physical examination, special investigations, and additional information from other sources. The process can be initiated at the first meeting, but further appointments will usually be necessary to complete a detailed assessment.

In the history, the patient's current and previous pattern of drug use should be established, including routes of administration, tolerance and withdrawal symptoms, previous treatment and reasons for relapse. The doctor should note medical complications including abscesses, hepatitis, overdoses and convulsions; psychological problems including anxiety, depression, drug induced psychosis or suicidal behaviour; social problems such as relationship difficulties and family disruption; and legal problems including prison sentences or outstanding court cases. The doctor should ask about injecting and sharing of needles, and unsafe sexual practices, and assess the extent of the patient's knowledge about Human Immunodeficiency Virus (HIV) and hepatitis transmission.

The examination should include signs of intoxication or withdrawal, new or old needle marks, jaundice, skin infections, hepatomegaly, lymphadenopathy and cardiac murmurs.

Investigations should include a full blood count, liver function tests and tests for hepatitis B and C. HIV testing should be considered but this must only be done after the patient has received adequate pre-test counselling. A urine sample can be taken and a full drug screen requested to confirm the exact nature of drugs recently taken.

Additional information can often be obtained from the patient's previous doctor or from family members where appropriate. In the United Kingdom (UK), information may also be obtained from the local Family Health Service Authority and the Home Office Addicts Index can be contacted to ensure that the patient is not already receiving treatment elsewhere. Any doctor in the UK who comes in contact with a person addicted to certain controlled drugs (mainly opioids and cocaine, listed in the British National Formulary) has a statutory obligation to notify the Home Office in writing within seven days.

Treatment

Most drug misusers want to stop (Glanz & Taylor, 1986a). Some may be initially unwilling or unable to contemplate giving up. For these patients the primary health care team should try to help them reduce the harm associated with drug use (harm minimisation) and to treat any concurrent medical complications. The risks associated with injecting should be discussed. They should be encouraged to adopt alternative routes of administration or at least avoid sharing equipment. Issues concerning safer sex should also be covered, and non-immune individuals should be offered hepatitis B immunisation.

Prescribing for the opiate user

Prescribing a substitute opiate drug should only be considered if there is clear evidence of physical dependency. Giving methadone for example to an occasional non-dependent opiate user can actually lead to dependence or overdose. The combination of diphenoxylate and atropine ('Lomotil') and thioridazine in reducing dosage for seven days, together with simple reassurance can often provide adequate relief from mild withdrawal. The use of dependence producing drugs such as diazepam for symptomatic relief is best avoided. Dihydrocodeine is not recommended because its short action necessitates frequent administration and the tablet form can be crushed and misused by injection.

Patients with established physical dependence on opiate drugs may need an opiate substitute to help them to reduce their use and minimise injecting behaviour. Methadone is the drug of choice because of its long duration of action and because its oral liquid preparation makes it unsuitable for injection or diversion to the black market. It should therefore not be given as tablets or injections.

The dose of methadone which will keep the patient free from withdrawal but not lead to gross intoxication is called the stabilisation dose. Conversion tables exist which convert doses of other opiates into methadone equivalents as a rough guide, but remember patients may exaggerate the quantity of drug used and the purity of street heroin can vary greatly. To assess the required dose, give the patient up to 20 mg of methadone initially, see him daily for the next few days, and titrate the dose in increments of 10 mg against objective evidence of withdrawal. In practice, most opiate addicts need a total daily dose of 40 mg–60 mg.

After a few days, a gradual reduction in dose of methadone should commence, agreed with the patient. A rapid withdrawal might be achieved over two or three weeks by a reduction of 5 mg every second or third day. A more gradual withdrawal over a longer period of a few months would involve tapering the dose by 5 mg every week or fortnight. Towards the end, withdrawal is often more troublesome. The patient should be seen on a weekly basis and random urine testing should be undertaken throughout the treatment period. Withdrawal programmes lasting more than a few months should only be used in consultation with a specialist treatment unit.

During treatment, methadone should be prescribed on a daily basis and arrangements made with a local pharmacist for dispensing, to help prevent overdose or diversion to the black market. The patient should be warned that prescriptions cannot be dispensed in advance or in arrears, and that 'lost' methadone will not normally be replaced. In the UK general practitioners can arrange for daily dispensing for a period of up to two weeks by using the prescription forms FP10 (MDA) which are available from Family Health Service Authorities. Under the Misuse of Drugs Regulations 1985, doctors prescribing methadone must conform with certain legal requirements which will be found in the British National Formulary.

If a general practitioner decides to prescribe a substitute, then a drug treatment contract should first be agreed with the patient. Some doctors find it helpful to write out and get the patient to sign such a contract. The contract should specify the agreed goals of treatment, the frequency of attendance at the surgery, and the withdrawal schedule or rate of reduction with dates and amounts.

Lapses into illicit drug use occur, especially at the beginning of treatment when the patient is adjusting to a new lifestyle. Isolated occurrences can be used as an opportunity to learn how to prevent further lapses. However, with repeated relapse, or continuous use of other drugs, the general practitioner may decide to discontinue prescribing for the patient. Referral to a community drug team or local drug dependence clinic should be sought. 'Shared care' between general practitioner and drug specialist service might be considered at this stage. Individuals with a long history of chaotic drug use, those using a number of different substances simultaneously and those with severe medical or psychiatric complications are difficult to deal with in general practice and should always be referred to a specialist unit.

Sedative misuse and dependence

The general practitioner can make a significant contribution to the prevention of drug dependency by being aware of the dependence-producing potential of certain drugs and by improving prescribing practice – for example, by adopting guidelines on benzodiazepine prescribing (Ghodse & Khan, 1988; Russell & Lader, 1993). Review by the primary health care team of patients on long-term benzodiazepine prescriptions will often reveal evidence of dependence (Ghodse, 1995a).

Patients with benzodiazepine problems can be divided into two distinct groups. The first consists of poly-drug misusers who are part of the drug subculture and misuse a wide variety of other substances. They frequently use very high doses, often by injection, and obtain their supply illicitly or from numerous different sources. Treatment within the primary care setting is seldom appropriate for these patients who should be referred to a specialist service.

The second group consists of patients prescribed benzodiazepines for anxiety or depression over long periods of time. The average general practitioner can expect to have about 50 long-term benzodiazepine users (Russell & Lader, 1993). Of these up to 40% will experience physical withdrawal symptoms, although it is not possible to predict which patients will. The clinical features of the benzodiazepine syndrome are listed in Box 13.8. Onset of withdrawal occurs 2–10 days after reduction of the benzodiazepine and depends on the particular preparation's elimination half-life.

Benzodiazepines should never be stopped abruptly but be gradually reduced over time. For some patients, simple advice alone, from primary health care staff, to gradually reduce and stop their benzodiazepines, will be effective. If this brief intervention proves unsuccessful a more structured withdrawal programme can be worked out with the patient.

The patient should be transferred from short-acting compounds such as lorazepam or temazepam, to an equivalent dose of diazepam (Box 13.9). The diazepam should then be gradually reduced,

Anxiety symptoms
Anxiety
Apprehension
Tremor
Sweating
Insomnia

Psychological symptoms
Perceptual distortions
Abnormal body sensations (e.g. crawling in the skin)
Abnormal sensations of movement
Hypersensitivity to stimuli (e.g. hyperacusis, photophobia)
Depersonalisation (feelings of unreality)
Depression

Somatic symptoms
Ataxia (unsteadiness)
Pain
Paraesthesia (e.g. pins and needles)
Visual disturbances (e.g. blurred vision)
Flu-like symptoms
Gastro-intestinal symptoms

Major complications
Paranoid psychosis
Delirium
Epileptic seizures

Box 13.8 *Benzodiazepine withdrawal symptoms.*

Drug	Dose
Diazepam	5 mg
Chlordiazepoxide	15 mg
Loprazolam	500 micrograms
Lorazepam	500 micrograms
Oxazepam	15 mg
Temazepam	10 mg
Nitrazepam	5 mg
Flunitrazepam	2 mg
Flurazepam	15 mg

Box 13.9 *Approximate doses of benzodiazepines equivalent to 5 mg diazepam.*

according to what the patient can tolerate. Ideally, the duration of the withdrawal schedule should neither be too short (less than six weeks) nor too long (more than six months). A guide would be to reduce the dose by 10% every fortnight. The rate of reduction can often be more rapid initially, slowing down later as withdrawal becomes more troublesome. When doses become quite small towards the end, the patient may need to cut up their tablets. The patient should be seen fortnightly and progress closely monitored. Sometimes withdrawal symptoms may not appear until after a number of reductions.

As withdrawal progresses underlying neurotic symptoms may re-emerge and these may need appropriate interventions. A clear explanation of the nature of the withdrawal syndrome should be given to the patient and family, and any misconceptions corrected. Reassurance and instruction in simple relaxation techniques by primary health care staff will often be effective in helping the patient deal with withdrawal symptoms.

Post-withdrawal follow-up is essential as depression is common during this time and may require antidepressant medication (Ashton, 1987). More formal psychological interventions such as anxiety management, cognitive treatments (see Chapters 11 and 17), or even group therapy may be possible within the practice.

Other drug misuse

Stimulant drugs such as amphetamines and cocaine are widely abused and produce a sense of well-being, increased energy and confidence, suppressing appetite and reducing the need for sleep. Heavier use can produce restlessness, irritability, suspiciousness and even frank psychosis. Stimulants can be taken orally or snorted but are also often injected. 'Crack' is a smokable form of cocaine which is considered to be highly addictive.

However, although stimulants can produce marked psychological dependence, they are not usually associated with major physical withdrawal symptoms. They can therefore be stopped abruptly and the prescribing of substitute stimulants is not usually appropriate. Withdrawal, however, can be followed by a period of extreme exhaustion, depression, agitation and in some cases suicidal behaviour.

Patients using stimulant drugs should be informed about the risks of dependence and HIV infection and be advised to stop. Those continuing to inject should be discouraged to do so and advised about safe sexual practices. Patients should be informed about withdrawal symptoms and how to cope with them, for example, by getting increased sleep for a few days and avoiding self-medication with other drugs.

Lysergic acid diethylamide (LSD) and 'dance' drugs such as

ecstasy (methylene-dioxy-methamphetamine, MDMA) are often used in a recreational manner at parties, dance clubs, and discos. Physical dependence does not occur but these drugs are not free from risks. Panic attacks and psychotic episodes ('bad trips') may follow the use of these drugs and recently deaths from severe dehydration and hyperpyrexia have been associated with the use of ecstasy (Henry, 1992).

Volatile substance abuse or glue sniffing involves inhalation of gases or vapours in order to produce a state of intoxication not unlike drunkenness. Most solvent users are young teenagers and, for most, use will be experimental or occasional, with only one in ten becoming regular users. Nevertheless, there are over 100 deaths in Great Britain each year from volatile substance abuse and many of these are in first-time users. Many children may not be aware of the risks and the general practitioner is well placed to inform and advise both children and parents. Tell-tale signs which may aid early identification include unusual or secretive behaviour, appearance of drowsiness or intoxication, the smell of solvents on the body or clothes, a periorbital facial rash, or recurrent upper respiratory tract inflammation.

Resources for primary health care staff

It has been suggested that general practitioners would be more willing to treat drug users if they received more support, adequate back-up, and better training (Glanz & Taylor, 1986a; Bell, Cohen & Cremona, 1990; Ghodse, 1995). A similar attitude appears to apply in the case of willingness to treat heavy drinkers (Thom & Tellez, 1986). However, there will often be a wide variety of supports and resources available to primary health care teams from both the statutory and the voluntary services.

Health promotion units and organisations such as Alcohol Concern can be a source of educational material for patients and their families. The Medical Council on Alcoholism produces a handbook for general practitioners called *Hazardous Drinking* (Pollak *et al.*, 1990) and one for nurses and health visitors entitled *Alcohol and Health* (Hartz, Plant & Watts, 1990). The Department of Health publications *Drug Misuse and Dependence; Guidelines on Clinical Management* (DOH, 1991a) and *Substance Misuse Detainees in Police Custody; Guidelines for Clinical Management* (DOH, 1994) provide clear and practical guidance for non-specialist doctors including general practitioners.

Multidisciplinary community alcohol teams and community drug teams can be a valuable support to the primary health care staff by offering advice, assessment, joint management ('shared care'), and training for staff. Placing trained counsellors within a practice may be a particularly effective method of facilitating early recognition and intervention, and for providing on-the-job training for practice staff. A innovative project of this type *Addiction Prevention in Primary Care* has been established by St George's Hospital Medical School for the London boroughs of Wandsworth, Merton and Sutton (Ghodse, 1995*b*).

Many districts will have specialist units to which the more severely affected individuals can be referred. Alcoholics Anonymous and Narcotics Anonymous provide support groups for affected individuals while Al-Anon and Alateen offer help to their families. The opportunities are there for primary health care teams to become more involved today in the prevention of alcohol and drug misuse. Attendance at locally organised workshops and seminars may help update the knowledge and skill of the team, while certain centres (including St George's Hospital Medical School) now offer more formal certificate and diploma courses in substance misuse.

References

Advisory Council on the Misuse of Drugs (1993). *AIDS and Drug Misuse Update*. London: HMSO.

Anderson, P., Wallace P. & Jones, H. (1988). *Alcohol Problems: Practical Guides for General Practice 5*. Oxford: Oxford Medical Publications.

Ashton, H. (1987). Benzodiazepine withdrawal: outcome in 50 patients. *British Journal of Addiction*, **82**, 665–71.

Babor, T. F., Ritson, E. B. & Hodgson, R. J. (1986). Alcohol-related problems in the primary health care setting: a review of early intervention strategies. *British Journal of Addiction*, **81**, 23–46.

Babor, T.F., de la Fuente, J.R., Saunders, J. & Grant, M. (1992). *AUDIT The Alcohol Use Disorders Identification Test: Guidelines for Use in Primary Health Care*. Geneva: World Health Organisation.

Bell, G., Cohen, J. & Cremona, A. (1990). How willing are general practitioners to manage narcotic misuse? *Health Trends*, **2**, 56–7.

Bien, H.B., Miller, W.R. & Tonigan, J.S. (1993). Brief interventions for alcohol problems: a review. *Addiction*, **88**, 315–35.

Cohen, J. & Schamroth, A. (1989).General practice management of drug misusers. *The Practitioner*, **233**, 1471–4.

Cutler, S. F., Wallace P.G. & Haines A.P. (1988). Assessing alcohol consumption in general practice – a comparison between questionnaire and interview. *Alcohol and Alcoholism*, **23**, 441–50.

Department of Health (1991*a*). *Drug Misuse and Dependence: Guidelines on Clinical Management*. London: HMSO.

Department of Health (1991a). *The Health of the Nation – A Consultative Document for Health in England.* London: HMSO.

Department of Health (1994). *Substance Misuse Detainees in Police Custody; Guidelines for Clinical Management.* London: HMSO.

Douds, A.C. & Maxwell, J.D. (1994). Alcohol and the heart: good and bad news. *Addiction,* **89,** 259–61.

Elander, J., Porter, S. & Hodson, S. (1993). What role for general practitioners in the care of opiate users? *Addiction Research,* **1,** 309–22.

Ghodse, A.H. (1982). Living with an alcoholic. *Postgraduate Medical Journal,* **58,** 636–40.

Ghodse, A.H. (1995a). *Drugs and Addictive Behaviour: A Guide to Treatment.* 2nd edn. Oxford: Blackwell Science.

Ghodse, A.H. (1995a). A matter of substance. *The Health Service Journal,* **105,** 31.

Ghodse, A.H. & Khan, I. (1988). *Psychoactive Drugs: Improving Prescribing Practices.* Geneva: World Health Organization.

Glanz, A. & Taylor, C. (1986a). Findings of a national survey on the role of general practitioners in the treatment of opiate misuse: extent of contact with opiate misusers. *British Medical Journal,* **293,** 427–30.

Glanz, A. & Taylor, C. (1986b). Findings of a national survey on the role of general practitioners in the treatment of opiate misuse: views on treatment. *British Medical Journal,* **293,** 543–5.

Hartz, C., Plant, M. & Watts, M. (1990). *Alcohol and Health – A Handbook for Nurses, Midwives and Health Visitors.* London: The Medical Council on Alcoholism.

Henry, J.A. (1992). Ecstasy and the dance of death. *British Medical Journal,* **305,** 5–6.

Hoeksema, H. L. & de Bock G. H. (1993). The value of laboratory tests for the screening and recognition of alcohol abuse in primary care patients. *The Journal of Family Practice,* **37,** 268–76.

Lloyd, G.G., Chick J. & Crombie E. (1982). Screening for problem drinkers among medical in-patients. *Drug and Alcohol Dependence,* **10,** 355–9.

Marlatt, G. A. & George W. H. (1984). Relapse prevention: introduction and overview of the model. *British Journal of Addiction,* **79,** 261–73.

Mayfield, D., McLeod, G. & Hall, P. (1974). The CAGE questionnaire: validation of a new alcoholism screening instrument. *American Journal of Psychiatry,* **131,** 1121–3.

Office of Population Censuses and Surveys. (1992). *General Household Survey.* London: HMSO.

Pollak, B. (1989). Primary health care and the addictions: where to start and where to go. *British Journal of Addiction,* **84,** 1425–32.

Pollak, B., Smith A. & Wilson D. G. (1990). *Hazardous Drinking – A Handbook for General Practitioners*. London: The Medical Council on Alcoholism.

Richards, T. (1988). Drug addicts and the general practitioner. *British Medical Journal*, **296**, 1082.

Royal College of General Practitioners (1986). *Alcohol – A Balanced View*. London: Royal College of General Practitioners.

Royal College of Physicians (1987). *A Great and Growing Evil: The Medical Consequences of Alcohol Abuse*. London: Tavistock Publications.

Royal College of Psychiatrists (1986). *Alcohol: Our Favourite Drug*. London: Tavistock Publications.

Russell, J. & Lader, M.H. (1993). *Guidelines for the Prevention and Treatment of Benzodiazepine Dependence*. London: Mental Health Foundation.

Saunders, J.B., Aasland, O.G., Babor, T.B., de la Fuente, J.R. & Grant, M. (1993). Development of the alcohol use identification test (AUDIT). WHO collaborative project on the early detection of persons with harmful alcohol consumption. *Addiction*, **88**, 791–804.

Saunders, W.M. & Kershaw P.W. (1980).Screening tests for alcoholism – findings from a community study. *British Journal of Addiction*, **75**, 37–41.

Thom, B. & Tellez, C. (1986). A difficult business: detecting and managing alcohol problems in general practice. *British Journal of Addiction*, **81**, 405–18.

Wallace, P. G. & Haines, A. P. (1985). Use of a questionnaire in general practice to increase recognition of patients with excessive alcohol consumption. *British Medical Journal*, **290**, 1949–52.

Waller, T. (1993). *Working with General Practitioners*. London, Institute for the Study of Drug Dependence.

[14] Early detection of psychosis in primary care: initial treatment and crisis management

Tom Burns

Introduction

Tidy-minded health service planners often suggest a division of labour between primary and secondary care where 'neurotic' disorders are managed by general practitioners and 'psychotic' ones are handed over to the specialist mental health team. This attractive bureaucratic solution is, as any experienced general practitioner will know, no match for the real world. Many 'neurotic' disorders are far from simple and may require the full resources of a specialist mental health service. The contribution of general practitioners to the care of individuals with psychotic illnesses living in the community was clearly demonstrated in Murray-Parkes, Brown & Monck's (1962) survey of schizophrenic patients in London. Twelve months after discharge, only 56% were still in contact with a psychiatrist, while 70% had had recent contact with their general practitioner. Despite the increasing emphasis on community care and the expansion of mental health teams over the last 30 years the situation is virtually unchanged today. Twelve months after discharge from a West Lambeth mental hospital only 52% of patients with schizophrenia were found to be still in contact with a psychiatrist, while 57% were in contact with their general practitioner (Melzer et al., 1991). Only 60% of patients with chronic schizophrenia identified in setting up a case register in Camden had any continuing contact with specialist services (Pantelis, Taylor & Campbell, 1988).

Whilst some of this may be due to a failure of community mental health teams to commit resources effectively to their stated target group of the severely mentally ill (Sims, 1991), it may also reflect a realistic appraisal by the patient of his needs at different stages of his illness. There is growing recognition of the role of the general practitioner in the care of patients with psychosis, which is particularly important in early diagnosis and management of initial presentations (Burns & Kendrick, 1994).

What does psychosis mean?

The terms 'neurotic' and 'psychotic' are under considerable pressure. The two most recent classifications of psychiatric disorders, the American Psychiatric Association's Diagnostic and Statistical Manual DSM-IV (APA, 1994) and the WHO's 10th International Classification of Diseases (World Health Organisation, 1992) relegate the terms to symptom descriptions or qualifiers. This reflects difficulties in defining them in a consistent manner or matching them to the evolving understanding of psychiatric disorders.

While the finer points of taxonomy within psychiatry may make the terms unfashionable they remain in regular use both within mental health and general practice. Psychosis is used to indicate those severe mental illnesses characterised by a loss of reality testing. What is common to them is that their characteristic distortions and misperceptions are not modified by contradictory external experience. Delusions (false, powerful and unshakeable beliefs) and hallucinations (sensory experiences without any external stimulus – most often hearing voices but also seeing things or feeling odd sensations in the body) are the dominant symptoms in most acute psychoses. The psychotic patient is totally convinced by his experiences, e.g. that his body *is* decaying, unlike the depressed patient who may say 'it's *as if* my body was decaying and I had no energy left'.

The psychoses fall roughly into three groups.

Delusional psychoses

These include schizophrenia and the paranoid psychoses. The characteristic symptoms of acute schizophrenia are hallucinations (usually of voices talking to, or about, the patient) and delusions, which are often persecutory but can be quite fantastic. Specific enquiry can reveal so-called 'passivity phenomena' where the patient experiences his thoughts or actions being controlled from without (e.g. by hypnotism or telepathy). This may be associated with 'thought disorder' where the logical flow or form of thinking is disturbed. While these latter features are highly valued by psychiatrists for distinguishing between schizophrenic and paranoid psychoses they are of considerably less practical importance than the emergence of negative symptoms (apathy, emotional blunting and self-neglect). These develop in schizophrenia over time but not in the other psychoses to anything like the same degree. A discrepancy between the patients' expressed beliefs and their behaviour is common in schizophrenia – for example, a patient may accept admission to hospital for food and shelter despite being convinced that he has great wealth, or accept medicine while denying that he is ill. This is not always so and a careful clinical judgement based on familiarity with the patient is needed.

Affective psychoses

Psychotic depression is distinguished by the presence of delusions, and more rarely, hallucinations congruent with the depressed mood. It usually poses no diagnostic problem because of the self-reproachful and guilt-laden picture. Mania and hypomania are commoner. Here lack of reality testing reveals itself in grossly deficient judgement. The patient is elated and overactive, often bursting with optimism and over-confidence. There is an almost total resistance to recognising that there is anything wrong at all. Delusions and hallucinations are frequent but are not invariable.

Organic psychoses

These psychoses range from progressive dementias through to brief confusional states resulting from prescription drugs (e.g. high-dose steroids and anti-parkinsonian agents) or from alcohol or street drugs (e.g. cocaine, ecstasy and amphetamine). The management of dementias is outside the scope of this chapter. Brief psychotic episodes in the elderly associated with polypharmacy are increasingly reported. For most of these the general practitioner's main role is to maintain a high index of suspicion and to remove the offending agent as quickly as is safely possible. Drug- or alcohol-induced paranoid disorders follow similar, albeit briefer, courses to their functional equivalents and will not be dealt with separately.

Is the onset of psychosis predictable?

Psychotic illnesses usually present in early adulthood. There is usually no clue to predict the onset, but there is evidence suggesting that developmental abnormalities may be present long before symptoms are manifest. Some children who will later develop schizophrenia have a history of abnormal behaviour during their school age years.

Done and colleagues (1994) from the Clinical Research Centre in Harrow Middlesex examined data from the National Child Development Study (NCDS), a long-term follow-up study of children born in 1958, monitoring their physical, educational and social development. Using the national Mental Health Inquiry, they identified all NCDS subjects who had been psychiatric inpatients between 1974 and 1986. The 40 adults identified with schizophrenic illnesses and 35 with affective psychosis were compared with 1914 randomly selected members of the cohort who had never been admitted for psychiatric treatment. At the age of seven children of both sexes who developed schizophrenia later in life had been rated by their teachers as showing more social maladjustment than controls. This was more so for boys and related to over-active and disruptive behaviour. At both seven and 11 pre-psychotic (affective) children differed little from normal controls. The authors concluded that abnormalities of social adjustment are detectable in childhood in some people who are going to develop psychotic illness later.

It is *not* possible, however, to conclude from this study that children who show disruptive behaviour or excessive withdrawal in childhood will necessarily go on to develop schizophrenia themselves, even with a strong family history. The behaviours identified are very common and certainly not specific to any recognisable pre-schizophrenic syndrome. This is important to remember when counselling the relatives of patients with schizophrenia who have young children.

Importance of early recognition

In the United Kingdom the general practitioner remains the main point of entry into mental health services for psychotic individuals for a number of good reasons. The ease of access and non-stigmatising nature of general practice recommend it to early presentation. Consulting the general practitioner under the pretext of a minor physical worry is common for psychological problems (Bridges & Goldberg, 1985). It is particularly helpful when the patient's developing illness is confusing and hard to put into words (e.g. non-specific unease at the start of a psychosis).

This ease of access extends to families, and sometimes neighbours, who feel that they can approach the general practitioner about the patient. This is particularly important because many patients lack insight into their developing illness. Family approaches are also very common when patients with established illness are relapsing. Quite often these consultations take the form of offering some token complaint and relying on the general practitioner's intuition to pick up that something else is in the air. A mother's concerns about withdrawal and recent 'strangeness' of her son may be the only clue to the insidious onset of schizophrenia.

A number of factors are known to be associated with a poorer prognosis in schizophrenia, including poor premorbid attainment, an early and gradual mode of onset, the absence of affective features and male gender. The question of whether the duration of symptoms prior to treatment also affects the prognosis was addressed by a research team from New York (Loebel *et al.*, 1992). Fifty-four patients with schizophrenia and 16 with schizoaffective disorder were followed for three years in their first episode of illness. The duration of both non-specific behavioural changes and specific psychotic symptoms prior to treatment was assessed by interviews with patients and their families. This was related to outcome in terms of time to remission of acute psychosis as well as the degree of symptom relief after treatment. The mean duration of symptoms prior to initial treatment was 52 weeks, preceded by a mean of 99 weeks of non-specific behavioural changes. Duration of illness before treatment was indeed found to be significantly associated with both time to, and degree of, remission. The authors speculated that the longer the illness is allowed to progress before neuroleptic treatment is started, the more damage is suffered, making the disorder more resistant to treatment. They concluded that in the United States, patients can remain untreated for long periods despite substantial symptoms – an average of three years in this study.

The situation should be better in the UK with wider access to primary care. However, Johnstone *et al.* (1986) in a study of 253 patients referred in their first episode of schizophrenia to North-wick Park Hospital, found that, while 71 (28%) were admitted within two months of the onset of psychosis, as many as 66 (26%) had been unwell for more than a year before admission. Many relatives described difficulty in obtaining appropriate assessment and in arranging adequate management. In 46 cases (18%), nine or more contacts were made with health professionals before admission and in frustration relatives often made repeated appeals to non-medical services, such as self-help groups.

It is important for these reasons to strive to engage patients in treatment as soon as symptoms develop. This has implications for general practitioners' responses to families requesting help with their relatives with early schizophrenia.

With mania, the benefits of early recognition (usually via the family) are even more obvious. It is often in the early stages of elation, with disinhibition and poor judgement, that patients spend thoughtlessly and may severely damage their reputations. This early stage may also be the one hope of obtaining voluntary compliance with medication.

Schizophrenic patients consult their general practitioners frequently but often for physical rather than psychological problems (Nazareth & King, 1993). When a physical complaint seems bizarre, distinguishing delusions from exaggerated anxieties of serious illness (e.g. constipation as the first sign of cancer) can be very difficult. The delusional or bizarre quality is often in the patient's understanding of the complaint. For example, psychotic-ally depressed individuals present with real constipation but only if questioned directly about its cause will delusions about internal rot and decay be revealed. The delusional origins are often best explored by asking the patient directly what they think is causing the illness.

General practitioner treatment of first episodes

Having detected the onset of a first episode psychosis it is worth seeking an early specialist opinion. Nearly all patients with psychoses have been in contact with the specialist services at some stage. Most general practitioners surveyed in South West Thames Health Region (Kendrick *et al*, 1991) were willing to be involved in the care of the long-term mentally ill (41% were prepared to coordinate it), but over 90% considered that the secondary mental health services should be involved. However, the patient may not accept the referral and most general practitioners have had to manage hypomanic episodes or initiate treatment for schizophrenia on their own. The severity of the disorder and degree of risk may leave no option but to involve the specialist services. More often, however, it is a complex clinical judgement, weighing the benefits of establishing early treatment by a doctor whom the patient trusts against possibly muddying the clinical picture and treatment with limited resources.

Discussing the case with the consultant psychiatrist on the telephone before starting treatment has multiple benefits:

1. It allows the general practitioner to clarify diagnostic and management issues in his own mind with discussion of management principles and checking drug doses. Most general practitioners (and psychiatrists) are used to patients habituated to high dose antipsychotics. A dose of 100 mg chlorpromazine thrice daily (tds) in a drug-naive patient may be very sedative and generate resistance to treatment. Starting lower (e.g. 50 mg in the morning (mane) and 100 mg at night (nocte)) with an increase after two to three days is preferable.

2. Agreeing a time-scale for assessing the success or otherwise of the initial treatment plan avoids things drifting.

3. It alerts the specialist team to the problem and primes them for urgent intervention should this be required in the future. It may be possible to arrange flexible input between the teams (e.g. the community psychiatric nurse could visit the patient to monitor side-effects and initiate engagement). Being consulted early generally ensures a more positive response from the team.

4. A jointly agreed treatment plan (e.g. using a drug regime familiar to the specialist team) makes the assessment by the psychiatrist, if it comes, much less confusing. The clinical picture *will* have been altered by the drugs and it seriously complicates the task if the psychiatrist is unfamiliar with those used.

5. It avoids recriminations if the treatment should run into problems, e.g. if in mania the initial treatment (perhaps a modest dose of antipsychotic) fails to control the illness but only modifies the symptoms resulting in a protracted and frustrating situation for all involved.

Liaison

An established relationship between general practitioner and the community mental health team is necessary if patients with severe disorders are to be treated in primary care. The precise arrangements will differ in different parts of the country. Sectorised mental health services cover over 80% of Britain's population (Johnson & Thornicroft, 1993) and do at least ensure identified responsibility for any given patient. Sectorised services are challenged by the development of general practitioner fundholding (Kendrick, 1994) where many practices have insisted upon a more variable pattern of services. Sectors based on practices rather than street lists are developing, although sometimes linkage between practices and secondary services is based entirely on specific contracts. Whatever system is operated there must be clear understanding between general practitioner and psychiatrist. Establishing closer links than the purely formal will also improve the capacity of the primary health care team to initiate and sustain treatment for severe disorders. Various liaison links between mental health teams and primary health care teams have been described (Strathdee & Williams, 1984; Tyrer, 1984; Strathdee, 1988). They are generally considered time well-spent, generating better working relationships and improved care for patients. Work at St George's Hospital Medical School indicates that the care of psychotic patients formed the main focus for such liaison meetings with a group of local general practitioners, despite constituting only a minority of referrals.

Affective psychoses

The risk to the patient of delay is the overwhelming consideration for initiating treatment without a specialist opinion. With hypomania the likelihood of gaining co-operation diminishes rapidly in the early phase of the disorder. It is almost always best to try and initiate treatment with antipsychotics as soon as possible. The general practitioner should stick to a drug he knows well and aim for a rapid escalation from a low starting dose. Haloperidol, widely used in inpatient care, is probably not a good choice in general practice because of the higher risk of dystonias in the early stages. Thioridazine and chlorpromazine are particularly suitable because of their mild sedative effects. Loading the dose at night is often the only option acceptable to patients who often admit to sleep disturbance while denying all other symptoms. This helps to 'sell' treatment to patients with limited insight.

Change in mental state is rapid in hypomania and the patient needs to be reviewed very frequently – preferably every second day in the first week or so. It is important to try and avoid conflict during this phase and gentle, persistent encouragement may prevail where insistence or the exercise of authority certainly will not. Hypomanic patients, despite an outward air of affability, are easily irritated. Regular contact with the general practitioner can creatively exploit the patient's expansive state. Sleep is one of the most useful indicators of treatment response. Aim to achieve a dose of antipsychotic which gives six to eight hours' uninterrupted sleep nightly. Some day-time drowsiness is a welcome sign if the patient will tolerate it. This usually heralds a noticeable reduction in elation and over-activity. It is important to monitor this stage closely as there can be a rapid reduction in energy and emergence of parkinsonian side-effects. Dosages need to be reduced carefully to avoid loss of symptom control. Anti-parkinsonian drugs, best avoided initially, may now be needed (e.g. orphenadrine 50 mg twice daily (bd)).

When the hypomania fades and some insight begins to return the patient may accept a referral to the psychiatrist. Although the worse may seem over, the general practitioner is still well advised to connect the patient with the mental health services (Box 14.1). Hypomania can run a protracted course and the patient also runs a high risk of becoming significantly depressed. Initiating lithium prophylaxis is best considered after a full and thorough review.

Delusional depression

This rarely presents a problem about referral on to the psychiatrist. Such patients are usually full of self-reproach and guilt and are unlikely to disagree with their doctor. If there is definite evidence of depressive delusions (usually grotesquely exaggerated guilt over some minor misdemeanour in the past, or a conviction of poverty

---

Avoid trying to pressurise or deceive the patient into seeing a psychiatrist.

Discuss the case with a psychiatrist on the telephone.

Attempt to involve the community psychiatric nurse.

Try thioridazine or chlorpamazine intitially – outline the side-effects.

Prescribe anti-parkinsonian agents only if side-effects develop.

Sell the treatment as a remedy for sleep disturbance.

Allow 2–3 weeks before deciding how effective treatment has been.

Visit patients who fail to attend follow-up appointments.

Involve the secondary care team when the patient develops insight.

Box 14.1 *Treating the patient with psychosis who declines to see a psychiatrist.*

or terminal illness), the patient is less likely to respond to anti-depressants and electroconvulsive therapy may need to be considered, so it is best to refer directly without waiting for a trial of antidepressants.

Schizophrenia and paranoid disorders

There is usually less urgency to initiate treatment in these disorders. Often the illness will have been developing over several weeks or even months before consultation. In contrast to the roller-coaster experience of treating hypomania, the problem here is more often one of establishing and maintaining contact with the patient. Sometimes the patient may know that something is amiss but not know what. In some paranoid disorders (particularly late onset) there may be little outward sign of the illness and complex delusional systems can be uncovered by a chance remark:

e.g. A 72 year-old ex-actress had recently consulted her general practitioner for a minor gynaecological complaint. She had been on his list for two years but had never been to see him. Cheerful and outgoing, she was well groomed and denied other problems. A comment by the general practitioner about some recent vandalism in her neighbourhood led her to describe how she had moved house every 2–5 years for the last two decades because she 'knew' that a boyfriend from the early 1950s was still following her. She was deluded that he intended to punish her for allegedly informing the police on him over 40 years ago. She moved house every time she 'spotted his agents' in the neighbourhood.

With such patients, whose clinical picture is dominated by delusions and distressing hallucinations, there is often no significant emotional arousal or behavioural problems. It is possible to develop trust and a greater understanding of the illness in follow-up assessments. An appointment (e.g. at the end of the surgery) when more time can be spent exploring the issues and possibly introducing the idea of a psychiatric referral can help. If the patient resists, suggesting that they see 'another specialist', hoping they will assume it is a physician, usually ends in grief and should be avoided. With a physical component in the presentation, stressing the interplay of anxiety and physical ill-health is more helpful.

If possible, consult the psychiatrist before starting antipsychotics. Start with small doses (e.g. chlorpromazine 100 mg nocte, trifluoperazine 5 mg bd) and slowly work up to full therapeutic doses (e.g. chlorpromazine 150 mg tds, trifluoperazine 15 mg bd) in several stages observing the patient weekly. Using much higher doses has no more rapid antipsychotic effect, and the risk of sedation and extrapyramidal effects is greatly increased. Routinely prescribing anti-parkinsonian agents is best avoided.

Antipsychotics are not good hypnotics so if the patient is anxious and has disturbed sleep a hypnotic such as temazepam 10–20 mg should be prescribed. Families become understandably anxious when the patient is up and about at night, and ensuring some sleep for the patient will give the family a chance to rest.

When prescribing antipsychotics it is essential to outline the anticipated side-effects. If they are not mentioned, they may be misinterpreted for a worsening of the illness and in any case undermine trust in the doctor. The anticholinergic effects (dry mouth, blurred vision, postural hypotension) are inevitable initially and patients need to be reassured that they will soon fade. Extrapyramidal effects (stiffness and tremor) develop more slowly and can be reduced with orphenadrine or procyclidine. Akathisias (subjective and objective restlessness, particularly of the legs) are experienced by many patients and are very difficult to deal with. Beta blockers and benzodiazepines can help but it is best to avoid them if possible. Changing to a different antipsychotic can sometimes help (akathisias are much less likely with chlorpromazine or thioridazine than with trifluoperazine). Acute dystonias are rare but if they are going to occur do so early. They are commoner in younger males and more so in ethnic minority patients. An acknowledgement of the risks, reassurance that, although distressing, they are not dangerous, and clear instructions about how to get help (e.g. through the surgery or Accident and Emergency Department) are essential.

Antipsychotic drugs take weeks to achieve their maximum benefit (any immediate impact is by reduction in arousal from their sedative properties). Using doses above British National Formulary recommended levels, or chopping and changing drug treatment, will rarely hasten the clinical response.

New drugs

There are a number of newer, so-called 'atypical', antipsychotics now available. They are characterised by their low risk for extrapyramidal side-effects and tardive dyskinesia. The best known is clozapine, which has been demonstrated to be effective in a proportion of patients with treatment resistant schizophrenia. Because of the risk of agranulocytosis, it can only be initiated from hospital at present. Risperidone benefits from the same freedom from extrapyramidal effects without the need for blood tests, although it has not been demonstrated to be significantly more effective than standard antipsychotics. The absence of extrapyramidal side-effects with risperidone makes it considerably more acceptable to most patients and drowsiness is minimised by employing a structured dosage schedule for the first three days' treatment.

These newer drugs are considerably more expensive than traditional neuroleptics, however, so it is important to think through and agree a policy, preferably together with the local psychiatrist, on their use as first line agents. First episode schizophrenics should remain on medication for at least two years so these decisions are very significant. It is highly likely that important advances in this area will be made over the next few years with the prospect of being able to treat schizophrenia without exposing patients to the risk of tardive dyskinesia.

In some cases (with a clear, recent onset and a strong possibility of precipitation by drugs or overwhelming physical or psychological stress), it may be enough simply to observe the patient drug-free for a week or so. If an illness is treated successfully with antipsychotics it is still best to obtain a specialist opinion. This allows a broader needs assessment and also an opinion about how long to persist with treatment. With brief or spontaneously remitting disorders, the reason for doing so may be less obvious:

e.g. A 23 year-old man with a florid paranoid psychosis was brought to the hospital by the police. He had assaulted his girlfriend and smashed the television which he believed had been broadcasting pornographic pictures of her and a workmate. He responded rapidly to treatment with trifluoperazine, regained full insight and, though remorseful and quite depressed, insisted on returning to live with his girlfriend. Both she and his mother were keen to have him back home. There was no previous recorded psychiatric history and he was virtually unknown to his general practitioner with whom he had been registered for four years. His general practitioner had been unable to obtain records from his previous private doctor who had retired. Four weeks after discharge the patient jumped in front of a train. In the course of the suicide audit his previous general practitioner notes were eventually tracked down. These recorded a brief paranoid disturbance when the patient was 17, followed by a prolonged and severe depressive episode which had been managed entirely in primary care and was unknown to those involved in the later breakdown.

What to say to the patient and family (Box 14.2)

The onset of a psychotic disorder gives rise to anxiety in both patient and family. How serious is it? Will he make a complete recovery? Is it in the family ? What the general practitioner says depends on the questions asked, the level of understanding displayed by the family, and the doctor's level of certainty. The lists of prognostic factors learnt in medical school are of little help. The family (and later the patient) wants an individualised judgement about the likelihood of a further breakdown, how long he will have to stay on medication, the possibility of a return to work, and the

---

Listen carefully to the family's particular concerns.

Be as honest as possible but not brutal with specific labels.

Emphasise the importance of stress and its avoidance.

Emphasise the importance of drug treatment.

Raise the possibility of psychosocial interventions (see Chapter 19).

Box 14.2 *What to say to the family.*

prospects for independent living. Such certainty can rarely be acquired in the first breakdown.

While the general practitioner may experience great pressure to answer questions, it is more important at this stage to listen. Let the parent, spouse or carer say what they think has happened and what their worries are. Misconceptions about the nature and causation of mental illnesses abound, and it is impossible to reassure or adequately inform until one understands the specific concerns. The family may equate a diagnosis of schizophrenia with lifetime incarceration or dangerousness. A psychotically depressed woman's family assumed that she could never be left alone for the rest of her life after a suicide attempt despite her full recovery with electroconvulsive therapy.

It is best to be as honest as possible. To co-operate with a demanding treatment regimen, the patient needs to acknowledge that his disorder is serious. The benefits of recognising and legitimising the patient's experiences and behaviour as 'an illness' cannot be over-emphasised. It can prevent attaching blaming and criticisms from family members which exacerbate the breakdown. It also reassures the patient that he is not the first to have these experiences and that the doctor knows what he is doing. Using terms such as 'paranoid schizophrenia' and 'manic depression', however, pose problems because of their loose and often stigmatising use in general speech.

I tell the patient and family that this is a 'psychiatric illness' and usually call it a psychotic disorder. I emphasise that there are treatments available and in the first instance these will rely on medicines to reduce anxiety and arousal. It is useful to underscore the relationship between stress and the breakdown and to emphasise that the patient may be experiencing this stress in a strange and unfamiliar way which means that he cannot recognise it. As well as medicines, he needs to take it a bit easier (e.g. stay off work or college, reduce contact with family members initially).

If the family insist on a label, then it is crucial to indicate the wide range of outcomes which are possible. It is important to be fairly optimistic at this stage, while acknowledging the impossibility of confident prediction.

Aetiology is rarely straightforward in psychotic illnesses. Most patients and families find it helpful to have an explanation of the process in terms of arousal and stress leading to chemical or neurotransmitter imbalance in the brain. It is still necessary to stress that child-rearing practices do not cause psychosis and that past individual events (no matter how dramatic) are unlikely to be truly causal.

Even in the first breakdown it is important to introduce the concept of maintenance treatment and wider psychosocial interventions. These are dealt with more fully by Strathdee and Kendrick and Kuipers (Chapters 18 and 19). Alluding to them, while acknowledging the central role of medication at the start of treatment, fosters engagement. A purely pharmacological approach to mental health problems is out of step with current social attitudes.

Use of the Mental Health Act

Compulsory admission for assessment of treatment of mental illness in England and Wales is governed by the Mental Health Act (1983). Section 2 or Section 4 of the Act can be applied where: '(a) the patient has a mental disorder (mental illness, arrested or incomplete development of mind, or psychopathic disorder) which warrants detention in hospital for assessment' and '(b) the patient should be so detained in the interests of his own health or safety or to protect other persons.'

The Act does not apply if there are viable alternatives to detention in hospital, or the patient agrees to go voluntarily. Applying a section should always be avoided if at all possible.

Section 2 (Admission for assessment for 28 days)

This is applied by the Approved Social Worker (ASW), on the recommendation of the consultant psychiatrist or other 'Section 12' approved doctor, and a second doctor who should preferably be a general practitioner with prior knowledge of the patient. No more than five days must elapse between the two doctors' examinations of the patient.

Section 4 (Admission in an emergency, for 72 hours)

This allows the general practitioner alone to admit the patient, but should be used only in a genuine emergency, where there is significant risk of immediate harm or a need for physical restraint, and where it is not possible, or there is not time, to obtain a second medical opinion. In the absence of the ASW, only the 'nearest relative' can make the application for admission under Section 4, and then only if they have seen the patient within 24 hours. The nearest relative is, in order of preference: the spouse (including common-law spouse after 6 months of cohabiting), oldest child, parent, oldest sibling, grandparent, grandchild, uncle or aunt, and nephew or niece. The patient must be seen by a Section 12 approved doctor within 72 hours.

The Act is different in Scotland, is soon to be amended and probably will be subject to widespread revision within the next few years. General practitioners, like psychiatrists, need to keep abreast of those parts which they regularly use. The ASW is invariably the most knowledgeable about the details of the Act and can easily be consulted by telephone.

Interpretation of the Act

The most common area of dispute when applying the Act is over interpretation of the idea of a 'risk to health'. This *does not* mean physical danger (which is only a requirement for an admission for assessment in an emergency, Section 4). It means any serious risk to the patient's health – including their mental health. It therefore includes continuation or deterioration of their psychosis if treatment is not started.

The decision to admit must balance the severity of the disorder (including distress to patient and carers as well as disorganised behaviour) and the likelihood that admission will help, against overriding the patient's express wishes and the distress and stigma that a compulsory admission can involve. Luckily, the approved social worker is specifically charged with protecting the patient's rights and exploring alternative solutions. As the general practitioner is likely to know the patient and his circumstances best, his contribution is particularly valuable in assessing the severity of the disorder and the risk to health imposed. The psychiatrist should, in consultation with the general practitoner, know more about the likelihood of inpatient care affecting the course of the illness.

Compulsory admissions are often fraught occasions with family distress, pressure from neighbours and the police, etc. Once the decision is made to admit, there is little achieved by prolonging the interview. The longer it goes on, the more exhausted and intolerant all involved may become. The general practitioner can often draw upon his acknowledged authority and established relationship with the patient in a way that the psychiatrist rarely can (Burns & Kendrick, 1994). It is important in these crisis situations to remember the longer-term perspective. A complete breakdown in the general practitioner–patient relationship is rare after such an admission. A brief visit to the ward to find out how a patient is doing can often serve to rebuild bridges.

Box 14.3 lists the important items to be carried in the doctor's night bag.

Medication

Tablets

Chlorpromazine 25 mg, haloperidol 1.5 mg, diazepam 5 mg, lorazepam 1 mg (tablets have a bag-life of around one year after dispensing, unless they are in blister packs, which may last up to five years).

Injections

Haloperidol 5 mg, diazepam 10 mg, procyclidine 10 mg (injections usually have a bag-life of around 2–3 years).

Section forms

Pink forms 5 and 7 should be carried in case Section 4 needs to be applied. The forms for Section 2 should be brought along by the duty ASW.

Telephone numbers

Duty ASW, duty consultant psychiatrist, police, ambulance.

British National Formulary

Always check the dose for any individual patient.

Box 14.3 *What to carry in the general practitioner's night bag.*

Conclusion

The average general practitioner will see a new case of psychosis only once every four to five years, and the care of patients with psychotic illnesses is unlikely to constitute more than a small proportion of his total mental health workload. These patients can, however, be a rewarding group with whom to work. Many of their needs fit well the style and approach of general practice – continuity over time, a family focus, a problem solving approach, short non-stressful consultations and ease of access.

Establishing effective liaison with the mental health services (Strathdee, 1988) should complement the established service offered by general practitioners, ensuring greater familiarity with the patient and with the relevant community mental health team. The results should be less anxiety associated with the inevitable crises and compulsory admissions which have traditionally dominated the general practitioner's view of psychosis. Greater job satisfaction should result from supporting and improving the quality of life of one of the most severely disabled groups in our society.

References

American Psychiatric Association (APA). (1994). *Diagnostic and Statistical Manual of Mental Disorders*. 4th edn. Washington DC: American Psychiatric Association.

Bridges, K. & Goldberg, D. (1985). Somatic presentations of DSM-3 psychiatric disorders in primary care. *Journal of Psychosomatic Research*, **29**, 563–9.

Burns, T. & Kendrick, T. (1994). Schizophrenia. In *Psychiatry and General Practice Today*. Pullen, I., Wilkinson, G., Wright, A. and Gray, P., eds. Royal College of Psychiatrists and Royal College of General Practitioners.

Done, D.J., Crow, T.J., Johnstone, E.C. & Sacker, A. (1994). Childhood antecedents of schizophrenia and affective illness: social adjustments at ages 7 and 11. *British Medical Journal*, **309**, 699–703.

Johnson, S. & Thornicroft, G. (1993). The sectorisation of psychiatric services in England and Wales. *Social Psychiatry and Psychiatric Epidemiology*, **28**, 45–7.

Johnstone, E.C., Crow, T.J., Johnson, A.L., & Macmillan, J.F. (1986). The Northwick Park study of first episodes of schizophrenia I: presentation of the illness and problems relating to admission. *British Journal of Psychiatry*, **148**, 115–20.

Kendrick, T. (1994). Fund-holding and commissioning general practitioners. *Psychiatric Bulletin*, **18**, 196–9.

Kendrick, T., Sibbald, B., Burns, T. & Freeling, P. (1991). Role of general practitioners in care of long-term mentally ill patients. *British Medical Journal*, **302**, 508–10.

Loebel, A.D., Lieberman, J.A., Alvir, J.M.J., Mayerhoff, D.I., Geisler, S.H. & Szymanski, S.R. (1992). Duration of psychosis and outcome in first-episode schizophrenia. *American Journal of Psychiatry*, **149**, 1183–88.

Melzer, D., Hale, A.S., Malik, S.J., Hogman, G.A. & Wood, S. (1991). Community care for patients with schizophrenia one year after hospital discharge. *British Medical Journal*, **303**, 1023–6.

Mental Health Act 1983, London: HMSO.

Murray-Parkes, C., Brown, G.W. & Monck, E.M. (1962). The general practitioner and the schizophrenic patient. *British Medical Journal*, **1**, 972–6.

Nazareth, I.D. & King, M.B. (1993). Controlled evaluation of management of schizophrenia in one general practice: A pilot study. *Family Practice*, **9**, 171–2.

Pantelis, C., Taylor, J. & Campbell, P. (1988). The South Camden Schizophrenia Survey. An experience of community-based research. *Bulletin of the Royal Colllege of Psychiatrists*, **12**, 98–101.

Sims, A. (1991). Even better services: a psychiatric perspective. *British Medical Journal*, **302**, 1061–3.

Strathdee, G. (1988). Psychiatrists in primary care: the general practitioner's viewpoint. *Family Practitioner*, **5**, 111–15.

Strathdee, G. & Williams, P. (1984). A survey of psychiatrists in primary care: the silent growth of a new service. *Journal of the Royal College of General Practitioners* **34**, 615–18.

Tyrer, P. (1984). Psychiatric clinics in general practice: an extension of community care. *British Journal of Psychiatry*, **145**, 9–14.

World Health Organisation (1992). *International Classification of Disease* (10th revision) (ICD 10). Geneva: WHO.

Part three

Limiting disability and preventing relapse

[15] Tertiary prevention of childhood mental health problems

Jeremy Turk

Introduction

The aims of tertiary prevention are to reduce the complications and disability associated with established disorders, particularly those which have become chronic. Thus tertiary prevention includes not only active intervention aimed at the presenting condition itself but also rehabilitation to reduce potential secondary problems (Henderson, 1988).

Tertiary prevention in child mental health relies heavily on the family; tight-knit extended families where the members are available to help each other are ideal. Parents also need ready access to comprehensive professional and welfare support in the community to help them cope with their children's disability.

Impairment, disability and handicap

Central to the concept of tertiary prevention is an understanding of the concepts of impairment, disability and handicap. The World Health Organisation International Classification distinguishes these three different levels of the consequences of disease. Impairment means loss or abnormality of psychological, physiological or anatomical structure or function – body parts or systems do not work. Disability is the resulting loss or restriction of the ability to perform an activity – the things people cannot do which they would normally be expected to do. Handicap is the disadvantage resulting from impairment or disability for a given individual, that limits or prevents the fulfilment of roles in life which would normally be achieved, taking into account age, sex and social and cultural factors.

Disability is a continuum. Hence prevalence rates depend on the chosen threshold of severity above which people are counted as disabled. Disabilities are usually chronic and multiple. Behavioural disabilities are most common in children. In Great Britain there are approximately 360 000 children under the age of 16 who have one or more disabilities (Bone & Meltzer, 1989). This figure represents just over 3% of all children, more boys than girls. Less than 2% of disabled children live in communal establishments.

Tertiary prevention strategies aim to minimise disability and prevent handicaps despite the persistence of impairment. Where the underlying impairment is well understood, then very specific medical interventions may be adopted to prevent the consequences. Thus dietary restriction of phenylalanine in phenylketonuria and thyroxine supplementation in congenital hypothyroidism prevent complications developing whilst the underlying metabolic abnormalities remain unaffected. In other conditions, however, the aetiology remains obscure or is multifactorial, for example, childhood depression. As well as medical treatment, tertiary prevention will therefore usually include psychological, educational, family and social aspects. Primary health care professionals need to be aware of what interventions are available for their young patients and their families, and will often be involved in these interventions themselves.

Preventive interventions – medical

Inborn errors of metabolism

Children with phenylketonuria or galactosaemia can be helped to develop normally by the early institution of restrictive diets minimising intake of the substrate which would otherwise accumulate at toxic levels (Hayes et al., 1988; Fishler et al., 1989). Dietary restriction in phenylketonuria is required well into adolescence to prevent slowing of cognitive development (Smith, Beasley & Ades, 1991). Blood phenylalanine levels are correlated with both intelligence and behaviour (Smith, Beasley & Ades, 1990). Mothers with phenylketonuria must also keep to strict low phenylalanine diets while pregnant to ensure normal fetal development (Drogari et al., 1987). Similarly, daily thyroxine supplementation prevents the adverse consequences of congenital hypothyroidism on intelligence (New England Collaborative, 1990), giving testosterone in Klinefelter syndrome improves behaviour in many cases (Nielsen, Pelsen & Stensen, 1988) and folic acid supplementation in children with fragile X syndrome may ameliorate the associated hyperactivity, poor concentration, and impulsive tendencies (Turk, 1992).

General practitioners and health visitors must be aware of the importance of continuing such diets or supplements and be willing to prescribe where necessary and to support parents in maintaining them for many years.

Hyperactivity

It is now clear that some children suffer from a specific central nervous system deficit in attentional skills (Zametkin & Rapoport,

1987) with a genetic basis (Goodman & Stevenson, 1989). It results in poor concentration, restlessness, fidgeting, and marked impulsiveness. Functional brain scanning has confirmed underperfusion of the frontal areas and corpus striatum in affected individuals (Lou *et al.*, 1989). The primary biologically determined features of the disorder are associated with secondary emotional and behavioural problems including low self-esteem, depression, conduct disorders and family relationship problems. Follow-up studies confirm that these children are at risk of later relationship difficulties, substance misuse and antisocial tendencies (Hechtman & Weiss, 1986).

A substantial body of literature supports the use of stimulants such as methylphenidate (Ritalin) and dexamphetamine (Dexedrine) in the treatment of children with hyperactivity and attention deficit disorders (Taylor, 1986). Controversy has surrounded the prescription of these medications in the United Kingdom despite their common usage in North America. General practitioners may be asked to prescribe under specialist supervision.

Early referral for specialist diagnosis of suspected hyperactivity is crucial to the institution of appropriate medical treatment as part of a therapeutic package including psychological, educational, and family interventions.

Parents may raise the issue of avoiding food additives in the prevention of childhood hyperactivity with general practitioners and health visitors. This may be of value occasionally but is usually a placebo effect (Taylor, 1984). Blind comparisons with a normal diet, and double-blind challenges, have yielded contradictory findings. However, single case studies do show a few children to behave much worse with additives than placebo. A sensible approach is to take note of ubiquitous dietary psychotropic agents such as caffeine. A sceptical but interested and supportive approach with parents is important to avoid the treadmill of progressively more distasteful diets. Be open regarding the likely lack of value, be willing to help evaluate effects of the diet and keep open the question of psychological treatments.

The issue of fad therapies is one for concern. Many are not without financial or physical risk to the child and family. The main deleterious effects are listed in Box 15.1.

Prevention of suicide

Adolescents with serious depressive conditions are at risk of attempted and completed suicide (Rao *et al.*, 1993). Primary health care professionals should be aware of the common variations in the presentation of depression in young people which contrast with adult depressive disorders (Box 15.2).

If assessment indicates mild depression as an appropriate reaction to circumstances, then all that is required may be regular meetings

Toxicity

Interference with better documented methods of therapy

Expense

Time

Alienation of the child

Family stress

Unrealistic raising of hope and expectations

Box 15.1 *Deleterious effects of fad therapies.*

Irritability and social withdrawal are particularly common.

Of young people with depressive disorders, 20% also have a conduct disorder.

Nearly 50% of young people with depressive disorders have anxiety.

Box 15.2 *Development variations in the manifestation of depression in young people.*

with child and parents, sympathetic discussion and encouraging support. However, severe depression accompanied by endogenous features (psychomotor retardation, diurnal mood variation, poor appetite, early morning waking) does not usually respond well to psychological interventions. In such cases antidepressant medication is indicated, even where there is an 'understandable' cause for the depression, though the research evidence for the efficacy of antidepressants in young people is at present inconclusive (Harrington, 1992).

Selective serotonin reuptake inhibitors (e.g. fluoxetine, fluvoxamine, paroxetine) are recommended because of their lack of cardiovascular side-effects. Exceptionally severe depression may require more traditional tricyclic antidepressants, lithium, or in-patient psychiatric treatment. Other problems such as impaired peer relationships, conduct problems and family difficulties must be tackled in conjunction with the above. Interest is growing in the possible use of cognitive psychotherapeutic approaches in depression (McAdam, 1986), eating disorders (Turk, 1993) and psychological disturbance more generally (Kendall, 1981).

Preventive interventions – educational

The cornerstone of effective educational provision for children with disabilities or chronic psychiatric problems, in order to prevent further problems from developing, is full assessment leading to a statement of special educational needs (the so-called 'statementing process'). This is outlined in the UK Education Act of 1981, and emphases the needs of each child rather than diagnostic labels.

Health Authorities have an obligation to notify the Local Education Authority (LEA) when they suspect a child may have special educational needs (SEN). The process of statementing should be a collaborative one between parents and professionals. Parents should be reminded that they have an important say in their child's school placement and that they should not feel themselves to be passive recipients of professional advice.

The 1993 Education Act and Code of Practice emphasise further the responsibility of every school ('special' or otherwise) to have a policy and service for their pupils with special educational needs for which they will have received a specific budgetary allowance and for which they will be accountable. Each school must have a special educational needs coordinator. In part, this is a response to the growing demand for children with disabilities and chronic disorders to be educated within mainstream schools. However, there is a noticeable change in the emphasis on statementing. The new Code of Practice has as one of its principles, that most children with special educational needs will be in mainstream schooling, with no statement. Furthermore many children with statements will be in mainstream schools as well (Bentley, Russell & Stobbs, 1994). Box 15.3 outlines the five-stage model of assessment and provision.

The timetable for assessment and statementing should not normally exceed 26 weeks. Where consensus between parents and professionals regarding assessments and statements is simply unobtainable, parents have the right of appeal to an SEN tribunal allowing a quick and independent review. A special educational needs guide for parents is available (Department for Education, 1994).

Early intervention

Early enrichment programmes (e.g. Head Start) can compensate for social deprivation and enhance cognitive development in individuals who would otherwise have mild learning disability. Their use in more severely disabled children is less clear. In these subjects the resulting changes in parental attitudes and expectations are probably of greater importance (Clarke & Clarke, 1986).

The Portage home intervention project has been the subject of much recent enthusiasm and service development in most districts

Stage 1
Class or subject teachers identify or register a child's special educational needs, and consulting the school's SEN coordinator take initial action

Stage 2
The school's SEN coordinator takes lead responsibility for gathering information and for coordinating the child's special educational provision, working with the child's teachers

Stage 3
Teachers and the SEN coordinator are supported by specialists from outside the school

Stage 4
The LEA considers the need for a statutory assessment and, if appropriate, makes a multidisciplinary assessment

Stage 5
The LEA considers the need for a statement of special educational needs and, if appropriate, makes a statement and arranges, monitors and reviews provision

Box 15.3 *The five-stage model of assessment and provision for children with special educational needs.*

(Shearer & Shearer, 1972). Weekly home visits allow joint professional and parent decisions regarding developmental short-term goals and training methods to be undertaken in the ensuing week by the parent. While attractive conceptually, the approach is not free from criticism. Evaluation studies have often been of poor design and benefits have proved difficult to confirm scientifically. Parental satisfaction remains high though.

Not surprisingly, it seems that the severity of disability is a major factor determining the outcome of early educational intervention (Guralnick, 1991). There is little or no discernible long-term effect on linguistic or cognitive skills of children with biologically determined learning disabilities such as Down's syndrome. However, positive spin-offs in terms of parental perceptions of support and feelings of receiving direction should not be underestimated.

Preventive interventions – psychological

Parental counselling and the breaking of bad news

Parental understanding of the nature and implications of their child's disability is crucial to the early acceptance and institution of appropriate remedial and preventive intervention. How bad news is shared and who does it are important issues. Parents want to be told the truth, however painful, and earlier rather than later. Time is essential and multiple meetings are required in order to combat the inevitable shock and denial (Cunningham, Morgan & McGrucken, 1984). Counselling by a well-informed person is essential. Both over- and under-optimism by the informant can be extremely upsetting in the longer term (Carr, 1985).

The term counselling describes a wide-ranging supportive approach whereby the professional assists the family in adjusting to its new and unexpected situation in a number of differing ways. Counselling has educational and psychotherapeutic components. In disability work the counsellor should have sufficient working knowledge of the disabling condition to help educate the family about the disorder's nature, its cause (if known) and its likely effects developmentally. Gaps in the family's knowledge need to be addressed and myths refuted. Contrary to earlier beliefs that a search for the cause of a child's disability was a sign of psychological non-acceptance, it is now acknowledged that awareness of the diagnosis and aetiology is of great importance both practically and psychologically (Box 15.4). In addition, the counselling must have psychotherapeutic benefit for the family.

Psychotherapeutic counselling (see Chapter 8) often involves non-directive support aimed at facilitating the family's task of reflecting on their predicament and developing their own

---

The individual and family's basic right to know.

Relief from uncertainty regarding cause of disabilities.

Facilitation of grief resolution.

Focusing towards the future.

Possible genetic counselling for the extended family.

Instigation of interventions relevant to strengths and needs.

Potential for identifying with, and belonging to, a support group.

Box 15.4 *Reasons for giving parents a diagnosis.*

perspective of their situation and how to cope with it. To be truly supportive, the counsellor must be a warm, genuine and understanding individual with an unconditional respect (even if not approval) for the family's stance. The ability to empathise, rather than just sympathise, describes an attempt to truly understand how the family must be feeling rather than merely expressing concern – to see how the world must look to them. Although the ventilation of feelings is important, this alone is usually not enough to facilitate change. Discussion must be directive as well – coaxing the family towards a problem-solving approach, whereby pathways to potential solutions to the difficulties they will face can be clarified and tested out.

An essential component of the counsellor's skills must be an understanding of the bereavement and grieving process. The family will tend to go through a series of psychological stages reflecting their grief at the loss of the anticipated idealised child and the arrival of the child with disabilities (Bicknell, 1983).

Denial is common and varies from a momentary inability to understand or acknowledge the news ('shock') to long-term refutation of the child's disabilities and needs. Subsequent protest and anger is often directed to the breaker of bad news but may also be directed against the self as guilt and depression with irrational self-blame for events seen as having contributed to the problem. Searching may be internal ('soul-searching') or more concrete, e.g. 'shopping around' for multiple professional opinions or trying out many fad therapies of dubious potential benefit. Usually these phases are replaced by the slow gaining of a new individual and family identity ('adaptation').

The phenomenon of 'chronic sorrow' has been recognised whereby any reminders of the disabled child's problems repeatedly rekindle grief feelings (Wikler, Wasow & Hatfield, 1981). Such events usually emphasise the child's differences from others, e.g. falling behind a younger sibling developmentally, needing a statement of special educational need, or returning to a dependent life at home after schooling.

In breaking bad news, messages need to be clear, brief, understandable and repeated. There must be ample time for the family to reflect and respond without the professional feeling they should be intervening ('therapeutic silences'). A follow-up written account of the discussion, factual information imparted, and practical details, e.g. of support groups and allowances, should be provided. Additionally, other involved professionals should be updated to prevent duplication of effort and maximise efficiency of multidisciplinary support. Hall, Hill & Elliman (1994) describe a useful checklist of important aspects relating to the breaking of bad news to parents regarding their child's disability (Box 15.5).

Parents want to be told:
- *as soon as professionals are suspicious*
- *in privacy*
- *without interruptions*
- *together, or with a grandparent or friend if an unsupported parent*
- *simply and slowly*
- *at least twice*
- *in writing as well as verbally*

Arrange a follow-up visit

Provide information on parent organisations or parent contact

Be a good counsellor

Listen for unspoken questions, e.g. regarding life expectancy or possible genetic implications

Offer practical advice on what the parents can do to help

Facilitate an appropriate second opinion if this is desired

Deal with other practical issues, e.g. education and immunisation, when parents want to discuss them

Understand the bereavement reaction but beware of the wide range of human responses to grief

Box 15.5 *Breaking bad news to parents regarding their child's disability.*

Psychological therapies

Psychological therapies may be one-to-one (individual) or with others (family, group). In addition their focus can be primarily one's feelings, conscious or otherwise (psychoanalytic), one's thoughts (cognitive), or one's actions (behavioural). These approaches are far from being mutually exclusive. Most psychotherapists use elements from more than one approach. There is good evidence that the therapist's personal attributes are as important as the school of philosophy he purports to belong to (Shapiro, 1969).

The importance of these approaches within tertiary prevention in child psychiatry arises from the predominance of psychological over physical treatment methods and the emphasis on family relationships and attitudes. They not only allow for, but rely on, involvement of the child's parents, siblings, caretakers, and teachers. These psychotherapeutic approaches are usually out-patient based. The aim is to preserve and enhance normal psycho-social development and to relieve suffering.

Individual psychoanalytic psychotherapy describes the well-established intensive one-to-one approach whereby the child meets alone with the therapist regularly over a long period of time. This approach is usually coupled with supportive work between mother and psychiatric social worker. It is usually saved for complex, longstanding emotional and personality difficulties due to its expense and the need for extremely frequent clinic attendances by both child and parent. Despite the relative paucity of outcome research, it is still a popular form of therapy. Individual psycho-therapy in fact covers a spectrum ranging from counselling to extensive transference work (Trowell, 1994).

Play therapy is a useful form of individual psychotherapy with young children (Axline, 1964). The application of many elements do not require extensive analytic training. The content of a child's play can give hints to preoccupations, anxieties, adverse experiences and family behaviour. The approach is non-directive and reflective. For this reason, more impulsive children and those with a low frustration tolerance may find it annoying and difficult to comply with. For more thoughtful young people, it can be a liberating experience to have the time and space to ponder import-ant issues with an individual sufficiently detached emotionally from the close family.

Projective techniques in individual psychotherapy are more com-plicated and directive. They rely on the interpretive abilities of the therapist. One such approach, the squiggle game, requires the therapist and child to draw a squiggle on paper and then elaborate it. The content of the child's resulting picture can then be used as a starting point for discussion.

Group psychotherapy in young people is reserved mainly for adolescents, especially those with social difficulties. It is a common form of therapy on inpatient psychiatric units. Just as important is the group structuring of the therapeutic milieu in inpatient and day patient units.

Family therapy has gained enormous popularity over the last few decades (Barker, 1986). The approach is frequently viewed as synonymous with child guidance and child psychiatry services. This is neither surprising nor necessarily inappropriate, given the family's status as the most important system within which the child lives. However, once again there is relatively little evidence for its efficacy or indications. Benefits have been found in the manage-ment of physical illness (asthma, diabetes, gastrointestinal prob-lems), eating disorders in pre-adolescence, and family relationship difficulties. There are a variety of schools of family therapy each with their gurus and followers. The more general principles of bringing all family members together to reflect on the problem, and to view the child as having a problem within the family rather than being a problem child in isolation, are of equal, if not greater, importance than the specifics of particular therapeutic schools.

Behavioural psychotherapy and behaviour modification programmes based on simple operant principles are some of the commonest and some of the best proven psychotherapeutic approaches available for young people (Hill, 1989). They are particularly applicable to the primary care setting, can be undertaken by parents, teachers, or youth workers, and are used extensively in inpatient and outpatient settings and residential facilities. With children, an obvious necessity is to invoke parents as cotherapists and to include some form of reinforcement schedule in the programme to maximise the child's co-operation.

In essence, behaviour modification approaches consist of the manipulation of positive or negative consequences of the child's behaviour in a systematic fashion in order to increase or decrease the frequency or intensity of that behaviour (Box 15.6). General principles include the continuing need to consider family, friends, teachers and important other people to the child. There has to be awareness of the child's developmental level as it affects understanding of the programme, age appropriateness of goals and rewards, and the need for the child to maintain a sense of dignity and control. Frequent readily attainable rewards are necessary, that can be easily withdrawn, as well as a specific personal programme, with understanding of what is making children do what they do in particular settings, at certain times and with specific people. This can be achieved through a functional analysis of behaviour using an 'ABC' chart (Kanfer & Saslow, 1965). This consists of three vertical columns labelled antecedents, behaviour, and consequences. By documenting the problem behaviour, common themes can be discerned and appropriate interventions developed (Box 15.6).

Examples of behavioural approaches with children include graded exposure and modelling for phobias. This approach, also known as systematic desensitisation (see Chapter 11), consists of a hierarchy of tasks of increasing difficulty which allow the individual to overcome the fear in a gradual stepwise fashion.

Exposure and response prevention for obsessive–compulsive disorders allows the young person to practise resisting the urge to think or do something, especially when in situations which aggravate the problem, for example conscious efforts not to shout out during quiet time in class, or sitting on one's hands to prevent fulfilling the urge to nail bite when anxious.

Alarms and dry bed training for enuresis are probably the most celebrated approaches, which will be very familiar to health visitors (see Chapter 9). Other commonly used behavioural techniques include shaping and training for skills building whereby successive

1. Define objectively which behaviours are problematic:
   (a) to the child
   (b) to the family

2. Prioritise these behaviours

3. Choose a behaviour likely to respond – not necessarily the most problematic

4. Undertake a functional analysis with comprehensive description of the behaviour (when, where, what, how, with whom), antecedents and consequences

5. Evolve a plan on the basis of the above findings for counteracting maladaptive behaviour and enhancing appropriate behaviours. Consider available methods of increasing and decreasing behaviours

6. Relate the above plan to each stage of the behavioural sequence in question

7. Ensure the plan is crystal clear to all involved. Ensure dissent can be voiced. Consider the practicality of the plan

8. Rate the response of the behaviour to intervention

9. React on the basis of trends over time – not individual events

10. Persist for a reasonable time considering possible reasons for success or failure

Box 15.6 *Steps in developing a behavioural programme.*

approximations to the desired behaviour are systematically re-inforced, and rapid exposure (flooding) with older adolescents and early school refusers. Relaxation and biofeedback for anxieties and panic attacks are more popular with older children.

The behavioural approach has proved to be one of the most successful of all for persistent nocturnal crying in babies (see Chapter 9). Removal of attention and reinforcement for nocturnal crying, including eye contact, hugs, kisses, and sweet drinks, coupled with regular checks to ensure the child's welfare, usually produces rapid and enduring extinction of the unwanted and troublesome behaviour.

Parental management training is an obvious extension of behavioural approaches, whereby the health professional tutors the

Advice to local education authorities on special educational needs

Advice to social services and courts on criminal and child protection matters including:
- *abuse*
- *advice on reception into care ('accommodation')*
- *adoption and fostering*
- *support for rehousing*

Box 15.7 *Important therapeutic environmental manipulations.*

parents in their efforts to become more proficient 'behavioural psychotherapists' with their offspring (Sutton, 1992).

Cognitive psychotherapy methods (see Chapter 17) are usually linked with behavioural approaches in for example, anger management, anxiety management, self-esteem building and impulse control ('stop and think'). Research evidence for benefits is sparse despite appreciation that very young children can benefit from help with underdeveloped, deficient or distorted cognitive strategies and constructs.

Environmental manipulation consists of the restructuring of the child's life environments. This approach is especially useful where problems are irremediable, and therefore has great relevance to tertiary preventative work. Environmental manipulations of particular note are listed in Box 15.7. Inpatient psychiatric admission for children and adolescents is usually reserved for intensive therapy or when it is impossible to contain the child at home.

Conclusions

The cornerstones of tertiary prevention must include:

(i) the early identification and evaluation of disturbance,
(ii) the early sharing of information with parents, while paying careful attention to the associated grief reaction,
(iii) the early instigation of a multidisciplinary therapy package including medical, psychological, educational and social components,
(iv) a nominated key worker who can develop a closeworking relationship with the child and family in order to help coordinate input and monitor progress.

Primary health care teams, in particular general practitioners and health visitors, need to be aware of what interventions modern multidisciplinary child mental health services can offer, and which children and families are likely to benefit. In addition primary health care professionals should be prepared to contribute to the long-term care and supervision of their young patients with established disabling conditions.

References

Axline, V. (1964). *Dibs: In Search of Self.* London: Gollancz.

Barker, P. (1986). *Basic Family Therapy.* London: Collins.

Bentley, A., Russell, P. & Stobbs, P. (1994). *An Agenda for Action.* London: National Children's Bureau.

Bicknell, J. (1983). The Psychopathology of Handicap. *British Journal of Medical Psychology*, **56**, 167–78.

Bone, M. & Meltzer, H. (1989). *The Prevalence of Disability among Children; OPCS. Surveys of Disability in Great Britain, report 3.* London: HMSO.

Carr, J. (1985). The effect on the family of a severely mentally handicapped child. In *Mental Deficiency: The Changing Outlook.* Clarke, A.M., Clarke, A.D.B. and Berg, J.M., eds. 4th edn. London: Methuen.

Clarke, A.M. & Clarke, A.D.B. (1986). Thirty years of child psychology: a selective review. *Journal of Child Psychology and Psychiatry*, **27**, 719–59.

Cunningham, C., Morgan, P. & McGrucken, R.B. (1984). Down syndrome: is dissatisfaction with disclosure of diagnosis inevitable? *Developmental Medicine and Child Neurology*, **26**, 33–9.

Department for Education (1994). *Special Educational Needs, A Guide for Parents.* London: HMSO.

Drogari, E., Smith, I., Beasley, M. & Lloyd, J.K. (1987). Timing of strict diet in relation to fetal damage in maternal phenylketonuria. *Lancet*, **ii**, 927–30.

Fishler, K., Azen, C.G., Friedman, E.G. & Koch, R. (1989). School achievement in treated PKU. children. *Journal of Mental Deficiency Research*, **33**, 493–98.

Goodman, R. & Stevenson, J. (1989). A twin study of hyperactivity-II. The aetiological role of genes, family relationships and perinatal adversity. *Journal of Child Psychology and Psychiatry*, **30**, 691–709.

Guralnick, M.J. (1991). The next decade of research on the effectiveness of early intervention. *Exceptional Children*, **58**, 174–83.

Hall, D., Hill, P. & Elliman, D. (1994). *The Child Surveillance Handbook.* Oxford: Radcliffe Medical Press.

Harrington, R. (1992). Annotation: the natural history and treatment of child and adolescent affective disorders. *Journal of Child Psychology and Psychiatry*, **33**, 1287–302.

Hayes, A., Bowling, F.G., Fraser, D., Krimmer, H.L., Marrinan, A. & Clague, A.E. (1988). Neonatal screening and an intensive management programme for galactosaemia: early evidence of benefits. *Medical Journal of Australia*, **149**, 21–5.

Hechtman, L. & Weiss, G. (1986). Controlled prospective fifteen year follow-up of hyperactives as adults: non-medical drug and alcohol use and anti-social behaviour. *Canadian Journal of Psychiatry*, **31**, 557–67.

Henderson, A.S. (1988). *An Introduction to Social Psychiatry*. Oxford: Oxford Medical Publications.

Hill, P. (1989). Behavioural psychotherapy with children. *International Review of Psychiatry*, **1**, 257–66.

Kanfer, F.H. & Saslow, G. (1965). Behavioral analysis – an alternative to diagnostic classification. *Archives of General Psychiatry*, **12**, 529–38.

Kendall, P.C. (1981). Cognitive–behavioral interventions with children. In: *Advances in Clinical Child Psychology*, vol 4. Lahey, B.B. and Kazdin, A.E., eds. New York: Plenum Press.

Lou, H.C., Henriksen, L., Bruhn, P., Borner, H. & Nielsen, J.B. (1989). Striatal dysfunction in attention deficit and hyperkinetic disorder. *Archives of Neurology*, **46**, 48–52.

McAdam, E.K. (1986). Cognitive behaviour therapy and its application with adolescents. *Journal of Adolescence*, **9**, 1–15.

New England Congenital Hypothyroidism Collaborative (1990). Elementary school performance of children with congenital hypothyroidism. *Journal of Pediatrics*, **116**, 27–32.

Nielsen, J., Pelsen, B. & Srensen, K. (1988). Follow-up of 30 Klinefelter males treated with testosterone. *Clinical Genetics*, **33**, 262–9.

Rao, U., Weissman, M.M., Martin, J.A. & Hammond, R.W. (1993). Childhood depression and risk of suicide: preliminary report of a longitudinal study. *Journal of the American Academy of Child and Adolescent Psychiatry*, **32**, 21–7.

Shapiro, A.D. (1969). Empathy warmth and genuineness in psychotherapy. *British Journal of Social and Clinical Psychology*, **8**, 350–61.

Shearer, M. & Shearer, D.E. (1972). The Portage project: a model for early childhood education. *Exceptional Children*, **36**, 210–17.

Smith, I., Beasley, M. & Ades, A.E. (1990). Intelligence and quality of dietary treatment in phenylketonuria. *Archives of Disease in Childhood*, **65**, 472–8.

Smith, I., Beasley, M. & Ades, A.E. (1991). Effect on intelligence of relaxing low phenylalanine diet on phenylketonuria. *Archives of Disease in Childhood*, **66**, 311–16.

Sutton, C. (1992). Training parents to manage difficult children. *Behavioural Psychotherapy*, **20**, 115–39.

Taylor, E. (1984). Diet and behaviour. *Archives of Disease in Childhood*, **59**, 97–8.

Taylor, E.A. (1986). Childhood hyperactivity. *British Journal of Psychiatry*, **149**, 562–73.

Trowell, J. (1994). Individual and group psychotherapy. In *Child and Adolescent Psychiatry: Modern Approaches* Rutter, M., Taylor, E. and Hersov, L., eds. Oxford: Blackwell Scientific.

Turk, J. (1992). Fragile X syndrome and folic acid. In *1992 International Fragile X Conference Proceedings*. Hagerman, R.J. and McKenzie, P., eds. pp. 195–200. Dillon, Colorado: Spectra Publishing.

Turk, J. (1993). Cognitive approaches to the treatment of eating disorders in children. In *Childhood Onset Anorexia Nervosa and Related Eating Disorders*. Lask, B. and Bryant-Waugh, R., eds. pp. 177–190. Hove: Lawrence Erlbaum.

Turk, J., Hagerman, R.J., Barnicoat, A. & McEvoy, J. (1994). The fragile X syndrome. In *Mental Health and Mental Retardation – Recent Advances and Practices*. Bouras, N., ed. pp. 135–153. Cambridge: Cambridge University Press.

Wikler, L., Wasow, M. & Hatfield, E. (1981). Chronic sorrow revisited: parent vs. professional depiction of the adjustment of parents of mentally retarded children. *American Journal of Orthopsychiatry*, **51**, 63–70.

Zametkin, A.J. & Rapoport, J.L. (1987). Neurobiology of attention deficit disorder with hyperactivity: where have we come in 50 years? *Journal of the American Academy of Child and Adolescent Psychiatry*, **26**, 676–86.

[16] Tertiary prevention: longer-term drug treatment in depression

Eugene Paykel

Longer-term outcome in depression

With modern treatment, the immediate outcome of episodes of depression is relatively good. Follow-up studies show that most patients improve considerably within a few months of presentation, although in a proportion remission is delayed or there are residual symptoms and a small number of patients remain severely ill and treatment resistant. It takes some years before longer term outcome can be evaluated after introduction of therapeutic advances. The antidepressants came into use just before the beginning of the 1960s, and for some time it was the good short term outcome that was most apparent. However in recent years it has become apparent that the longer-term outcome beyond immediate remission is far less satisfactory.

Relapse or recurrence?

It has become customary in the literature to distinguish between early and late symptom return (Frank *et al.*, 1991). The term *relapse* is used for an early return of symptoms, within the first six to nine months. This can plausibly be seen as return of the original episode in which the symptoms have been suppressed by treatment, but the underlying biological process may not have recovered. The term *recurrence* is used to describe later symptom return which it is assumed represents occurrence of a new episode. The distinction, although useful, is not hard and fast.

Psychiatric follow-up studies

There have been many short-term and longer-term follow-up studies in depression (Coryell & Winokur, 1992). Many are out of date in that they antedate modern treatment. In a widely quoted short-term follow-up under modern treatment conditions, involving subjects from a large American collaborative study, 63% of patients recovered within the first four months, although 26% still had not done so at one year (Keller *et al.*, 1982*a*). However, 24% of recovered patients relapsed within three months of recovery and 30% within a year (Keller *et al.*, 1982*b*). In a recent follow-up in Cambridge of a more representative sample (Ramana *et al.*, 1995), 45% of the sample had remitted within three months of initial interview and 70% within six months. However, 40% of those who remitted relapsed in the next ten months.

Another problem which emerges in these studies is that of *partial remission* with residual symptoms which persist and fluctuate, causing considerable disability and family problems. In a Cambridge follow-up study, residual symptoms were present at remission in 32% of the sample. These subjects showed a very high relapse rate in the next ten months, of 76% (Paykel *et al.*, 1995). This ominous prognostic significance has also been found in another naturalistic study (Faravelli *et al.*, 1986), in follow-up studies of cognitive therapy and in drug discontinuation trials.

Longer-term studies confirm these problems. In two recent follow-up studies over approximately 16 years (Lee & Murray 1988; Kiloh, Andrews & Neilson, 1988) approximately 60% of subjects were readmitted at least once. Among those not readmitted, 20% showed either mild–moderate chronic illness, or very slow recovery from the index episode. Overall, between 11% and 25% showed very poor outcomes with chronic severe disorder and handicaps. Suicide and other mortality rates were increased. In a similar 12-year follow-up from Edinburgh (Surtees & Barkley, 1994), findings were comparable, as they were in a similar Canadian study (Lehmann *et al.*, 1988).

These were all studies of psychiatrically treated samples, usually admitted to hospital, and often from referral centres in which more resistant cases might be treated. Studies in general practice would be more representative and might show a better outcome. Unfortunately, there have been few follow-up studies. In a three and a half-year study from The Netherlands (Ormel *et al.*, 1993), there was substantial improvement but residual symptoms and disability were common.

Predicting chronicity

In follow-up studies, chronicity has been found to be associated with longer prior illness, personality neuroticism, a positive family history, and female sex (Paykel, Klerman & Prusoff, 1974; Keller *et al.*, 1986; Weissman, Prusoff & Klerman, 1978; Hirschfeld *et al.*, 1986; Scott, Barker & Eccleston, 1988; Scott, 1988). Relapse has been found related to occurrence of stressful life events and absence of social support in the follow-up period (Paykel & Cooper, 1992), high expressed emotion, (Vaughn & Leff, 1976; Hooley, Orley & Teasdale, 1986, and see Chapter 19); older age of onset and more previous episodes (Keller *et al.*, 1983).

Implications for prevention

These findings on follow-up raise the importance of longer-term drug treatment in tertiary prevention of relapse, recurrence and disability. This chapter will focus on unipolar depression and on use of antidepressants, since these are the common situations in general practice. The chapter by Scott (see Chapter 17) in this volume deals with psychological therapies in unipolar disorder, and they will not be discussed here. Patients with bipolar disorder (the modern term for manic depressive disorder) also show a particularly recurrent course in long-term follow-up studies (Coryell & Winokur, 1992). Many do well on lithium but a proportion do not. Although it is less common than unipolar depression, the disability associated with this disorder can be very great.

Longer-term controlled trials of antidepressants

Continuation and maintenance treatments

Parallel to the distinction between relapse and recurrence it has now become customary to distinguish two kinds of longer-term drug treatment in depression. The term *continuation treatment* is used to refer to continuation of antidepressants for periods of the order of six months after acute treatment, to prevent relapse. The term *maintenance treatment* refers to longer drug therapy to prevent recurrence. There is strong evidence for the benefit of antidepressants in long-term use.

Table 16.1 summarises controlled trials of antidepressants in continuation therapy. The key studies were published mainly in the 1970s and examined, in depressives responding to initial treatment, the effects on early relapse of continuation of tricyclic antidepressant for approximately six months, as opposed to its early withdrawal. Further studies were carried out in the 1980s, including studies of monoamine oxidase inhibitors. All the studies showed that high relapse rates in patients withdrawn early from antidepressants were substantially reduced (halved or better) by continuing for at least six months.

Table 16.2 sets out comparisons of maintenance of antidepressants and placebo in longer-term controlled trials for prevention of recurrence published up to 1993. More studies of newer drugs have been undertaken since. Most of the studies have shown considerable benefit from antidepressants, although recurrence rates have sometimes nevertheless been substantial. Antidepressants found superior to placebo in the Table include imipramine, maprotiline, dothiepin, phenelzine, zimeldine, fluoxetine, and sertraline. Probably all the antidepressants which produce remission also produce long-term benefit, so the choice depends on what has produced acute benefit in this patient.

Some caveats are required. Most of these studies were carried out in patients who had responded to the acute treatment with the antidepressant in question. Hence the studies had selected those particularly likely to benefit from further treatment and to experience symptom return when it was withdrawn. Also, many of the maintenance trials have been carried out in patients who have already had previous recurrences and who are known therefore to have a high likelihood of further attacks. The studies therefore exaggerate the recurrence rates to be expected. Trials in less selected samples might not show as much benefit.

How long should treatment continue?

The optimal length of treatment is not proven by these studies. This really requires comparison of withdrawal at different time points after recovery. It has become a general recommendation that routine continuation after response should be for about six months, and this corresponds to the length of most studies. A recent United States recommendation has been for four months after complete remission of all symptoms (Prien, 1992). This is based on evidence that there are high rates of relapse when drugs are withdrawn in the presence of residual symptoms (Mindham, Howland & Shepherd, 1973; Prien & Kupfer, 1986; Georgotas & McCue, 1989).

Study	Drug	Relapse rate Placebo	Relapse rate Drug
Discontinuation designs			
Tricyclics			
Mindham et al., 1973	Amitriptyline/ Imipramine	50%	22%
Klerman et al., 1974; Paykel et al., 1975	Amitriptyline	29%	12%
Coppen et al., 1978	Amitriptyline	31%	0%
Stein, Rickels & Weisse, 1980	Amitriptyline	69%	28%
Prien, Klett & Caffey, 1973	Imipramine Lithium	73%	32% 30%
Prien et al., 1984	Amitriptyline	38%	5%
Prien & Kupfer, 1986	Lithium Imipramine and lithium	38%	11%
MAO inhibitors			
Davidson & Raft, 1984	Phenelzine	100%	14%
Harrison et al., 1986	Phenelzine	100%	20%

Table 16.1 *Controlled trials of antidepressant continuation in prevention of relapse*

For longer-term maintenance in those who require it, the evidence is less clear. Some patients may require very lengthy or indefinite maintenance. Kupfer *et al.* (1992) found, in highly recurrent patients, that withdrawal of imipramine after as long as three years was followed by high recurrence rates, which were markedly reduced by continuing the maintenance treatment.

Study	Drug	Relapse rate Placebo	Relapse rate Drug
Tricyclics			
Prien et al., 1973	Imipramine	85%	20%
	Lithium		14%
Prien et al., 1984	Imipramine	71%	41%
	Lithium		57%
	Combination		31%
Kane et al., 1982[b]	Imipramine	83%	100%
	Lithium		29%
	Combination		13%
Glen, Johnson & Shepherd, 1984	Amitriptyline	89%	50%
	Lithium		42%
Rouillon et al., 1989	Maprotiline 75 mg	35%	16%
	Maprotiline 37.5 mg		24%
Georgotas & McCue, 1989[b]	Nortiptyline	63%	54%
	Phenelzine		13%
Frank et al., 1990	Imipramine	78%	22%
	Interpersonal psychotherapy		64%
	Combination		24%
Old Age Depression Interest Group, 1993	Dothiepin	61%	40%
MAO inhibitors			
Georgotas & McCue, 1989	Phenelzine (see above)		
Robinson et al., 1991	Phenelzine 60 mg	81%	26%
	Phenelzine 45 mg		33%
Newer drugs			
Bjork, 1983	Zimeldine	84%	32%
Montgomery et al., 1988	Fluoxetine	57%	26%
Doogan & Caillard, 1992	Sertraline	41%	8%

[a] Length 1–3 years.
[b] No significant difference.

Table 16.2 *Maintenance trials of antidepressants in prevention of recurrence published up to 1993* [a]

Lithium and other drugs

Unipolar depression

Lithium has been shown to be superior to placebo in maintenance treatment of unipolar depressives (Baastrup et al., 1970; Coppen et al., 1971; Prien et al., 1973; Fieve, Kumbaraci & Dunner, 1976; Kane et al., 1982). Most of the studies have been in the long-term treatment of severely ill hospitalised patients, and it does have a place in such patients, particularly where antidepressant maintenance has failed to control the disorder. In practice, this decision is likely to be taken by the hospital clinic. The much more common situation in general practice is of long-term maintenance use of the antidepressant which has produced acute remission.

Bipolar depression

There have been numerous controlled trials of lithium in bipolar disorder. The evidence that it acts prophylactically to produce substantial reductions in recurrence rates is very strong and well established (Abou-Saleh, 1992; Prien, 1992).

Carbamazepine

Some patients respond only partially or not at all to lithium maintenance. Estimates of this proportion vary, depending on the setting. There is now an established role for carbamazepine in bipolar disorder. A number of controlled trials have shown benefit (Post, 1992). The effects appear to be less dramatic than for lithium, and carbamazepine is more often used as an adjunct, added to lithium, than alone.

Valproate

A more recent recruit to bipolar therapeutics is another anticonvulsant, sodium valproate. There are fewer controlled trials as yet, but overall the evidence of benefit is persuasive (Post, 1992). Because of side-effects, this is a third-line drug, after carbamazepine.

Other drugs

Antidepressants must be used with care in bipolar disorder. They are of benefit, and are often required in depressed bipolars, but they run the risk of precipitating mania (Paykel, 1994). Tricyclics may be particularly prone to precipitate rapid cycling, although the evidence is not conclusive. Antidepressants should therefore be used with cover by lithium. Monoamine oxidase inhibitors may be preferable, although there is not good evidence. Neuroleptics may also be of benefit in resistant bipolars, since they do not precipitate depression and may help to control mood elevation. They should, however, be avoided where possible because of the risks of

---

Unipolar disorder
   Antidepressants
      Tricyclic and related drugs
      Selective serotonin reuptake inhibitors
      Monoamine oxidase inhibitors
      Other newer antidepressants
   Lithium

Bipolar disorder
   Lithium
   Anticonvulsants
      Carbamazepine
      Sodium valproate

Box 16.1 *Drugs used in the longer-term treatment of depression.*

producing tardive dyskinesia. Drugs used in the longer-term treatment of depression are listed in Box 16.1.

Clinical guidelines

A number of clinical guidelines have been published in recent years, and these assist in the formulation of recommendations for longer-term drug treatment in general practice (Paykel & Priest, 1992; Prien, 1992). The recommendations are summarised in Box 16.2.

Continuation treatment
   Continue acute antidepressant treatment for four to six months after the symptoms have completely remitted, before reducing the dose
   Withdraw slowly, over a further two months
   If symptoms recur, resume the full dose, for a further nine to twelve months

Maintenance treatment
   Indicated for a history of several recurrences, especially if severe
   Discuss with the patient and the family where appropriate
   The decision should usually involve a psychiatrist
   Treatment should usually be for three years for unipolar depression and five years for bipolar depression, before trying a gradual withdrawal.

Box 16.2 *Clinical guidelines for the longer term use of antidepressants.*

Continuation treatment

Continuation of an antidepressant after acute response is now well established as routine in psychiatric practice. It should also be the usual routine in general practice, unless there is persuasive evidence that the response is non-pharmacological, e.g. occurring on very low dose, developing very early after treatment commencement, or closely related in timing and context to reversal of a major stress, e.g. where partners in a broken relationship have been united. Continuation is particularly important where there has been partial remission with residual symptoms, or a history of previous relapse or recurrence, but should not be limited to these situations.

As a general rule the *dose* used for continuation should initially be the same as that which has produced acute response. After two to three months this may be reduced if side-effects are a problem, but the reduction should be by only a small amount, as there is a risk of symptom return if blood levels become too low.

The usual *length* of an antidepressant course before the commencement of withdrawal should be about six months after response. The patient should also have been free of residual symptoms for four months. Withdrawal is then better carried out slowly, over two months, to minimise the risk of relapse. There is also an occasional physiological withdrawal syndrome on stopping tricyclics, probably due to loss of the atropinic effect which is a side-effect and manifesting in malaise, coryza-like symptoms and diarrhoea. This only occurs on very abrupt stopping from comparatively high doses, is easily reversed by restarting the drug, and should not be confused with symptom return.

Treatment of relapse

In some patients, withdrawal will be followed by return of depressive symptoms. Where withdrawal has been slow, this may sometimes occur while the patient is still on a low dose. This phenomenon usually does reflect a genuine relapse, and if symptoms persist, is an indication for resumption of full dose, followed by continuation for a further period of nine months to a year. Some of these patients relapse again on later drug withdrawal, and become candidates for long-term maintenance.

Maintenance treatment

Longer-term maintenance is indicated where there have been several recurrences, particularly if recent. Various recommendations for initiating maintenance have been formulated, such as two episodes in two years or three episodes in five years (Prien, 1992). This will also depend on the severity of episodes, whether they are long in the past or recent, their potential impact on the patient's personal life, family life and career, which can vary at different points in the life cycle, and the patient's own views and willingness to commit himself or herself to prolonged drug treatment. Discussion is required with the patient and where appropriate the family, and a joint decision is appropraite. This is a point at which a psychiatric opinion will also be valuable.

In bipolar disorder, which is more often recurrent and can wreck the patient's personal life through the disinhibition accompanying mania, the threshold will be lower. There is a case for at least relatively short-term maintenance following a single episode of mania, if admission has been required.

For most unipolar depressives the maintenance treatment choice will be an antidepressant; for most bipolars, lithium. Again, therapeutic doses of antidepressant are required, of the same order as those needed for acute treatment in the particular patient. The length of maintenance is harder to specify, as it depends on the previous history, but it will usually be at least three years for unipolars and five years for bipolars, and it will often be longer. Unless there is clear evidence from previous history that further recurrence has followed drug withdrawal, withdrawal should be tried at some point. Withdrawal of antidepressants, lithium, or other drugs after long-term maintenance should always be gradual. Some unipolars and many bipolars will require lifetime maintenance.

Compliance

Patients are often understandably reluctant to take drugs long-term. There are many studies documenting poor compliance in depression, as in many other psychiatric and physical disorders. Patients commonly fear the addictive potential of psychotropic drugs, often confusing antidepressants with benzodiazepines. Tricyclic antidepressants and lithium do not produce pleasant feelings, other than the relief of mood disorder in those who suffer from it. Most people who take them do not like their side-effects and prefer to be off them. The absence of any street market is the most persuasive evidence of their absence of addictive potential.

Studies of compliance in general indicate that the best results are where patients are well informed, able to make their own judgements, and have a good relationship and therapeutic alliance with the prescribing doctor. Drugs are not the whole treatment for depression. Psychosocial, psychotherapeutic and cognitive therapies are also important (see Chapter 17). These do not usually substitute for antidepressants but supplement them, producing benefit in personal adaptation which antidepressants cannot, and assisting symptom remission and avoidance of relapse where antidepressants are incompletely effective.

290   E. PAYKEL

References

Abou-Saleh, M.T. (1992). Lithium. In *Handbook of Affective Disorders*. Paykel, E.S., ed. 2nd edn. pp. 369–385. Edinburgh: Churchill Livingstone.

Baastrup, P.C., Poulsen, J.C., Schou, M., Thomsen, K. & Amdisen A. (1970). Prophylactic lithium: double blind discontinuation in manic-depressive and recurrent-depressive disorders. *Lancet*, **ii**, 326–30.

Bjork, K. (1983). The efficacy of zimeldine in preventing depressive episodes in recurrent major depressive disorders – a double blind placebo-controlled study. *Acta Psychiatrica Scandinavica*, **68**, 182–9.

Coppen, A., Noguera, R., Bailey, J., Burns, B.H., Swani, M.S., Hare, E.H., Gardner, R. & Maggs, R. (1971). Prophylactic lithium in affective disorders. *Lancet*, **ii**, 275–9.

Coppen, A., Ghose, K., Montgomery, S., Rao, V.A.R., Bailey, J. & Jorgensen A. (1978). Continuation therapy with amitriptyline in depression. *British Journal of Psychiatry*, **133**, 28–33.

Coryell, W. & Winokur, G. (1992). Course and outcome. In *Handbook of Affective Disorders*. Paykel, E.S., ed. 2nd edn. pp. 89–108. Edinburgh: Churchill Livingstone.

Davidson, J. & Raft, D. (1984). Use of phenelzine in continuation therapy. *Neuropsychobiology*, **11**, 191–4.

Doogan, D.P. & Caillard, V. (1992). Sertraline in the prevention of depression. *British Journal of Psychiatry*, **160**, 217–22.

Faravelli, C., Ambonetti, A., Pallanti, S. & Pazzagli, A. (1986). Depressive relapses and incomplete recovery from index episode. *American Journal of Psychiatry*, **143**, 888–91.

Fieve, R.R., Kumbaraci, T. & Dunner, D.L. (1976). Lithium prophylaxis of depression in bipolar I, bipolar II and unipolar patients. *American Journal of Psychiatry*, **133**, 925–9.

Frank, E., Kupfer, D.J., Perel, J.M., Cornes, C., Jarrett, D.B., Maccinger, A.G., Thase, M.E., McEachran, A.B. & Grochocinski, V.J. (1990). Three year outcomes for maintenance therapies of recurrent depression. *Archives of General Psychiatry*, **47**, 1093–99.

Frank, E., Prien, R.F., Jarrett, R.B., Keller, M.B., Kupfer, D.J., Lavori, P.W., Rush, A.J. & Weissman M.M. (1991). Conceptualisation and rationale for consensus definitions of terms in major depressive disorder. Remission, recovery, relapse and recurrence. *Archives of General Psychiatry*, **48**, 851–5.

Georgotas, A. & McCue, R.E. (1989). Relapse of depressed patients after effective continuation therapy. *Journal of Affective Disorders*, **17**, 159–64.

Glen, A.I.M., Johnson, A. I. & Shepherd, M. (1984). Continuation therapy with lithium and amitriptyline in unipolar depressive illness: a randomised double-blind controlled trial. *Psychological Medicine*, **14**, 37–50.

Harrison, W., Rabkin, J., Steward, J.W., McGrath, P.J., Tricamo, E. & Quitkin, F. (1986). Phenelzine for chronic depression: a study of continuation treatment. *Journal of Clinical Psychiatry*, **47**, 346–9.

Hirschfeld, R.M.A., Klerman, G.L., Andreasen, N.C., Clayton, P.J. & Keller, M.B. (1986). Psycho-social predictors of chronicity in depressed patients. *British Journal of Psychiatry*, **148**, 648–54.

Hooley, J.M., Orley, J. & Teasdale, J.D. (1986). Levels of expressed emotion and relapse in depressed patients. *British Journal of Psychiatry*, **148**, 642–7.

Kane, J.M., Quitkin, F., Rifkin, A., Ramos-Lorenzi, J.R., Nayak, D.P. & Howard, A. (1982). Lithium carbonate and imipramine in the prophylaxis of unipolar and bipolar II illness. *Archives of General Psychiatry*, **39**, 1065–9.

Keller, M.B., Shapiro, R.W., Lavori, P.W. & Wolfe, N. (1982a). Recovery in major depressive disorder: analysis with the life table and regression models. *Archives of General Psychiatry*, **39**, 905–10.

Keller, M.B., Shapiro, R.W., Lavori, P.W. & Wolfe, N. (1982b). Relapse in major depressive disorder: analysis with the life table. *Archives of General Psychiatry*, **39**, 911–15.

Keller, M.B., Lavori, P.W., Lewis, C.E. & Klerman, G.L. (1983). Predictors of relapse in major depressive disorder. *Journal of the American Medical Association*, **250**, 3299–304.

Keller, M.B., Lavori, P.W., Rice, J.P., Coryell, W. & Hirschfeld, R.M.A. (1986). The persistent risk of chronicity in recurrent episodes of nonbipolar major depressive disorder: a prospective follow-up. *American Journal of Psychiatry*, **143**, 24–8.

Kiloh, L.G., Andrews, G. & Neilson, M. (1988). The long term outcome of depressive illness. *British Journal of Psychiatry*, **153**, 752–7.

Klerman, G.L., DiMascio, A., Weissman, M.M., Prusoff, B. & Paykel, E.S. (1974). Treatment of depression by drugs and psychotherapy. *American Journal of Psychiatry*, **131**, 186–91.

Kupfer, D.J., Frank, E., Perel, J.M., Cornes, C., Mallinger, A.G., Thase, M.E., McEachran, A.B. & Grochocinski, V.J. (1992). Five-year outcome for maintenance therapies in recurrent depression. *Archives of General Psychiatry*, **49**, 769–73.

Lee, A.S. & Murray, R.M. (1988). The long-term outcome of Maudsley depressives. *British Journal of Psychiatry*, **153**, 741–51.

Lehmann, H.E., Fenton, R.R., Deutch, M., Feldman, S. & Engelsmann, F. (1988). An 11-year follow-up study of 110 depressed patients. *Acta Psychiatrica Scandinavica*, **78**, 57–65.

Mindham, R.H., Howland, C. & Shepherd, M. (1973). An evaluation of continuation therapy with tricyclic antidepressants in depressive illness. *Psychological Medicine*, **3**, 5–17.

Montgomery, S.A., Dufour, H., Brion, S., Gailledreau, J., Laqueille, X., Ferrey, G., Moron, P., Parant-Lucena, N., Singer, L., Danion, J.M., Beuzen, J.N. & Pierredon, M.A. (1988). The prophylactic efficacy of fluoxetine in unipolar depression. *British Journal of Psychiatry*, **153**, 69–76.

Old Age Depression Interest Group (1993). How long should the elderly take antidepressants? A double blind placebo-controlled study of continuation/prophylaxis therapy with dothiepin. *British Journal of Psychiatry*, **162**, 175–82.

Ormel, J., Oldenhiknel, T., Brilman, E. & van den Brink, W. (1993). Outcome of depression and anxiety in primary care: a three wave 3½ year study of psychopathology and disability. *Archives of General Psychiatry*, **50**, 759–66.

Paykel, E. S. (1994). The place of antidepressants in long-term treatment. In *Psychopharmacology of Depression*. Montgomery, S. A. and Corn, T. H., eds. pp. 218–239. Oxford: Oxford University Press.

Paykel, E.S. & Cooper Z. (1992) Life events and social support. In *Handbook of Affective Disorders*. Paykel, E. S., ed. pp. 149–170. Edinburgh: Churchill Livingstone.

Paykel, E.S., Klerman, G.L. & Prusoff, B.A. (1974). Prognosis of depression and the endogenous-neurotic distinction. *Psychological Medicine*, **4**, 47–64.

Paykel, E.S., DiMascio, A., Haskell, D. & Prusoff, B.A. (1975). Effects of maintenance amitriptyline and psychotherapy on symptoms of depression. *Psychological Medicine*, **5**, 67–77.

Paykel, E.S., Ramana R., Cooper Z., Hayhurst H., Kerr J. & Barocka A. (1995). Residual symptoms after partial remission: an important outcome in depression. *Psychological Medicine*, **25**, 1171–80.

Post, P.M. (1992). Anticonvulsants and novel drugs. In *Handbook of Affective Disorders*. Paykel, E. S., ed. 2nd edn., pp. 387–417. Edinburgh: Churchill Livingstone.

Prien, R.F. (1992). Maintenance treatment. In *Handbook of Affective Disorders*. Paykel, E.S., ed. 2nd edn. pp. 419–435. Edinburgh: Churchill Livingstone.

Prien, R.F. & Kupfer D.J. (1986). Continuation drug therapy for major depressive episodes: how long should it be maintained? *American Journal of Psychiatry*, **143**, 18–23.

Prien, R.F., Klett C.H. & Caffey E.M. (1973). Lithium carbonate and imipramine in prevention of affective episodes. *Archives of General Psychiatry*, **29**, 420–5.

Prien, R.F., Kupfer, D.J., Mansky, P.A., Small, J.G., Tuason, V.B., Voss, C.B. & Johnson, W.E. (1984). Drug therapy in the prevention of recurrences in unipolar and bipolar affective disorders. *Archives of General Psychiatry*, **41**, 1096–104.

Ramana, R., Paykel, E.S., Cooper, Z., Hayhurst, H., Saxty, M. & Surtees, P.G. (1995). Remission and relapse in major depression: a two year prospective follow-up study. *Psychological Medicine*, **25**, 1161–70.

Robinson, D.S., Lerfald, S.C., Bennett, B., Laux, D., Devereux, E., Kayser, A., Corcella, J. & Albright, D. (1991). Continuation and maintenance treatment of major depression with the monoamine oxidase inhibitor phenelzine: a double-blind placebo-controlled discontinuation study. *Psychopharmacology Bulletin*, **27**, 31–9.

Rouillon, F., Phillips, R., Serrurier, D., Ansart, E. & Gerard, M.J. (1989). Rechutes de dépression unipolaire et efficacité de la maprotiline. *L'Encéphale*, **15**, 527–34.

Scott, J. (1988). Chronic depression. *British Journal of Psychiatry*, **153**, 287–97.

Scott, J., Barker, W.A. & Eccleston, D. (1988). The Newcastle Chronic Depression Study: patient characteristics and factors associated with chronicity. *British Journal of Psychiatry*, **152**, 28–53.

Stein, M.K., Rickels, K. & Weisse, C.C. (1980). Maintenance therapy with amitriptyline: a controlled trial. *American Journal of Psychiatry*, **137**, 370–71.

Surtees, P.G. & Barkley, C. (1994). Future imperfect: the long-term outcome of depression. *British Journal of Psychiatry*, **164**, 327–41.

Vaughn, C.E. & Leff, J.P. (1976). The influence of family and social factors on the course of psychiatric illness: a comparison of schizophrenic and depressed neurotic patients. *British Journal of Psychiatry*, **129**, 125–37.

Weissman, M.M., Prusoff, B.A. & Klerman, G.L. (1978). Personality in the prediction of long-term outcome of depression. *American Journal of Psychiatry*, **135**, 797–800.

[17] Tertiary prevention in depression: cognitive therapy and other psychological treatments

Jan Scott

Introduction

The interventions described in this chapter are psychological treatments which aim to induce remission in acute depressive disorders and prevent further episodes. Both *relapse* (early symptom return) and *recurrence* (a new illness episode) are common: at least 50% of patients with a first episode of depression have a further attack (see Chapter 16). Even higher recurrence rates (75% within 5 years) are reported for those with incomplete recovery from the index episode or with a previous history of depression (Elkin *et al.*, 1989). About 16% of sufferers develop chronic depression (Scott, 1988). Mortality rates from suicide and other causes are also increased in those with depression.

The above issues highlight the need for effective tertiary prevention. The role of pharmacotherapy in the acute, continuation, and maintenance phases of the treatment of depression has been well studied, and clinical guidelines have been developed (Chapter 16). High rates of recurrence are particularly common if antidepressants are withdrawn early, where the individual has a history of previous episodes, or where psychosocial problems are present (Frank *et al.*, 1990; Scott & Paykel, 1995). This has led to increased interest in psychological approaches to treatment.

Although psychological treatments have not been evaluated as extensively as drug therapy, data is emerging on good clinical practice in the use of these interventions in the acute episode (Scott, 1995) and in the prevention of relapse (Ludgate, 1994). This chapter identifies the role and characteristics of effective psychological treatments of depression. It reviews cognitive therapy, one of the most popular approaches, from a clinical and research perspective and concludes by examining the adaptation of cognitive therapy to primary care settings.

Why use psychological treatments in primary care?

Clinician and patient factors

As shown in Box 17.1, there are several reasons why psychological interventions may be the treatment of choice for certain patients in the primary care setting. An increasing number of depressed individuals do not wish to be prescribed medication for psychological problems. The general practitioner may also wish to avoid medication. Mild depression does not respond particularly well to drugs, and depression superimposed on underlying personality disorder also responds less favourably. In other cases, clinicians may be wary of prescribing drugs because of poor compliance, potentially dangerous interactions with other medications, or because the patient is particularly sensitive to drug side-effects or at risk of deliberate self-harm through overdosage.

In patients with moderate or severe depressive disorders, psychotherapy may be used as an adjunct to pharmacotherapy. Drug treatment is often required initially to relieve acute biological symptoms and stabilise the patient's mental state so they can engage in a psychological approach. It may then be possible to tackle the psychosocial problems that precipitated or maintained the depressive episode, or which increase the risk of early relapse. Alterna-

---

Psychologically minded patients
   Particularly where automatic negative thoughts are easily identified

Medication is unsuitable
   The patient declines to try it
   Poor compliance
   Unacceptable side-effects
   Non-response to drugs
   Potential drug interactions
   Risk of overdosage

Mild depression

Presence of personality dysfunction

Low self-esteem

Interpersonal problems

Social problems
   e.g. unemployment

Box 17.1 *When to think of psychological treatments.*

tively, non-response to all other appropriate therapies may mean that a psychological approach is the only option left untried.

A possible preventive role

The shift in emphasis towards prevention and cost-effectiveness has also increased interest in the potential role of psychological therapies. Although recognisable improvements occur more rapidly with pharmacotherapy, drugs are only effective whilst an individual continues to take them. In psychological therapies such as cognitive therapy, the goal is to produce permanent and specific changes in coping strategies. The effects of such interventions may therefore be more durable and may have a greater impact on the risk of relapse in the longer term.

Characteristics of effective psychological treatments

The selection of a psychological approach for acute and prophylactic treatment of depression is best restricted to therapies with a track record established in randomised controlled clinical trials (US Department of Health & Human Sciences (US DHHS), 1993). The most widely researched approach is cognitive therapy. In a smaller number of studies interpersonal therapy has also been shown to be effective, but it has remained largely a research rather than a clinical tool. Most other psychotherapies, such as short-term dynamic therapies, have not been subjected to empirical investigation so their efficacy has not been proven, nor disproven.

Research suggests (Zeiss, Lewinsohn & Munoz, 1979; Kornblith et al., 1983; Teasdale, 1985) that a psychological approach is likely to be effective in depression if:

(i)   it is based on a clear model,
(ii) the interventions are well planned and logical, and
(iii) the patient gains a sense of self-efficacy (see Box 17.2).

Both cognitive therapy and interpersonal therapy share these characteristics. The model of depression put forward is readily understood both by clinicians and more importantly by patients of different intellectual capacities. The treatment programmes can be described clearly in therapy manuals which promote consistency in their application. These problem-solving, goal-directed approaches may be particularly attractive for health professionals working in primary care: clear targets can be set and change can be monitored more readily than with less specific counselling approaches. Also, cognitive therapy and interpersonal therapy are by definition short-term (less than 20 sessions), giving a cost–benefit advantage over many psychotherapies (particularly psychodynamic approaches).

The therapy has a well-planned rationale and is highly structured

Plans for producing change are made in logical sequences

Feedback and support reinforce change and encourage independent use of the skills to produce change

Improvement is attributed to the individual's skill (rather than the therapist's)

The therapy gives the individual a greater sense of self-efficacy

Box 17.2 *Characteristics of effective psychological therapies.*

Cognitive theory of depression

Although several forms of cognitive therapy exist, the most widely researched is the cognitive restructuring model developed by Beck (1976, 1983 Beck *et al.*, 1979). His theory states that:

> An individual's emotional response to an event or experience is largely determined by the conscious meaning placed upon it.

Thus, it is not simply what happens to an individual, but how they perceive what has happened to them that becomes critical. This fits with clinical experience, as only one in ten people who experiences a significant loss actually develops clinical depression. The cognitive model tries to identify individual mediating factors which may account for the observed differences in response to stress.

Early experiences

Beck suggested that early learning experiences lead to the development of underlying beliefs (termed 'schemata') which the individual uses to construct subjective reality. Although we may not realise it, we constantly refer back to these beliefs to make sense of our day-to-day experiences. Individuals vulnerable to depressive disorders are thought to have developed dysfunctional beliefs (usually because their 'rules' are too extreme or rigid). In later life, these schemata may be activated by critical events or incidents that mesh with the person's belief system.

For example, an individual whose early experiences lead them to believe that '*In order to be happy, I have to be liked by everyone*', may become depressed after experiencing rejection. Alternatively, someone who believes that '*In order to be happy, I have to be successful in everything I do*', may become depressed if they fail to gain promotion at work. The common characteristic of beliefs that increase the risk of depression is that they are too global (being liked

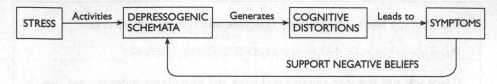

Fig. 17.1 *A diagrammatic representation of the Cognitive Model of depression.*

by everyone or being successful at everything) and unlikely to be achievable.

The 'negative cognitive triad'

As shown in Fig. 17.1, the theory suggests that once a maladaptive schema is activated it gives rise to involuntary negative automatic thoughts and these in turn lead to depressed mood (Fennell, 1989).

It is well recognized clinically that depressed individuals frequently interpret events, even positive or neutral ones, in negative ways. Such negative views of themselves ('I'm useless'), their world ('Everything is bad around me') and their future ('The future is hopeless'), known as the *negative cognitive triad*, have a further adverse effect on their mood and make the individual more depressed and more prone to interpret their future experiences in a negative way.

Illogical thinking

Negative automatic thoughts are maintained because of systematic errors in information processing (such as overgeneralisation or all-or-nothing interpretations). These render the individual 'blind' to contradictory evidence, or distort their interpretation so that it fits with their belief system. Thus, a vicious cycle develops in which lowering of the mood increases the intensity of negative thinking, which leads to further depression of mood and behavioural disturbance.

Cognitive therapy

Essential characteristics

Cognitive therapy is a short-term problem-solving therapy in which the patient and therapist jointly explore the patient's ideas and beliefs. The essential characteristics are shown in Box 17.3.

It is time-limited – a course of therapy lasts approximately 10–20 sessions (of about 45 minutes each).

It is structured – each session has an agenda.

It is collaborative – the therapist and patient are seen as equal partners in the therapeutic relationship.

It is problem orientated and focused on the 'here and now'.

It is a 'scientific' approach – thoughts and schemata are regarded as hypotheses to be tested out (not as facts).

It is an educational approach – the aim is to teach the patient specific problem-solving and compensatory skills for present and future use.

Between-session homework is a vital part of therapy ensuring transfer to skills from therapy to real life situations.

It is based on a coherent conceptualisation of the individual's problems which is shared with the patient.

Box 17.3 *Essential characteristics of cognitive therapy.*

Use in depression

One of the initial aims of cognitive therapy is to expose links between events, thoughts and feelings, and examine the way these influence (and are influenced by) the individual's behaviour. The therapy aims to alleviate the acute symptoms of depression through the use of behavioural (action orientated) techniques such as *activity scheduling, mastery and pleasure ratings,* and *graded task assignment* (breaking complex tasks down into manageable subtasks). Verbal techniques initially focus on identifying negative automatic cognitions and developing alternative constructions (Beck *et al.*, 1979). Later in cognitive therapy, the aim is to help the patient identify and change underlying dysfunctional schema. The core techniques are listed in Box 17.4.

Initial assessment

The first task in cognitive therapy is to identify the problem list and to negotiate jointly the targets of treatment. It is often helpful to categorise the person's problems into intrapersonal (e.g. low self-esteem), interpersonal (e.g. marital disharmony), and basic functioning (e.g. difficulty coping with work). The problems are then ranked in order of priority. The more depressed the individual, the more likely it is that the early targets will be behavioural

---

Behavioural techniques
   Weekly activity scheduling
   Mastery and pleasure ratings
   Graded task assignments

Cognitive techniques
   Eliciting automatic thoughts
   Testing automatic thoughts
   Identifying and modifying schemata

Box 17.4 *Core techniques in cognitive therapy.*

change (how to act or how to cope) with the gradual introduction of cognitive techniques.

Teaching the patient about the cognitive model

The second core task in cognitive therapy is to understand how early experiences have led to the development of the patient's particular dysfunctional beliefs and to explain what critical incidents have reactivated these beliefs and led to the current depressive episode. This conceptualisation is shared with the patient, and the therapist tries to develop the patient's curiosity to discover things about themselves.

Misunderstandings

A major misconception about cognitive therapy is that it is some form of 'positive thinking' where negative thoughts are simply replaced by positive ones. The therapy is not simply a collection of cognitive and behavioural techniques that can be applied in a 'blanket' (give them everything) or 'cook book' style (a little of this, a splash of that). The therapy, as opposed to the use of individual techniques, actually has a very distinctive style and comprises a carefully coordinated package of verbal and behavioural interventions (Fennell, 1989). This means that the use of the interventions listed in Box 17.4 varies with both the specific problems and hypothesised underlying beliefs identified for that particular depressed individual. In cognitive therapy the choice of intervention is not random, the decision as to which particular technique to employ is made on the basis of the cognitive conceptualisation.

Cognitive therapy and prevention of relapse

The development of more adaptive beliefs, and practising new behaviours based on modified assumptions, have always been critical components of cognitive therapy. However, researchers are currently examining additional changes to the practice of cognitive therapy that specifically address the issue of relapse prevention (Wilson, 1992).

Techniques in relapse prevention

Ludgate (1994) suggests a number of strategies which are likely to be helpful in reducing the risk of relapse, particularly if they are included in the therapeutic process from the outset rather than being relegated to the final few sessions in a short-term psychotherapy.

These techniques include: gradually increasing patient responsibility for between session homework tasks; fostering generalisation of skills to a wide variety of situations through 'overlearning' (repeated reinforcement and retraining in cognitive therapy techniques); gradually reducing the frequency of sessions over time; educating the patient regarding expectations for their future functioning; discussing the need for and benefits of maintenance activities; identifying any barriers to undertaking self-maintenance therapy; identifying any likely obstacles to continued progress; anticipating and planning for setbacks through the development of lists of early warning signs and symptoms and through 'cognitive rehearsal' of coping strategies; enlisting the help of significant others; and modifying the environment to reduce external stress factors. Some of these approaches are already part of good clinical practice and the other interventions are easily added to the model.

The aims of these measures are to:

1. increase the patient's sense of control;
2. teach self-monitoring to make the patient aware of their own early warning symptoms of relapse;
3. identify 'high risk' situations when relapse is more likely and develop a hierarchy of coping strategies and emergency plans (which include identifying when professional help will be sought);
4. help motivate the patient to continue to use the skills taught in therapy so that they can undertake effective self-management despite symptom fluctuations.

Type of maintenance therapy

In 'anti-relapse' work the need for continued use of the therapy techniques is highlighted. Three styles of maintenance cognitive therapy are described which require decreasing levels of therapist input (Ludgate, 1994).

Continuation therapy

In complex or more difficult to treat episodes of depression, regular but less frequent cognitive therapy sessions (usually 4–6 weekly) continue to be held with the therapist.

Booster sessions

This is standard practice in cognitive therapy. The patient returns once or twice in the six months after discharge for a 'refresher course'. The aim is to monitor progress and check out with the therapist any problems they have in applying their skills to new situations. Recently group 'booster' sessions have been advocated (Ludgate, 1994).

Self-maintenance

The patient organizes time to do 'self-therapy'. They formally monitor their use of cognitive therapy after discharge using diaries and set aside protected time to do sessions on their own.

Cognitive therapy – at least as good as drug treatment?

The majority of outcome research regarding psychological treatments of depression has focused on the efficacy of cognitive therapy in reducing acute symptoms. For convenience, the studies reviewed here are divided into three categories: meta-analytic studies of outcome in acute depression, follow-up studies, and research on combination treatments.

Acute depression

Earlier studies of individual cognitive therapy on both sides of the Atlantic demonstrated that it was at least as effective and acceptable as antidepressant drugs or 'treatment as usual' in non-psychotic outpatient unipolar depressives, both in primary care and hospital outpatient settings (for a review see Scott, 1995). Furthermore, there was a tendency for cognitive therapy to have lower drop-out rates than drug treatments (Hollon, Shelton & Davis, 1993). Whilst most of these studies can be criticised for the failure to include pill–placebo control groups and for the relatively small sample sizes (Scott, et al., 1994), meta-analyses of treatment studies of acute depressive episodes suggest that cognitive or behavioural approaches show superiority over insight-orientated or dynamic therapies (Dobson, 1988; Robinson, Berman & Neimeyer, 1990).

However, these early reviews excluded studies of interpersonal therapy (Andrews & Garvey, 1981). The most recent meta-analytic study of 29 carefully selected randomised controlled trials for acute major depression (US DHHS, 1993) incorporated Interpersonal Therapy studies including the three-centre National Institute of Mental Health (NIMH) study (Elkin et al., 1989). It was found that overall, the recovery rates using individual cognitive therapy (50%) and interpersonal therapy (52%) were not significantly different, but that brief psychodynamic therapies were less potent (35%).

Relapse prevention

There are few sophisticated follow-up studies examining the role of cognitive therapy in the prevention of relapse (the length of follow-up is so far insufficient to comment on its effects on recurrence rates). Earlier publications comprise naturalistic follow-ups of pharmacological or cognitive therapy treatment responders with differing methodologies and varying lengths of follow-up (see Scott, 1995). In general, patients treated with cognitive therapy, either on its own or in combination with drugs, had better outcomes than patients treated with pharmacotherapy alone. Relapse rates ranged from 15–55% in cognitive therapy treated patients and 50–80% in pharmacotherapy-treated patients. More recent follow-up studies (Evans et al., 1992; Shea et al., 1992) have overcome some of the previous methodological problems, particularly regarding adequate maintenance pharmacotherapy (Hollon et al., 1993; Scott, 1995). Evans et al. (1992) demonstrated that the relapse rate in the cognitive therapy group (20%) was not significantly different from that in the drug continuation treatment group (27%) but was less than half that of the patients who had drug treatment withdrawn at the time the depression remitted (50%). These findings support a trend identified in the NIMH follow-up (Shea et al., 1992) with reduced relapse rates and a lower proportion of patients returning to treatment in the cognitive therapy treated group.

Combined pharmacotherapy and cognitive therapy

Data on whether the use of a combination of cognitive therapy and pharmacotherapy bestows any additional benefit over either treatment alone is inconclusive. The combination may be advantageous in severe or partially remitted chronic depressions (Hollon et al., 1993; US DHHS, 1993). Most studies showed a non-significant trend for a higher response rate and lower relapse rate (an increment of 10–15% in absolute terms) in those receiving a combination of pharmacotherapy and cognitive therapy as opposed to either treatment alone.

Practical issues in primary care

Is cognitive therapy a realistic option?

Research largely confirms the efficacy and acceptability of cognitive therapy in the treatment of depression. However, this does not mean it can be promoted as an alternative treatment in primary care without question. The realities of day-to-day clinical practice suggest a number of issues still need to be resolved. For example, in the research studies quoted cognitive therapy was undertaken by therapists who received specialist training and ongoing supervision in this approach. As yet no study has looked at the use of cognitive therapy by members of the primary health care team as opposed to its use by trained therapists working in the primary care setting.

A major difficulty for primary care professionals is the relative lack of availability of specialist cognitive therapists in many parts of Britain. Also, cognitive therapy requires more time to be spent with the patient than treatment with pharmacotherapy. To justify the use of this approach, it would be necessary to demonstrate either that cognitive therapy is more cost effective in the long term (Scott & Freeman, 1992) or that it uniquely benefits certain sub-groups of patients (Clark, 1989). The former issue may be resolved when more comprehensive data on the prevention of relapse and recurrence are available. With respect to the latter issue, clinical impression suggests that psychologically minded individuals with evidence of cognitive dysfunction who wish to be active in their treatment may do well with cognitive therapy.

Research efforts to identify clearly those depressed individuals who will respond differentially to psychological as opposed to pharmacotherapy have been disappointing (Scott, 1995). At present, Teasdale's (1985) view that cognitive therapy seems to work best for patients who 'get depressed about being depressed' is as helpful as any other published criteria. If treatment in the primary care setting is the preferred option, then the approaches outlined below may be of use.

Cognitive strategies for primary care professionals

Abbreviated cognitive therapy

To be able to develop a shorter version of cognitive therapy that would be attractive for use in the primary care setting, it is first necessary to identify the 'active ingredients' of the therapy. It has been shown that adherence to the cognitive therapy model and the therapist's level of expertise are significantly associated with improvement (DeRubeis & Feeling, 1990; Hollon et al., 1993).

Components of cognitive therapy associated with change in depression are the teaching 'hypothesis-testing' skills (examining and testing automatic thoughts and beliefs) and the use of between session homework tasks that practise these skills (Jarrett & Nelson, 1987; Twaddle & Scott, 1991). The patient's expectation that a particular treatment will work for them is also positively correlated with outcome (Sotsky et al., 1991).

Using all the above information, a pilot study using an abbreviated model of cognitive therapy (six sessions of 20 minutes each) was undertaken in Newcastle upon Tyne. The results suggested that this approach can be effective in the treatment of depression in primary care (Scott et al., 1993). However, it was clear that the therapist had to have a great deal of cognitive therapy expertise to make effective and efficient use of the time available. As training opportunities in cognitive therapy for primary care staff are limited, it is important to review other potential ways in which components of the cognitive therapy package may be used in treating depression in this setting.

'Psychoeducation'

At a basic level, educating patients about the nature of their disorder, ensuring that both the clinician and patient agree about the nature of the problem, identifying a list of target symptoms to be treated, exploring automatic negative thoughts about the proposed medication, and frequent supportive contacts are techniques likely to increase patient satisfaction and improve treatment compliance.

Adjunctive techniques

Minimal interventions using single cognitive therapy techniques (as listed in Box 17.5) can be employed by clinicians without extending the consultation session. Depressed patients receiving drug treatment often find using *activity schedules*, which can help get them going again, and identifying activities which they can accept give them some pleasure (*mastery and pleasure recording*) extremely

---

Cognitive therapy approach in interviews
  Take a problem-orientated approach
  Set targets for change
  Look at links between events, thoughts and feelings

Specific techniques
  Homework assignments between appointments
  Mastery and pleasure recording
  Event–thought–feeling diaries
  Graded task assignments
  Thought challenging techniques

Self-help books

Abbreviated cognitive therapy
  Six 20-minute sessions dealing with acute symptoms and teaching
  basic cognitive therapy techniques

Referral to a trained cognitive therapist
  (Fifteen to twenty 45-minute sessions)

Box 17.5 *Cognitive strategies for the primary health care team.*

helpful. Patients often comment that making a daily timetable reduces tension and distress and helps overcome inertia. It seems that simply structuring their day can be of great benefit.

Keeping a thought diary allows exploration of links between mood shifts and specific negative ideas. Writing the thought down seems to operate to distance the patient from the thought and allows them to take a more objective approach to challenging their ideas. Using individual techniques and a problem-solving approach allows the clinician to assess progress on a number of parameters. Furthermore, these techniques can be used after recovery from the acute episode to maintain well-being and increase the sense of self-control.

'Bibliotherapy'

Whilst the primary health care team may not be able to spend long periods of time undertaking cognitive therapy interventions, the use of educational books is of potential benefit in promoting a sense of self-efficacy or in teaching self-monitoring and self-management skills. Several researchers (Twaddle & Scott, 1991) have commented on patients who have rapidly adapted to the cognitive therapy approach after a small number of sessions supplemented by reading material. Many patients are able to understand and begin to use the techniques with minimal explanation. Alternatively, it may be possible to allocate the patient specific chapters of self-help books to read as 'homework assignments' and to build continuity between follow-up sessions at the surgery. Useful books are listed in Box 17.6.

Cognitive Therapy and the Emotional Disorders
   A. T. Beck. Pelican

Love is Never Enough
   A. T. Beck. Penguin

Coping with Depression
   Ivy Blackburn. Edinburgh: W. R. Chambers

Feeling Good: The New Mood Therapy
   David Burns. New Jersey: Signet

A New Beginning
   Gary Emery. New York: Touchstone

Mind over Mood
   Dennis Greenberger & Christine Padesky. New York: Guilford

---

Box 17.6 *Self-help books.*

Conclusions

There are many potential benefits arising from the use of cognitive and behavioural techniques in the primary care setting. However, employing these techniques in isolation must be clearly distinguished from the specific therapy package that constitutes cognitive therapy. The latter requires formal training, and interventions are selected on the basis of an underlying rationale (Fennell, 1989).

Extensive outcome research suggests that cognitive therapy is an effective treatment for non-psychotic mild to moderately severe unipolar depressive disorders, a population seen extensively in primary care settings. In addition, as cost–benefit analysis becomes a major concern of health service purchasers and providers, the time-limited nature of this approach, combined with the evidence that it may reduce relapse rates, is likely to lead to an increase rather than a decrease in its use in the future (Scott & Freeman, 1992).

Limitations

Hollon and colleagues (1993) commented that, if cognitive therapy (without maintenance sessions) reduces the risk of relapse to the level obtained with maintenance pharmacotherapy, this will be the first time any form of antidepressant treatment has been shown to have an effect beyond the point of termination of the intervention. However, before enthusiasm for psychological approaches overtakes clinical common-sense, it is worth noting that only 38% of patients who are offered cognitive therapy find the treatment acceptable, respond to it at three months and remain well at two years (Evans *et al.*, 1992). The figure for patients receiving pharmacotherapy is very similar (31%). It seems that clinically, the early introduction of a treatment which is acceptable to that particular patient and which has established efficacy during the acute phase of the depression, combined with more rigorous attention to aftercare, are the most effective preventive strategies currently available (Scott & Paykel, 1995).

References

Andrews, G. & Harvey, R. (1981). Does psychotherapy benefit neurotic patients? A re-analysis of the Smith, Glass and Miller data. *Archives of General Psychiatry*, **38**, 1203–08.

Beck, A. T. (1976). *Cognitive Theory and the Emotional Disorders*. pp. 47–132. New York: International Universities Press.

Beck, A. T. (1983). Cognitive therapy of depression: new perspectives. In *Treatment of Depression: Old Controversies and New Approaches*. Clayton, P. and Barrett J., eds. pp. 265–284. New York: Raven Press.

Beck, A. T., Rush, A. J., Shaw, B. F. & Emery, G. (1979). *Cognitive Therapy of Depression*. New York: Guilford Press.

Clark, D. (1989). Cognitive therapy for depression and anxiety: is it better than drug treatment in the long term? In *Dilemmas and Difficulties in the Management of Psychiatric Patients*. Hawton, K. and Cowen, P., eds. Oxford: Oxford University Press.

DeRubeis, R. & Feeling, M. (1990). Determinants of change in cognitive therapy of depression. *Cognitive Therapy and Research*, **14**, 469–82.

Dobson, K. (1988). A meta-analysis of the efficacy of cognitive therapy for depression. *Journal of Consulting and Clinical Psychology*, **57**, 414–19.

Elkin, I., Shea, M., Watkins, J., Imber, S., Sotsky, S., Collins, J., Glass, D., Pilkonis, P., Leber, W., Docherty, J., Fiester, S. & Parloff, M. (1989). National Institute of Mental Health treatment of depression collaborative treatment program. *Archives of General Psychiatry*, **46**, 971–82.

Evans, M., Hollon, S., DeRubeis, R., Piasecki, J., Grove, W., Garvey, M. & Tuason, V. (1992). Differential relapse following cognitive therapy and pharmacotherapy for depression. *Archives of General Psychiatry*, **49**, 802–8.

Fennell, M. J. (1989). Depression. In *Cognitive Behaviour Therapy for Psychiatric Problems: A Practical Guide*. Hawton, K. Salkovskis, P., Kirk, J. and Clark, D., eds. pp. 167–234. Oxford: Oxford University Press.

Frank, E., Kupfer, D., Perel, J., Cornes, C., Jarrett, D., Mallinger, A., Thase, M., McEachran, A. & Grochocinski, V. (1990). Three-year outcomes for maintenance therapies in recurrent depressions. *Archives of General Psychiatry*, **47**, 1093–9.

Hollon, S., DeRubeis, R., Evans, M., Wiemer, M., Garvey, M., Grove, W. & Tuason, V. (1992). Cognitive therapy and pharmacotherapy for depression: singly and in combination. *Archives of General Psychiatry*, **49**, 774–81.

Hollon, S., Shelton, R. & Davis, D. (1993). Cognitive therapy for depression: conceptual issues and clinical efficacy. *Journal of Consulting and Clinical Psychology*, **2**, 270–5.

Jarrett, R. & Nelson, R. (1987). Mechanisms of change in cognitive therapy of depression. *Behaviour Therapy*, **18**, 227–41.

Kornblith, S., Rehm, L., O'Hara, M. & Lamparski, D. (1983). The contribution of self-reinforcement training and behavioural assignments to the efficacy of self-control therapy for depression. *Cognitive Therapy and Research*, **6**, 499–528.

Ludgate, J. (1994). Cognitive behaviour therapy and depressive relapse: justified optimism or unwarranted complacency? *Behavioural and Cognitive Psychotherapy*, **22**, 1–12.

Newton, J. & Craig, T. (1991). Prevention. In *Community Psychiatry*. Bennett, D. and Freeman, H., eds. pp. 488–516. Edinburgh: Churchill Livingstone.

Robinson, L., Berman, J. & Neimeyer, R. (1990). Psychotherapy for the treatment of depression: a comprehensive review of controlled outcome research. *Psychological Bulletin*, **108**, 30–49.

Scott, A. & Freeman, C. (1992). Edinburgh primary care depression study: Treatment outcome, patient satisfaction, and cost after 16 weeks. *British Medical Journal*, **304**, 883–7.

Scott, C., Scott, J., Tacchi, M. J. & Jones, R. H. (1993). Abbreviated cognitive therapy for depression: a pilot study in primary care. *Behavioural and Cognitive Psychotherapy*, **22**, 57–64.

Scott, J. (1988). Review article: chronic depression. *British Journal of Psychiatry*, **153**, 287–97.

Scott, J. (1995). Depression. In *Clinical Topics in Psychotherapy*. Tantum, D., ed. London: Gaskell Press. In Press.

Scott, J. & Paykel, E. S. (1995). Depression: risks and possibilities for prevention. In *Handbook of Preventative Psychiatry*. Raphael, G. and Burrows, G., eds. London: Elsevier.

Scott, J., Moon, C., Blacker, C. & Thomas, J. (1994). The current literature: the Edinburgh primary care depression study. *British Journal of Psychiatry*, **164**, 410–15.

Shea, M. T., Elkin, I., Imber, S., Sotsky, S., Watkins, J., Collins, J., Pilkonis, P., Beckham, E., Glass, D., Dolan, R. & Parloff, M. (1992). Course of depressive symptoms over follow-up. *Archives of General Psychiatry*, **49**, 782–7.

Sotsky, S., Glass, D., Shea, M., Pilkonis, P., Collins, J., Elkin, I. *et al.* (1991). Patient predictors of response to psychotherapy: findings in the NIMH treatment of depression collaborative research programme. *American Journal of Psychiatry*, **148**, 997–1008.

Teasdale, J. (1985). Psychological treatments of depression: how do they work? *Behaviour Research and Therapy*, **23**, 157–65.

Twaddle, V. & Scott, J. (1991). Cognitive theory and therapy of depression. In *Adult Clinical Problems: A Cognitive-Behavioural Approach*. Dryden, W. and Rentoul, R. eds. pp. 56–85. London: Routledge.

US Department of Health & Human Sciences [US DHHS] (1993). *Depression in Primary Care: Treatment of Major Depression*. Depression Guideline Panel. pp. 71–123. Rockville: AHCPR Publications.

Wilson, P. (1992). Depression. In *Principles and Practice of Relapse Prevention*. Wilson, P., ed. pp. 128–156. London: Guilford Press.

Zeiss, A., Lewinsohn, P. & Munoz, R. (1977). Non-specific improvement effects in depression using interpersonal skills training, pleasant activity schedules, or cognitive training. *Journal of Consulting and Clinical Psychology*, **47**, 427–39.

[18] The regular review of patients with schizophrenia in primary care

Geraldine Strathdee and Tony Kendrick

Introduction

Major changes in the medical care of people suffering from schizophrenia have taken place in the last 30 to 40 years. With the advent of the major tranquillisers in the 1950s, psychiatrists were able for the first time to treat the severe symptoms of hallucinations and delusions, which meant that patients who would formerly have remained in hospital long term could be discharged (Brown, Murray-Parkes & Wing, 1961). This improvement in treatment, combined with the recognition that institutional life in itself seemed to exacerbate the lack of motivation and social withdrawal of many long-stay patients (Wing & Brown, 1970), has contributed to a fall of over 100 000 in the psychiatric hospital inpatient population in England from its peak of 150 000 in the mid-1950s.

Since the mid-1970s UK government policy has been to continue to discharge patients from the old large mental hospitals and eventually to close them altogether, replacing them with a network of health and social services in each district, including general hospital psychiatric units, day hospitals, community psychiatric services and local authority residential, day care and social support services (Department of Health and Social Security, 1975).

Since the shift from hospital care into the community, most people suffering from schizophrenia now spend nearly all their lives outside hospital. This presents a challenge to general practitioners.

The central role of the general practitioner

There are a number of reasons why the general practitioner should play a central role in the care of patients with chronic schizophrenia.

The general practitioner is the family's doctor

The general practitioner may well have seen the patient grow up and is likely to be familiar with the home circumstances. The relatives are usually patients of the practice too, and the effects of the illness on all the family will be immediately apparent to the general practitioner. The general practitioner has often earnt the respect of the family and will usually be the first port of call for help (see Chapter 14). Hunter (1978) found that families turned to their general practitioners more often than to the community psychiatric nurse when experiencing difficulties with their relatives with schizophrenia.

The general practitioner will inevitably become involved in the patient's psychiatric care

At the onset of the illness, nearly all patients with schizophrenia will require hospital admission and will therefore receive specialist care. However, after this initial hospitalisation, most patients return to the care of their general practitioners. In the longer term, many patients with schizophrenia lose all contact with specialist services and are looked after entirely in primary care (see Chapter 14). General practitioners have therefore been involved at least as frequently as psychiatrists in the care of patients with schizophrenia ever since the late 1950s. Whilst this involvement may often be limited to brief appointments for repeat prescriptions or sickness certificates, such contacts may in a large proportion of cases offer the only opportunity for assessment by a doctor.

Many community mental health teams do not offer 24-hour access

In some areas, case registers of patients with chronic schizophrenia and other long-term mental illnesses have been set up by the psychiatric services, and mental health teams attempt to maintain continuing contact with such patients over many years (Bamrah, Freeman & Goldberg, 1992). The relative contributions of the primary and secondary care teams in the long-term management of patients with schizophrenia will therefore vary from district to district. For a proportion of patients, the regular review of mental state and medication will be undertaken by the mental health team, with the community psychiatric nurse or other mental health professional acting as key worker in regular contact with the patient.

However, there is still a strong case to be made for the *personal* involvement of the general practitioner. First, the general practitioner needs to remain familiar with the patient's usual mental state, and patterns of relapse, in order to react effectively when problems develop. If the general practitioner does not see the patient himself, then he must rely on regular contact with the community psychiatric nurse. Self-evidently this strategy is at risk of communication failures. A crisis in a patient's care may happen at night or over a weekend when the community psychiatric nurse is off duty. Secondly, general practitioners, unlike many members of community mental health teams, usually practise in the same place for decades and are therefore in a good position personally to offer continuity of care in the long term. Thirdly, it is appropriate for the general practitioner to undertake the routine review of the majority of patients, especially those who are stable or in remission. This frees the psychiatric team to concentrate on the more complex problems of management, the most disabled patients, or those whose illnesses are least stable.

Patients with chronic schizophrenia have needs for physical care

Schizophrenia is associated with increased mortality rates from cardiovascular and respiratory diseases (Allebeck, 1989) and studies of patients with long-term mental illness have consistently found that a proportion of them have unmet needs for physical care (Brugha *et al.*, 1989). Patients with schizophrenia are entitled to physical care from their general practitioners, including preventive health care. Psychiatrists and community psychiatric nurses do not usually check blood pressures or take cervical smears, or offer help in tackling obesity or smoking.

The general practitioner is well placed to assess patients' needs for secondary care

In the 1990s new legislation on care in the community for vulnerable people made local authority social services departments responsible for ensuring that multidisciplinary assessments of the needs of people with disabling conditions are made, and called on general practitioners to contribute to these (Secretaries of State for Health, Social Security, Wales and Scotland, 1989). The government has reminded general practitioners that, under their terms of service they are obliged to refer patients needing specialist care and to give advice to those patients who might benefit from local authority social services. Where close working relationships are not already in place, the government wishes to see the development of clearly agreed local arrangements between general practitioners and social services for the assessment of patients' needs. General practitioners are therefore likely to be called on to become even more involved in the future in the assessment of patients with chronic schizophrenia.

Attitudes of general practitioners towards looking after patients with schizophrenia

General practitioners have not always welcomed the prospect of increased responsibility for patients with severe psychiatric disorders such as schizophrenia. General practitioners in Wales interviewed in 1961 said that they were apprehensive about a possible increase in the number of chronic psychiatric cases under their care, because they felt that their efforts with such patients often met with a poor or uncertain response (Rawnsley & Loudon, 1962). Only eight out of a sample of 69 general practitioners in Greater London interviewed in 1967 said that they would be willing to take on additional psychiatric patients and provide aftercare for them (May & Gregory, 1968).

One reason for general practitioners' negative attitudes to involvement in the care of chronic psychiatric patients might be that many have had very little training in their care. Less than one-third of general practitioners overall, and only 40% of new principals, have worked in a hospital psychiatry post (Kendrick et al., 1991; Styles, 1991). The majority of general practitioners have therefore had only a short training in psychiatry as medical students, after which they have had to learn about the care of psychiatric patients in the community whilst in service as general practitioner trainees and then as general practitioners.

However, there is evidence that general practitioners have become more positive about their involvement with patients with long-term mental illnesses like schizophrenia over the last 20 to 30 years, and that this has been associated with increased help from community mental health teams.

Working with community mental health teams – changing attitudes

There has been a large increase in the number of psychiatrists who spend some of their time working in general practitioners' surgeries, together with community psychiatric nurses, social workers and psychologists (Strathdee & Williams, 1984). This has increased the practical help and advice immediately available to primary care teams and in some cases increased their own confidence in dealing with mental illness. Strathdee (1988) found that general practitioners participating in liaison attachment schemes with psychiatrists working on their premises welcomed assessment and short-term treatment by the specialist, but did not regard long-term takeover of cases as optimum use of the consultant's time.

A survey of 369 general practitioners in South West Thames Region found that 90% were willing to share the care of long-term mentally ill patients with the psychiatrist. An encouraging 41% went further and said that they were prepared to organise their care with back-up from the psychiatric service only when necessary. However, almost none had any specific practice policies for the care of such patients and most agreed that some are brought to their general practitioner's attention only when a crisis develops in their care (Kendrick et al., 1991).

There is therefore a need for the kind of information presented in this chapter, which sets out what general practitioners should be doing when they see their patients with chronic schizophrenia, and when they might consider enlisting the help of psychiatric and social services to improve the care offered to this disadvantaged group. Chapter 20 sets out how general practitioners might organise their practices in order to offer the highest standards of continuing care to patients with chronic schizophrenia and other disabling long-term mental illnesses.

Multi-dimensional assessments

Before the advent of community psychiatric practice, psychiatrists tended to focus almost exclusively on the medical and medication aspects of a patient's care. It has been shown, however, that in the community many factors can influence the course and outcome of schizophrenia. These include the impact of life events such as loss of employment, break-up of relationships, bereavement, and other traumas (Brown & Birley, 1968), the attitudes and behaviour of relatives and carers towards the patient (Vaughn & Leff, 1976) and the quality of the patient's environment, including the opportunity to work and lead a rewarding life (Bennett, 1980). Therefore, any aspect of a patient's life which influences their mental state should be the legitimate concern of their doctor.

Box 18.1 delineates a 'good practice blueprint' for the review of a patient with chronic schizophrenia. This is a multidimensional assessment of physical, psychiatric, and social needs. It may not be possible to cover all these areas in one consultation, but they can all

---

Physical
Assessment of physical symptoms and signs
Advice on need for dental/chiropody/sight assessment
Preventive health care
Contraception

Psychiatric
Mental state assessment (concurrent depression)
Assessment of pre-morbid symptoms of relapse
Medication history and administration (tardive dyskinesia)
Relatives or other carers' attitudes and need for education

Social
Practical aids (benefits, bus pass)
Employment or daytime occupation
Social supports

Box 18.1 *A checklist for the consultation with a patient with schizophrenia.*

be covered in time, in the course of continuing contacts with the patient.

Communication problems

A number of problems may make the consultation difficult for the general practitioner and require extra time and effort to elicit a true picture of the mental state. The professional will recognise and tolerate a patient's inability to conform to accepted norms of behaviour.

Patients may be preoccupied with hallucinations or delusions which actively prevent them from responding to the doctor's questions. They may hold the delusional belief, for example, that the doctor is part of a conspiracy against them, or can read and criticise their thoughts. This can lead to difficult behaviours, rarely even violence. It may be difficult to avoid responding to the patient's feelings where these are powerful, but the doctor should beware expressing too much emotion. The doctor must try to separate himself in the patient's mind from the rest of a seemingly hostile world without colluding with the patient's delusions. It often takes some time to build trust. The doctor should make no assumptions and check the patient's understanding often.

The patient may suffer from poverty of speech, with long pauses between short utterances, and poor eye contact. The patient may be extremely passive. The doctor may need to be more active and ask very direct, closed questions.

It is remarkably easy to miss changes in symptoms in a patient one knows well. A study of the interaction of community psychiatric nurses and mental health social workers with patients with chronic schizophrenia revealed that symptoms could be missed in the absence of a specific search for them (Wooff & Goldberg, 1988). Interviews were often conducted with the language associated with an ordinary social enquiry, using rather general open-ended questions to which the patients tended to give reassuring responses that they were fine. When asked specific closed questions in the course of a subsequent diagnostic interview however, patients revealed hallucinations, delusions, anxiety and depression which had been missed by their usual key workers. This research has demonstrated the need for routine questioning in the regular review of patients with chronic schizophrenia.

Physical problems

Obesity may result from the side-effects of psychotropic drugs and a sedentary lifestyle. Many patients with chronic schizophrenia are smokers – they may have developed the habit during time spent in psychiatric wards where smoking is often a big part of the process of socialising between patients and between patients and staff. In some hospitals, cigarettes were even used as a kind of currency in token economies designed to reward patients for behaving in particular ways.

The kinds of problems which have frequently been found are listed in Box 18.2. Most can be dealt with entirely within primary care.

There is much anecdotal evidence that patients with chronic psychotic illnesses sometimes tolerate pain or other physical symptoms and do not present them to their doctors. Again, an open question such as 'How have you been feeling physically?' might be met with a bland statement that everything is fine. However, when closed questions are put symptoms might be revealed. Closed questions include, for example: 'Have you had any pains anywhere lately?', 'Have you any lumps anywhere', and 'Have you been bleeding from anywhere lately?' Once more, a checklist of items to cover might avoid missing important problems. For patients with long-standing illness, especially for the over-40s, the general practitioner might consider carrying out a battery of examinations and investigations – perhaps once every two years, regardless of a lack of complaints by the patient (Box 18.3). This is particularly relevant to general practitioners looking after patients who are so disabled as to require long-term support in group homes (Kendrick, 1994).

Circulatory problems
    High blood pressure
    Ischaemic heart disease
    Cerebrovascular disease

Respiratory problems
    Chronic bronchitis
    Chest infections

Obesity

Vision problems

Need for chiropody

Hearing problems

Drug side-effects
    Akathisia
    Oculogyric crises
    Parkinsonism
    Tardive dyskinesia

Box 18.2 *Physical problems of patients with chronic schizophrenia.*

Full physical examination
  BP
  Chest
  Skin
  Side-effects
  Urinalysis

Blood tests
  FBC and ESR
  T4

Chest X-ray

Electrocardiogram

Box 18.3 *Suggested routine screening of the older patient with schizophrenia.*

Mental state examination

The particular elements of the mental state which are relevant to the regular review of patients with chronic schizophrenia can be divided into the two categories shown in Box 18.4 (Crow, 1980).

Positive symptoms are the unusual experiences classic of an active psychotic process. The negative symptoms are associated with more long-standing illness and often cause relatives most concern. They are frequently attributed to the patient being 'lazy' or 'unmotivated' rather than being seen as an aspect of the illness. This has important implications for the education of relatives and their attitudes towards the sufferer.

Hallucinations

The commonest kind of hallucination is hearing voices, but somatic or tactile and visual hallucinations may occur too. The well-practised question used by psychiatrists is:

> Have there been times lately when you have heard noises or voices, or seen strange things, when no one was about and there was nothing else to explain it?

The impact of hallucinations on the patient's behaviour is the all-important factor; some patients have long-standing voices which do not trouble them; others are very distressed by them or pre-occupied with them for much of the time, and therefore may be in need of an increase or a change in medication.

Positive symptoms	Negative symptoms
Hallucinations	Poverty of speech
Delusions	Blunted emotions
Anxiety	Little motivation
Depression	Poor grooming and hygiene
	Poor social skills

Box 18.4 *Positive and negative symptoms.*

Delusions

Doctors sometimes find it difficult to find the right words to use to ask about delusions. They may be embarrassed, fearing that the patient might be offended by suggestions that they have beliefs which are false. Delusions of persecution may be obvious from the patient's behaviour, but they may be hidden too. Any such delusions may be revealed in response to a straight question such as:

> Have you had the feeling lately that people are talking about you or plotting about you or trying to hurt you?

Delusions of grandeur are less likely to be kept hidden, since the person often has a desire to make their importance known, but if no such delusions are obvious the doctor should still briefly check for them with a question such as:

> Is there anything special about you that would make anyone want to talk about you or hurt you?

A particularly distressing symptom for patients is 'thought broadcast', which is the delusion that anyone can read one's thoughts, that they may be written on one's forehead or that they are printed in the newspaper or heard on the television.

Again, the strength of the delusion is all important in deciding whether more treatment may be required. Some patients are very troubled by their delusions, and exhibit disturbed behaviour as a result. Others may keep false beliefs about the world to themselves for many years without ever acting on them.

Anxiety and depression

Although hallucinations and delusions are characteristic, the International Pilot Study of Schizophrenia (World Health Organisation, 1979) found that symptoms of depression and anxiety are also very common in schizophrenia. These may be due to distress caused by frightening and bizarre internal experiences. Depression may be present in its own right, or occur as a reaction to gaining insight into the chronic nature of the condition and the limitations it places on the patient's life. Depression can be difficult to detect in the context of negative symptoms and it is therefore very important to enquire specifically for symptoms during the consultation. These include sleep and appetite disturbance, crying, loss of concentration, and loss of enjoyment of life. The importance of detecting depression is that it will usually respond to the addition of an antidepressant drug.

Assessing suicide risk

Between 10% and 15% of people with schizophrenia eventually commit suicide, which is a very high risk. Studies suggest that the risks are higher for unemployed young male patients with good educational backgrounds and high expectations of performance, who are painfully aware of the effects of the illness on their achievements in life. They tend to have suffered chronic relapsing illnesses for some years and often commit suicide within a few weeks of hospital discharge (Roy, 1982). Before killing themselves, patients may discuss fears of mental disintegration and hopelessness for the future, and may well talk about doing it, with their relatives or their professional carers (Drake *et al.*, 1984).

Behaviour and appearance

The doctor should note postures, grimaces, flippant remarks, and loss of social restraint which might give clues to a change in mental state. Slowness and underactivity and lack of spontaneous speech may be negative symptoms of schizophrenia itself, or may be due to parkinsonian side-effects of neuroleptics, or due to superadded depression which will often respond to antidepressants. Self-neglect may be apparent from the state of the clothes, hygiene, and nutritional status. Irritability, hostile or aggressive behaviour are worrying signs which may indicate the need for an increase in medication with a major tranquilliser.

Working with the patient to prevent relapse

One useful paradigm for doctors involved in the care of patient with chronic illness is that of the diabetic patient (Fig. 18.1).

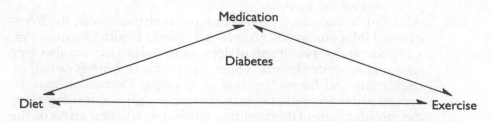

Fig. 18.1

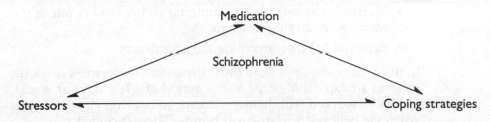

Fig. 18.2

The control of diabetes and the prevention of complications depends on the ability of the patient to balance food intake, exercise (energy expenditure) and medication. This is a useful model with which to compare the situation facing patients with chronic schizophrenia (Fig. 18.2).

A study in Manchester demonstrated that patients, relatives and carers can form a successful alliance, working together to recognise the progression of symptoms which occur when a patient is entering a period of relapse (Birchwood *et al.*, 1989). The following case history illustrates such a pattern:

Mrs P. was a single parent and medical secretary who had developed schizophrenia following the birth of her daughter six years previously. In the course of her illness she had been admitted as an in-patient eight times in a five-year period. Her daughter had been in care on these occasions and eventually a sympathetic employer had felt unable to continue her contract. Mrs P. had come to distrust medical care because her experience of illness was that she received high doses of medication, resulting in severe side-effects and had often been 'sectioned' and admitted to a locked ward at the local psychiatric hospital. On moving house, Mrs P. registered with a new general practitioner who had worked closely with a psychiatrist attached for one session weekly to the practice.

In response to the questions:
'How would you know if you were becoming ill? Is there a pattern which develops? Which symptoms come first?'
Mrs P. identified the following pattern to her relapses:

- Sleep disturbance for 2–3 nights
- Feelings of restlessness
- Inability to concentrate
- Feelings of anxiety and a vague sense of fear

- A tendency to withdraw and stay in her bedroom
- Lack of interest in personal care and food
- The start of 'voices'
- Bizarre behaviour such as dumping all her clothes out of the window, emptying dustbins
- Paranoid beliefs concerning the neighbours.

In many patients, such sleep disturbance and restlessness mark the onset of a relapse and occur over a period of a few days or weeks.

Mrs P. worked with her new doctor to develop clear strategies when she believed a relapse had begun. These included:

- An early consultation with the general practitioner (the practice receptionists had a list of patients who were to be given immediate appointments on request)
- Immediate intake of stelazine spansules 10 mg bd
- Discussion to identify possible stressors and work on coping skills.

Mrs P. was able to identify some of the stressors which precipitated relapse in her case. These included lack of sleep due to noisy neighbours playing loud music at night, anxiety when her social security payments were late, extra letters to type at work, concern when her daughter was bullied at school, and financial worries, for example, about paying for repairs to her washing machine.

Her coping strategies were to spend a quiet evening with her daughter at the home of a friend, have a few early nights listening to music at home, or telephoning a friend. When her auditory hallucinations became bothersome, she had strategies of distraction – taking a long bath, playing music loudly, going to play a ball game with her daughter in the park, or listening to the radio (see Box 18.5).

Stressors	Coping strategies
Loss of job	Withdrawal from situation
Difficult relationship	Chatting to a friend
Excessive socialising	Playing music
Stimulating environments, e.g. pubs, clubs	Long walks Stimulating activity
Financial problems	Sport
Housing problems	Art

Box 18.5 *Mrs P.'s stressors and coping strategies.*

Mrs P. had three relapses in the next ten years. It so happened that the only one requiring hospital admission was when her general practitioner, in whom she placed great trust, was on holiday.

Social needs (Box 18.6)

Finances

There is evidence that patients with long-term mental illness such as schizophrenia often fail to claim the benefits to which they are entitled (Marks, 1988). Finding one's way through the morass of social security benefits forms and rules is a difficult task even for people well used to the system. For patients who are suffering loss of concentration, anxiety and difficulty in thinking, the task is gargantuan.

Social Service departments or the Citizens' Advice Bureau can help patients claim income support or disability living allowance. A welfare benefits assessment package, recently developed at the Department of General Practice at St Mary's Hospital in London, provides a simple and effective means of clarifying if the patient is receiving appropriate benefits. Where a practice is able to establish liaison with a named social worker in the area office or mental health team, advice can be sought more readily. They may need more than this, however, if they have poor money management skills. The occupational therapist can help with this.

Finances

Housing

Employment

Daytime activity

Transport

Daily living skills
Self-care and hygiene
Cooking and shopping

Leisure pursuits

Social network

Box 18.6 *Review of daily living and social needs.*

Housing

The provision of secure, tenured, affordable housing is of importance in enabling the patient to develop a stable base from which to develop continuing relationships and utilise community resources. Again, where practices can form links with identified housing and estates officers, it may be possible to provide a stronger advocacy for the patient.

Employment

Schizophrenia may strike so early in life that the patient has not had time to gain any qualifications. Even where the person has managed to embark on a career, their illness may interfere with their ability to carry on and they may drift down the social scale and have to settle for jobs of less difficulty and therefore less financial reward.

Problems of illiteracy and lack of work skills can be tackled with remedial education and training, perhaps in sheltered workshops or employment rehabilitation centres. The job centre should be able to advise the general practitioner over the telephone. The Disablement Resettlement Officer is the person responsible.

Daytime activity and daily living skills

Where a person is unemployed, there is a need for structured daytime activity, such as attending a local authority day centre or psychiatric day hospital where occupational therapy can be offered. One of the difficulties facing individuals with long-term mental illnesses is an inability to transfer new skills into different settings. Where possible, therefore it is preferable for the patient to learn '*in vivo*' and in some areas mobile treatment teams work with patients to develop skills in the home setting.

Transport

The lack of transport has a bearing on many other aspects of social interaction and the ability to take up opportunities for day care, employment and leisure time activities. A bus pass may transform the situation for some patients.

Social network

The involvement of family and friends can be quickly ascertained by questions such as 'Is there anyone that you can really count on for help in a crisis?' and 'Is there anyone who really counts on you?' These are questions which, as well as revealing important information about the patient, also show the patient that the doctor is interested in them as a person and wants to gain insight into their quality of life and relationships. Such support is important in the prevention of social disability in schizophrenia (Chapter 19). Respite care is often important for the relatives, but may be better in the form of regular protected time each week rather than the occasional admission somewhere for two weeks' holiday.

Conclusion: realistic expectations for change in tertiary prevention

The doctor needs to be aware of what can be done for the problems which might be uncovered by going through the kinds of checklists described above, and where to refer for help. Many of the problems found will be longstanding and not amenable to sudden radical improvements. The primary health care team's expectations should be realistic and limited, to guard against feelings of frustration or hopelessness. Only one or two main problems should be tackled at a time. However, on the other hand, they should not assume that problems are necessarily intractable or hopeless and therefore not attempt to intervene. It is important to reassess repeatedly the need for further intervention or fresh review by the secondary care services.

References

Allebeck, P. (1989). Schizophrenia: a life-shortening disease. *Schizophrenia Bulletin*, **15**, 81–9.

Bamrah, J.S., Freeman, H.L. & Goldberg, D.P. (1992). Epidemiology of schizophrenia in Salford, 1974–1984. Changes in an urban community over ten years. *British Journal of Psychiatry*, **159**, 802–10.

Bennett, D.H. (1980). The chronic psychiatric patient today. *Journal of the Royal Society of Medicine*, **73**, 301–3.

Birchwood, M., Smith, J., MacMillan, F. *et al.* (1989). Predicting relapse in schizophrenia: the development and implementation of an early signs monitoring system using patients and families as observers, a preliminary investigation. *Psychological Medicine*, **19**, 649–56.

Brown, G.W. & Birley, J.L.T. (1968). Crises and life changes and the onset of schizophrenia. *Journal of Health and Social Behaviour*, **9**, 203–14.

Brown, G.W., Murray-Parkes, C. & Wing, J.K. (1961). Admissions and readmissions to three London mental hospitals. *Journal of Mental Science*, **107**, 1070–7.

Brugha, T.S., Wing, J.K., Brewin, C.R. *et al.* (1989). Physical health of the long-term mentally ill in the community: is there unmet need? *British Journal of Psychiatry*, **155**, 777–81.

Crow, T.J. (1980). Molecular pathology of schizophrenia: more than one disease process? *British Medical Journal* **280**, 66–8.

Department of Health and Social Security (1975). *Better Services for the Mentally Ill*. London: HMSO.

Drake, R.E., Gates, C., Cotton, P.G. *et al.* (1984). Suicide among schizophrenics. Who is at risk? *Journal of Nervous and Mental Disease*, **172**, 613–17.

Honig, A., Pop, P., Tan, E.S. *et al.*, (1989). Physical illness in chronic psychiatric patients from a Community Psychiatric Unit. Implications for daily practice. *British Journal of Psychiatry*, **155**, 58–64.

Hunter, P. (1978). *Schizophrenia and Community Psychiatric Nursing*. London: National Schizophrenia Fellowship.

Kendrick, T., Sibbald, B., Burns, T. & Freeling, P. (1991). Role of general practitioners in care of long-term mentally ill patients. *British Medical Journal*, **302**, 508–10.

Kendrick, T. (1994). General practitioner involvement in a group home. *Psychiatric Bulletin*, **18**, 600–3.

Marks, B.E. (1988). Social security benefits for the mentally ill. Uptake is low and information is sparse. *British Medical Journal*, **297**, 1148.

May, A.R. & Gregory, E. (1968). Participation of general practitioners in community psychiatry. *British Medical Journal*, **2**, 168–71.

Rawnsley, K. & Loudon, J.B. (1962). The attitudes of GPs to psychiatry. In *Sociology and Medicine. Sociological Review Monograph no 5*. Halmos, P., ed. University of Keele.

Roy, A. (1982). Suicide in chronic schizophrenia. *British Journal of Psychiatry*, **141**, 171–7.

Secretaries of State for Health Social Security, Wales and Scotland (1989). *Caring for People: Community care in the next decade and beyond*. London: HMSO.

Strathdee, G. (1988). Psychiatrists in primary care: the general practitioner viewpoint. *Family Practice*, **5**, 111–5.

Strathdee, G., Williams, P. (1984). A survey of psychiatrists in primary care: the silent growth of a new service. *Journal of the Royal College of General Practitioners*, **34**, 615–8.

Styles, W. McN. (1991). Training experience of doctors certificated for general practice. *British Journal of General Practice*, **41**, 488–91.

Vaughn, C.E. & Leff, J.P. (1976). The influence of family and social factors on the course of psychiatric illness: a comparison of schizophrenic and depressed neurotic patients. *British Journal of Psychiatry*, **129**, 125–37.

Wing, J.K. & Brown, G.W. (1970). *Institutionalism and Schizophrenia*. Cambridge: Cambridge University Press.

Wooff, K. & Goldberg, D.P. (1988). Further observations on the practice of community care in Salford: differences between community psychiatric nurses and mental health social workers. *British Journal of Psychiatry*, **153**, 30–7.

World Health Organisation (1979). *Schizophrenia: An International Follow-up Study*. Chichester: John Wiley.

[19] The prevention of social disability in schizophrenia

Elizabeth Kuipers

The importance of social factors in schizophrenia

Clinical course and social disability

Schizophrenia remains a mental illness characterised by a wide variety of outcomes (Shepherd et al., 1989). After a first episode around one quarter of sufferers will recover and need no further input. Another two-thirds will have a variable course with recurrent relapses. A final 10% will remain severely disabled and in need of continuing and high contact care from services. Women have a consistently better outcome than men. Unusually for a long-term illness, over the very long term (i.e. two to three decades from the 1950s) there has been a substantial improvement in recovery rates.

It is important to distinguish between clinical and social outcomes. A minority of patients continue to have medication resistant positive symptoms such as voices or delusional ideas which may be distressing. Estimates of the frequency of these phenomena range from around 5–7% (Leff & Wing, 1971), through 23% (Curson et al., 1985) to 55% (Harrow, Carone & Westermeyer, 1985; Harrow, Ratenbury & Stoll, 1988). There is also evidence that depression is found in a considerable number (25–40%) of those with psychosis (Hemsley, 1992; Johnstone et al., 1991), and that the suicide rate is around 10% (Hirsch, Walsh & Draper, 1982).

Social outcome is often linked to clinical outcome – a poorer clinical outcome is likely to lead to social impairment, but not inevitably so. Shepherd et al. (1989), found two-fifths of their sample to have no more than mild impairment after five years, although men were more impaired than women. Social disability was rated in relationships, sociability, leisure and work activities. Of these, clinical outcome was found to have most effect on work activities, although even here it accounted for only 30% of the variance. A few individuals were unimpaired in social functioning despite severe clinical morbidity, and vice versa. The importance of strong family ties and work opportunities was noted in those whose confidence and social competence were relatively unimpaired.

Thus from outcome studies, clear evidence exists for the importance of social factors both in clinical recovery and the prevention of social disability (Kuipers, 1994a). This theme will be the main focus of this chapter.

The range of social disabilities

The effects of severe mental illness on functioning are not always obvious. People with psychosis may have a range of 'positive' symptoms (hallucinations and delusions, see Chapter 18) which can interfere with thinking and concentration, and reduce the ability to tolerate social situations or complex relationships. Social networks are likely to be considerably decreased, from around 40 social contacts in 'normals' (Henderson, Byrne & Duncan-Jones, 1981) to between five and seven for those with long-term problems (Henderson, 1980; Cresswell, Kuipers & Power, 1992). Negative symptoms such as anhedonia (an inability to enjoy), apathy, poor motivation, poor self-care, and even self-neglect in some extreme cases, are common sequelae to an acute episode. These are rarely responsive to medication and are likely to remit only with relatively intense and structured social treatment over a two to three year time-span.

Other effects of severe mental illness include loss of confidence, low self-esteem, depressive and suicidal feelings (as discussed in Chapter 21), and guilt and anxiety about being a burden to carers. As schizophrenia mainly affects individuals in their early adulthood, there is an inevitable process of adjustment to reduced life achievements. If this is combined with poor insight, problems of unrealistic expectations may occur, combined with repeated failures as efforts to change are pitched too high.

The stigma of mental illness is still very much an issue, despite the efforts of self help and pressure groups such as the National Schizophrenic Fellowship (NSF) or MIND. to reduce it, and stigma can increase feelings of isolation and low self-worth. People may also have to cope with their vulnerability to relapse, the necessity of hospital admission, involuntary treatment and, at times, involvement with the legal and criminal justice systems. Many of these 'secondary' effects of schizophrenia (Wing, 1977) are potentially avoidable but only if the necessary help is easily available and accepted by the person concerned.

The likelihood of unemployment and reduced earnings potential means that considerable numbers of people with psychosis find themselves on benefits, having to cope with the complicated bureaucracy of claim forms and social services procedures. Further, many clients in long-term care have a variety of other difficulties which may, or may not, be related to the schizophrenia. These can include poverty, poor educational attainments, a range of other physical illnesses, and substance abuse. Finally, most sufferers will have been prescribed long-term medication. Coping with this fact, understanding the way medication works, and reducing side-effects, are all major issues that contribute to poor compliance and the possibility of an increased number of relapses.

Effects on carers

In the past, between 40% and 60% of patients have returned to live with their families after an episode of schizophrenia (Kuipers, 1993). In the era of care in the community, family members are even more likely to be involved as long-term carers. While some relatives are happy with this role, many feel unsupported and exploited by it. At least half the carers are likely to be elderly parents, normally mothers. Other include spouses, siblings or adult children, landladies or neighbours. Of long-term patients, 10% will have carers who are, or were, patients themselves. Thus families remain the main carers for people with schizophrenia and may be burdened by this role, both practically and emotionally (Fadden, Bebbington & Kuipers, 1987; Kuipers 1992). The degree of burden may be severe and can affect the carer's own well-being, particularly as caring is likely to last for a lifetime without respite (Lefley, 1987; MacCarthy et al., 1989). It is now well documented that having to support relatives with schizophrenia is likely to affect most aspects of family functioning. On the other hand, families potentially provide a 'normal' and caring environment for a patient, one in which social and clinical recovery can be considerably enhanced. The demands and costs of the caring role have to be recognised and balanced against its undoubted possible benefits for the patient in terms of support, company and recovery.

The burden faced by carers comprises a range of effects:

Carers are likely to face *restrictions in their social activities* (e.g. Mandelbrote & Folkard, 1961; Wing, Bennett & Denham, 1964; Waters & Northover, 1965) and have reduced social networks of their own (Anderson, Reiss & Hogarty, 1986). They may remain isolated in their own homes with few other social contacts (MacCarthy, 1988). The stigma of mental illness in the family is still widespread and may contribute to their social isolation (Kuipers et al., 1989).

Financial and employment difficulties are emphasised in a number of studies (e.g. Hoenig & Hamilton, 1966; Stevens, 1972). Because schizophrenia typically occurs in early adulthood and is likely to affect long-term earning and employment capacity, greater impact is felt where the patient had formerly been working (e.g. if carers are spouses) than in families where earning capacity and commitment were not yet established (e.g. parental carers). The loss of *potential* earnings is easy to underestimate, but at the very least the family's lifestyle is likely to be more impoverished than it would be otherwise.

Behaviour problems in patients are major correlates of burden (Lefley, 1987). The two areas that cause most difficulties are socially disruptive behaviour and negative symptoms such as social withdrawal (e.g. Creer & Wing, 1974; Gibbons et al., 1984, MacCarthy et al., 1989).

A wide range of *emotional responses* can be found in relatives who take on the caring role. They include anger, rejection, guilt, grief, loss, fears for the future, worry about a relative, vulnerability, stigma and feelings of isolation. The grief is comparable to a bereavement reaction and may follow a similar pattern and time course: shock, denial, anger, difficulty in accepting the person as they now are (Lefley, 1987). Things may not improve over time, since objective hardship may increase, as can resignation, which is associated with less objective stress, but may be detrimental to patients' functioning because too little is expected (MacCarthy et al., 1989).

The psychological impact on relatives of caring has only recently been assessed formally. When standard psychiatric measures are used such as the general health questionnaire (GHQ), (Goldberg & Hillier, 1979) or the present state examination (PSE) (Wing, Cooper & Sartorius, 1974), there is a consistent finding that about one-third of relatives have elevated levels of anxiety and depression associated with the caring role.

Expressed emotion (EE)

This is a measure of the reactions of relatives who live with schizophrenia to the person who has become unwell. It was developed by George Brown and colleagues in the 1950s and has been found to be a reliable and robust predictor of outcome in schizophrenia (Kavanagh, 1992), and in a range of other conditions including both mental and physical health problems (Kuipers, 1992, 1994b).

EE was developed to measure ordinary aspects of family life, but is unusual in focusing not only on the content of what is said, but also on the way it is expressed in the vocal aspects of speech such as speed, pitch and emphasis. Ratings are made from a tape recording of an interview with a carer and the most predictive ratings have been those of *criticism* and *emotional over-involvement*; high levels of either or both of these in a key relative have defined a family as 'high EE'. If a patient returns to live in such a family setting after an acute episode of schizophrenia, they are likely to have a significantly poorer outcome over the next nine months. In low EE families, relapse rates in the first year are around 20%, and in high EE families around 50%. This is over and above the effects of medication (Bebbington & Kuipers, 1994*a*).

We now know that carers make assumptions about patients when trying to deal with the day to day difficulties of living together. The most common is to think that a patient is being difficult or unhelpful and blame him or her for their behaviour (criticism). This is particularly likely if a person has many negative symptoms of schizophrenia as these are typically misunderstood and not seen as related to the acute attack or relapse. Alternatively, relatives may feel extremely worried, upset and concerned and try to alleviate this by taking over roles and functioning as if the person was a child again (emotional over-involvement). While this is an appropriate response to acute illness and loss of functioning, it is likely to impede social recovery by reducing opportunities for practising adult roles and behaviour, and overburdening a carer with more physically and emotionally demanding tasks.

A final aspect that is also important is being able to like and enjoy being with the patient (warmth). There is now an increasing amount of clinical evidence that families are particularly likely to promote recovery when there are high levels of warmth in carers.

A recent extension of the EE work has been to look at the overlap between relative and staff carers who often have to deal with similar behaviour problems and difficulties, although staff at least have holidays and time off. It was hypothesised that staff might have similar attitudes to relatives towards behaviour problems and difficulties, particularly in long-term care. This was indeed found to be the case in that over 40% of key worker staff had high EE ratings about at least one key patient (Moore, Ball & Kuipers, 1992). Some patients were particularly likely to be criticised especially those who were perceived as less warm and less likely to initiate interactions. In terms of outcome, a naturalistic study of two hostels, one with high EE staff interactions and one with low EE interaction, found poorer outcome in the former (Moore *et al.*, 1992). This has recently been confirmed by Snyder *et al.*, (1995) who found high levels of criticism in hostel staff associated with a poorer quality of life for residents.

Social intervention in schizophrenia

Offering help to carers

Living with carers may promote social recovery, reduce loneliness, maintain social networks and improve clinical outcome for sufferers. However, the costs, particularly for relatives, can be extremely high in terms of severe burden, increased levels of anxiety and depression, and high levels of both practical and emotional resources. In order to improve the quality of life for both patients and carers, families often benefit from the support and input of services, and may need specialised help if problems are very longstanding and intractable. However, there is now an established body of evidence that particular interventions are extremely helpful in improving outcome, reducing relapse rates to around 10% over 9 months, and also improving burden and social outcomes where these are measured (Leff *et al.*, 1982, 1985, 1989, 1990; Falloon *et al.*, 1982, 1985; Hogarty *et al.*, 1986; Hogarty, Anderson & Reiss, 1987; Tarrier *et al.*, 1988, 1989).

The techniques used in successful interventions are now relatively well established (Falloon *et al.*, 1985; Anderson *et al.*, 1986; Barrowclough & Tarrier, 1992; Kuipers, Leff & Lam, 1992). All of them stress the importance of establishing an equal partnership between professionals, carers and patients, and of recognising the expertise of carers on how to cope with difficulties. A more collaborative stance also allows professionals to take carers' viewpoints seriously and to act preventively rather than only in response to a crisis. Recent work shows that patients and carers themselves are well able to assess early signs of relapse (Birchwood *et al.*, 1989) and this can be extremely useful in helping to prevent more serious problems from developing.

Families are likely to need help with a range of issues and these are itemised in Box 19.1. In addition, spouses or partners will need help with the potential loss of their confidant(e), often combined with a need to change or share roles – outside work, housework, child care, etc. Adult children may need help coping with the poor parenting that they themselves received, and with feelings of guilt, loss and resentment.

There is an argument that all families caring for a relative with schizophrenia could benefit from help, and it is certainly true that a large proportion will be burdened, isolated and lack practical and emotional support. In order to reduce the burden of care, services need to offer a range of support and meet a variety of needs. Some caring groups such as partners or adult children will have additional requirements. Primary health care teams are particularly well placed to notice these needs and either provide or activate support such that patients' and relatives' quality of life is enhanced and not extinguished. However, the resources needed to offer support are not always available, and there are some clinical indications of families whose needs are most obvious (Kuipers *et al.*, 1992) (see Box 19.2).

In order to offer services to relatives, professionals must demonstrate that they respect relatives' views, opinions and expertise, and appreciate the burden of the care that they provide. This starting point is essential. For historical reasons, carers may well feel that professional services are inadequate and unhelpful, and reflect a

Understanding schizophrenia; what it is and what it means

Coping with day-to-day problems

Coping with symptoms of schizophrenia (negative and positive)

Emotional support to face and deal with long-term effects of schizophrenia, both on the patients and on themselves

Allowing patients appropriate roles in life, despite persistent disabilities, i.e. not over-protecting them, and allowing as much independence and adult functioning as possible

Worries about the future

The stigma and consequent isolation of those with mental illness

Continuity of care because the caring role can last a lifetime

Box 19.1 *Help that all carers may need.*

Relatives living with patients who relapse more often than once a year, despite being compliant with maintenance neuroleptics

Relatives who frequently contact staff for reassurance and help

Families in which there are repeated arguments, verbal and physical violence

Any family that calls in the police

A single relative, usually a mother, looking after a patient with schizophrenia on her own

Box 19.2 *Families with greatest needs.*

continuing failure to understand their difficulties. Thus, carers are often less than enthusiastic about offers of support and feel professionals may make things worse. Carers may agree with the patient on several counts:

- They may deny that mental illness is the problem.
- They may regard medication as unhelpful.
- They may feel services offer only inappropriate and crisis-orientated care – too little too late.

Because of these problems, offering care to families must be done with sensitivity and with the realisation that even though carers may resist offers of help and be difficult to engage in interventions, their need for support may be high. Although it would seem likely that offering help at the beginning of the caring role (i.e. after a first admission) would be preferable to offering it when attitudes and problems are more entrenched, there are difficulties with this. Clinical experience of work with first episodes of schizophrenia has been that denial and shock are very prevalent attitudes in carers, and because of the fact that some individuals will recover and not need further services, there is a reluctance from professionals to embark on intensive therapeutic measures.

Becoming involved with families after a second or third episode may actually be more beneficial; a patient's course of illness may be more obvious, problems will have recurred not disappeared, and families, including patients, may be more receptive to receiving help at this stage. Often a primary health care team will have been involved in the early episodes and so may be in a good position to help the family either link in with tertiary services or provide the link with longer-term psychiatric care.

The following areas are likely to be most useful for care teams to focus on with families.

Understanding schizophrenia

Many explanatory leaflets and booklets are now available. These can be discussed, preferably in the more relaxed setting of someone's home and any resulting questions can be answered. Such education is not a one-off process, and may need to be repeated many times. Patients' own views have to be dealt with sensitively. Their experience of symptoms can be tapped in order to help relatives understand them more clearly. By itself, information has limited impact on families (Cozolino et al., 1988). However, although it does not change long-term outcome, it is a useful starting point for later interventions, has high face validity for carers, and improves optimism.

Understanding medication

Clinical workers need to provide carers with consistent and practical advice about neuroleptics. There should be a clear and open discussion about the trade-off between side-effects and suppression of unwanted symptoms. The concept of prophylaxis is particularly difficult for lay people to understand. The way in which medication will be monitored should be discussed. Persuading carers of the benefits of medication may be crucial for gaining the acceptance of the patient.

Problem-solving

There is now considerable literature on how to help families solve problems (Kuipers *et al*, 1992; Falloon *et al*, 1993, Barrowclough & Tarrier; 1992). Many problems such as criticism are, in fact, to do with poor understanding of symptoms, particularly negative ones so that prior education is essential and the information must be repeated at this stage. It is important to ask all family members to list current problems and then to come to a consensus on the one problem that might be dealt with each time. Even very everyday issues such as who cooks the meals can be problematic and demonstrate how family functioning may have broken down into argument and frustration. Such mundane problems illustrate how families may have lost skills, e.g. listening to each other, negotiating a compromise, practising a solution. Family problem-solving sessions can begin to tackle all these issues. If a family can begin to experience a small success in problem-solving then the cycle of anger and resignation can begin to be replaced by more optimism and confidence and, most importantly, the underlying feelings of warmth and care may begin to return.

Emotional impact

Most of the manuals also deal with this. Relatives may need to be seen on their own to help them feel free to discuss negative aspects and the wide range of emotional responses they are likely to feel. Relatives' groups are also very helpful in providing models of coping, 'survival' techniques, and the normality of very extreme emotional states, such as grief and anger (Kuipers & Westall, 1992).

Overprotection

Some families have particular difficulties with allowing patients as much independence as possible despite continuing disabilities, and remove adult responsibilities so that the patient can be 'looked after' and recover. This is an understandable and caring response in the short term but, in the long term, social recovery is slowed and disabilities may increase.

If patients become 'stuck' in the childlike role, they may avoid adult roles and decisions and become increasingly burdensome. In some cases this can lead to a patient becoming verbally demanding and physically aggressive, particularly if a relative is small and frail and feels unable to say 'no' or to set other appropriate limits. Such problems are likely to need specialist help, such as dealing with anger, limit setting, negotiating more responsible roles for the patient and encouraging the carer to allow this. Carers may also need 'permission' to take up former interests and activities so that more balanced roles are available in the family.

Parents often have realistic *worries about the future*, about the care of the patients when they themselves become infirm or die. This is best discussed openly, while the carer is still fit, so that appropriate solutions can be faced earlier rather than later. However, some families, and some patients, are not able to deal with these issues until forced to do so.

Stigma

Carers themselves are likely to suffer stigma and may have reduced social networks. Joining a voluntary support group (such as the National Schizophrenia Fellowship) may help to alleviate this and provide an alternative source of emotional and practical help.

Continuity of care

Services should aim to provide continuity of care to relatives, despite staff or team changes. The key worker or care management system is particularly useful in this context. Services need to be geared to provide care at some level over many years, through telephone calls or meetings, and not just at crisis points. Regular contact allows preventive action to be taken much earlier, and can efficiently alert a clinical team to difficulties and problems. If patients disengage from services, carers may well be able to re-establish communication even in very difficult circumstances. The more open climate of care in the community, with the emphasis on user choice and information as a right, means that this need is more likely to be met than before. Involving relatives and patients in clinical meetings, discussing issues openly and accepting the validity of families' and clients' views, will ensure that long-term care plans are both feasible and realistic.

Respite

While the need for respite is clear, provision often depends on local and charitable initiatives. As hospital beds become scarcer, emphasis is now being put on 'respite houses' in the community. These services will need to be developed more routinely if they are to offer effective, planned help to families. Day care of various types also provides some respite for relatives, allowing them to spend time out of the house, and helping the sufferer to open up other roles apart from that of 'patient'. Relatives themselves may need 'permission' to take time off from caring, to take up interests, and to increase their social network. This alleviates the isolation and burden of the caring role, provides other contacts for support and gives a broader perspective on difficulties.

In some case, patients, carers and relatives will not be able to live together, however much respite is provided. In these situations it may be much better for staff to help negotiate reasonable alternatives, such as supported accommodation for the patient, rather than preserving a deteriorating relationship. Often, if alternatives are

faced and discussed before problems become intractable, independence can be fostered and carers' worries about the future can be
alleviated somewhat.

Offering help to the sufferer

In long-term schizophrenia, up to 20% of patients live alone and a
further 30% may live in a hostel setting. The staff may become like
a 'family' for a patient with consequent advantages and disadvantages. The latter are more usually due to critical or hostile attitudes
in staff rather than overprotection. For other patients, although
there may be family contact, either patient or relatives may decline
access to services. Thus there are substantial numbers of patients
who either may not have access to family care, whose family may
have rejected them as too problematic, or whose family may no
longer exist. Even those with good family support will also benefit
from individual help, and a range of social inputs will be likely to
prevent social disability and improve clinical outcome.

These include (Bebbington & Kuipers, 1994a,b):

- Dealing with residual symptoms – positive and negative
  symptoms, poor insight, poor concentration.
- Provision of structure and meaningful activity.
- Discussion of the emotional impact of schizophrenia – loss
  of self-esteem, reduced expectations, vulnerability.
- Dealing with other psychiatric symptoms – anxiety and
  depression, managing stress.

Cognitive–behavioural interventions

Many patients continue to suffer disabling and even distressing
positive symptoms such as hallucinations and delusions. Variation
in mental state may impair concentration and disrupt activities.
Insight may be poor or even non-existent so that offers of help or
support are rejected. Medication may be disliked and poorly understood which may contribute to or exacerbate the difficulties. New
cognitive behavioural interventions offer some evidence that medication resistant positive symptoms can be improved in psychosis.
These involve enhancing coping strategies, (Tarrier et al., 1993a,b)
and, more fundamentally, helping patients begin to review and
reassess the evidence for particular delusional ideas (Chadwick &
Lowe, 1990; Garety et al., 1994).

A particularly sensitive, empathic and sympathetic therapeutic
style is needed to do this, and such input must be done gradually
and in the context of a trusting therapeutic relationship, within
which psychotic thinking and experiences can be re-examined. The
aim is to establish the boundary of what is real, without arguing or

denying the validity of the patients' views, which are seen as equally valid but not shared.

Coping strategies

Coping responses that have been found to be useful tend to be idiosyncratic, but patients can be encouraged to try them in a more organised way, or to attempt new ones that they may not have discovered. Distraction, relaxation and social avoidance can all be useful, particularly if not taken to extremes (Tarrier *et al.*, 1993*a*). Recognising triggers for exacerbation or relapse is also useful, as most clients have a relapse 'signature' (Birchwood *et al.*, 1989) which is individual and if interrupted early can prevent a more severe breakdown (see Chapter 18). Once triggers are recognised, such as stressful social settings, an adaptive coping response can be encouraged and practised (such as only staying for a few minutes rather than waiting until the voices start). Such coping can also encourage feelings of control and mastery, rather than hopelessness and failure and will thus also begin to reduce problems of depression and low self-esteem.

Negative symptoms

These are the ones that carers find most difficult to deal with and the ones that are most responsive to social input. Lack of motivation, interest, self-care and social withdrawal (even day–night reversal) are all common aspect of long-term schizophrenia. They tend to respond to the following interventions.

Provision of structure and meaningful activity through a range of social and leisure activities can help improve interest and motivation, particularly if they are available at a range of times, in a local and approachable setting and if professionals are able to help to prompt and encourage attendance. The provision of a work environment is also important, although some people with schizophrenia regain employment or sheltered work, the function of work settings is at least as important. Work can provide meaningful activity that is normalising, allows a sense of achievement and self-esteem, and provides an alternative adult role in society to that of 'patient'.

Access to settings such as day care and day centres where occupational therapy is available and advice, counselling, company or a meal can be found, for those who drop in as well as those who attend regularly, is a vital aspect of enabling people with schizophrenia begin the process of social recovery.

Patients' understanding

Most severe illnesses are now recognised to have both an emotional and physical impact on the person who experiences them. In mental health, particularly in severe psychosis, the importance of discussing a patient's understanding, experience and ability to manage the problems, has taken longer to be recognised. Nevertheless, this is a crucial part of reducing social disability and enabling recovery to be as optimal as possible. The experience of acute schizophrenia is often very frightening and chaotic, so that even some discussion of what happened and what a patient understood about it can begin to help place events in context and to cope with the residual problems. More seriously, the fact of reduced expectations and achievements may be more difficult to accept and understand – poor insight is often blamed for this. The loss and change in circumstances that often accompany initial and subsequent episodes may be devastating; individuals may lose family, job, money and independence. They may subsequently have to face a completely changed lifestyle that they would not previously have chosen. Low self-esteem, lost confidence, fear of the future, are all understandable and common aspects of such events and may need to be discussed in some detail before an individual can begin to process what has happened, as well as how they will cope in the future.

Anxiety and depression

Depression and feelings of suicide are not uncommon accompaniments to schizophrenia and in view of the changes and losses often experienced are also not surprising. Less commonly recognised is anxiety or social avoidance. If it exists, it very often will be a trigger for renewed positive symptoms, and so its management may be especially important. Techniques such as recognising triggers, practising social encounters in a graded way, and utilising relaxation and distraction can all be useful in helping to reduce the impact of such difficulties.

Role of key workers or case managers

Primary health care teams and mental health teams now commonly include a range of professionals such as community psychiatric nurses, involved in the care of those with mental health problems. Despite the needs of those with schizophrenia, there may be a tendency for care to go first to the more articulate and rewarding clients and for the severely mentally ill to be more neglected. In primary care the role of community psychiatric nurses may be to take on such severely ill individuals and to make sure that they are linked in with local community mental health care teams. With the care programme approach now official policy, it is standard practice for a key worker to be allocated and this is likely for those with schizophrenia.

A key worker may have a range of responsibilities but one of the most important ones in this area is to make a relationship with the

Cognitive behavioural treatment for hallucinations and delusions

Identifying stressful situations and coping mechanisms

Provision of structure and meaningful activity

Supportive therapy and discussion of the impact of the illness

Relaxation and distraction techniques

Box 19.3 *Psychosocial interventions likely to help sufferers.*

patient that provides some continuity of care, enables a patient to be motivated and prompted (if negative symptoms are a problem), ensures monitoring of mental state and medication levels and coordinates the range of care necessary for both patient and carers. The role of the key worker is particularly crucial in severe mental illness because patients may be poorer at accessing specialist care and not recognise fully the range of needs that they have. It is recommended practice to incorporate the sufferer's aims and wishes into any care plan, involving and representing them at clinical team reviews, so that aims and goals can be revised as necessary. All those involved in purchasing care for severe mental illness should be aware of the potential value of social interventions (Box 19.3).

Conclusions

There is evidence of the effectiveness of a range of social treatments that can prevent and reduce social disability in patients, reduce burden in carers and improve the quality of life for individual and family members. While the needs of patients and carers may be extensive, provision of a range of appropriate services is likely to be extremely cost-effective in reducing the morbidity levels of both patients and carers, both now and in the future. Studies of the cost of social treatment suggests that even intensive input is easily recouped by reduced admission rates and days in hospital (Falloon *et al.*, 1985) and the accompanying reduction in stress levels and crises, for both carers and patients. Being prepared to take account of patient and carer needs in the community at an early stage is both a feasible and essential strategy in preventing long-term social disability in schizophrenia.

References

Anderson, C.M., Reiss D.J. & Hogarty G. E. (1986). *Schizophrenia in the Family: A Practitioner's Guide to Psychoeducation and Management*. New York: Guilford Press.

Barrowclough, C. & Tarrier, N. (1992). *Families of Schizophrenic Patients: Cognitive Behavioural Intervention*. London: Chapman and Hall.

Bebbington, P.E. & Kuipers, L. (1994a). The predictive utility of expressed emotion in schizophrenia: an aggregate analysis. *Psychological Medicine*, **24**, 707–18.

Bebbington, P.E. & Kuipers, L. (1994b). The social management of longstanding schizophrenia: the deployment of service resources. *The Clinician*, **12**, 17–29.

Birchwood, M., Smith, J., MacMillan F. *et al.*, (1989). Predicting relapse in schizophrenia: the development and implementation of an early signs monitoring system using patients and families as observers, a preliminary investigations. *Psychological Medicine*, **19**, 649–56.

Briera, A., Schreiber, J.L., Dyer, J. & Pickard, D. (1991). NIMH longitudinal study of chronic schizophrenia: prognosis and predictors of outcome. *Archives of General Psychiatry*, **48**, 239–46.

Chadwick, P. & Lowe F. (1990). The modification of delusional beliefs. *Journal of Consulting and Clinical Psychology*, **58**, 225–32.

Cozolino, L.J., Goldstein M.J., Nuechterlein, K.C. *et al.* (1988). The impact of education on relatives' varying in levels of EE. *Schizophrenia Bulletin*, **14**, 675–86.

Creer, C. & Wing. J.K. (1974). *Schizophrenia at Home*. Surbiton: National Schizophrenia Fellowship.

Cresswell, C.M. Kuipers, L. & Power, M.J. (1992). Social networks and support in long-term psychiatric patients. *Psychological Medicine*, **22**, 1019–26.

Curson, D.A., Barnes, T.R.E., Bamber, R.W., Platt, S.D., Hirsch, S.R. & Duffy, J.D. (1985). Long-term depot maintenance of chronic schizophrenic outpatients. *British Journal of Psychiatry*, **146**, 464–80.

Fadden, G.B., Bebbington P.E., & Kuipers, L. (1987). The burden of care: the impact of functional psychiatric illness on the patient's family. *British Journal of Psychiatry*, **150**, 285–92.

Falloon, I.R.H. (1985). Family management of schizophrenia. Baltimore: Johns Hopkins Press.

Falloon, I.R.H., Boyd, J.L., McGill, C.W., Ranzani, J., Moss, H.B. & Gilderman, A.M. (1982). Family management in the prevention of exacerbations of schizophrenia. A controlled study. *New England Journal of Medicine*, **306**, 1437–40.

Falloon, I.R.H., Boyd, J.L., McGill, C.W., Williamson, M., Razani, J., Moss, H.B., Gilderman, A.M. & Simpson, G.M. (1985). Family management in the prevention of morbidity of schizophrenia. Clinical outcome of a two-year longitudinal study. *Archives of General Psychiatry*, **42**, 887–96.

Falloon, I.R.H., Laporta, M., Fadden, G. & Graham-Hole, V. (1993). *Managing Stress in Families: Cognitive and Behavioural Strategies for Enhancing Coping Skills*, London: Routledge.

Garety, P.A., Kuipers., L. & Fowler D., *et al.*, (1994). Cognitive behaviour therapy for drug resistant psychosis. *British Journal of Medical Psychology*, **67**, 259–71.

Gibbons, J.S., Horn, S.H., Powell, J.M. *et al.* (1984). Schizophrenic patients and their families. A survey in a psychiatric service based on a district general hospital. *British Journal of Psychiatry*, **144**, 70–7.

Goldberg, D.P. & Hillier, V.G. (1979). A scaled version of the GHQ. *Psychological Medicine*, **9**, 139–46.

Harrow, M., Carone, B.J. & Westermeyer, J. (1985). The course of psychosis in early phases of schizophrenia. *American Journal of Psychiatry*, **142**, 702–7.

Harrow, M. Ratenbury, F. & Stoll, F. (1988). Schizophrenic delusions: an analysis of their persistence, of related pre-morbid ideas, and of other major delusions. In *Delusional Beliefs*. Oltmanns, T. and Maher, B., eds, NY: J. Wiley.

Hemsley, D. (1992). *Anxiety and Depression in Schizophrenia*. Personal communication.

Henderson, A.S. (1980). Personal networks and the schizophrenics. *Australian and New Zealand Journal of Psychiatry*, **14**, 255–9.

Henderson, A.S., Byrne, D.G. & Duncan-Jones, P. (1981). *Neurosis and the Social Environment*. Sydney. Academic Press.

Hirsch, S.R., Walsh, C. & Draper, R. (1982). Parasuicide: a review of treatment interventions. *Journal of Affective Disorders*, **4**, 299–311.

Hoenig, J. & Hamilton, M.W. (1966). The schizophrenic patient in the community and his effect on the household. *International Journal of Social Psychiatry*, **12**, 165–76.

Hogarty, G.E., Anderson, C.M., Reiss, D.J., Kornblith, S.J., Greenwald, D.P., Javma. C.D. & Madonia, M.J. (1986). Family psycho-education, social skills training and maintenance chemotherapy in the aftercare treatment of schizophrenia. One-year effects of a controlled study on relapse and expressed emotion. *Archives of General Psychiatry*, **43**, 633–42.

Hogarty, G.E., Anderson, C.M. & Reiss, D.J. (1987). Family psycho-education, social skills training, and medication in schizophrenia: the long and the short of it. *Psychopharmacological Bulletin*, **23**, 12–23.

Johnstone, E.C., Owens, D.G.C., Firth, C.D. & Leavy, J. (1991). Clinical findings: abnormalities of mental state and their correlates. The Northwick Park Follow-up Study. *British Journal of Psychiatry*, **159**, 21–5.

Kavanagh, D.J. (1992). Recent developments in expressed emotion and schizophrenia. *British Journal of Psychiatry*, **106**, 601–20.

Kuipers, L. (1992). Expressed emotion research in Europe. *British Journal of Clinical Psychology*, **31**, 429–43.

Kuipers, L. (1993). Family burden in schizophrenia: implication for services. *Social Psychiatry and Psychiatric Epidemiology*, **28**, 207–10.

Kuipers, L. (1994a) Social support and psychiatric disorder: research findings and guidelines for clinical practice. In *Social Support: Measurement, Intervention and Training Tasks*. Brugha, T., ed. Cambridge: Cambridge University Press.

Kuipers, L. (1994b). The measurement of expressed emotion: its influence on research and clinical practice. *International Review of Psychiatry*, **6**, 187–99.

Kuipers, L., Leff, J. & Lam, D. (1992). *Family Work for Schizophrenia: A Practical Guide*. London: Gaskell.

Kuipers, L., MacCarthy, B., Hurry, J. *et al.* (1989). Counselling the relatives of the long-term adult mentally ill. (ii) A low cost supportive model. *British Journal of Psychiatry*, **154**, 75–82.

Kuipers, L. & Westall, J. (1992). The role of facilitated relative groups and voluntary self help groups. In *Principles of Social Psychiatry*. Bhugra, D. and Leff, J., eds. London: Blackwell.

Leff, J.P. & Wing, J.K. (1971). Trial of maintenance therapy in schizophrenia. *British Medical Journal*, **3**, 599–604.

Leff, J.P., Kuipers, L., Berkowitz, R., Eberlein-Fries, R. & Sturgeon, D. (1982). A controlled trial of social intervention in schizophrenic families. *British Journal of Psychiatry*, **141**, 121–34.

Leff, J.P., Kuipers, L., Berkowitz, R. & Sturgeon, D. (1985). A controlled trial of social intervention in the families of schizophrenic patients: two year follow-up. *British Journal of Psychiatry*, **146**, 594–600.

Leff, J., Berkowitz, R., Sharit, N., Strachan, A., Glass, I. & Vaughn, C. (1989). A trial of family therapy versus a relatives' group for schizophrenia, *British Journal of Psychiatry*, **154**, 58–66.

Leff, J., Berkowitz, R., Sharit, N., Strachan, A., Glass, I. & Vaughn, C. (1990). A trial of family therapy versus a relatives' group for schizophrenia: a two-year follow-up. *British Journal of Psychiatry*, **157**, 571–7.

Lefley, H.P. (1987). Ageing parents as care givers of mentally ill adult children: an emerging social problem. *Hospital and Community Psychiatry.* **38**, 1063–70.

MacCarthy, B. (1988). The role of relative. In *Community Care in Practice.* Lavender, A. and Holloway, F., eds. London: Wiley & Sons.

MacCarthy, B., Lesage, A., Brewin C.R. *et al.* (1989). Needs for care among the relatives of long-term users of day-care. *Psychological Medicine,* **19**: 725–736.

McFadyen, J. (1991) Occupational therapy in the management of longstanding mental illness in the community. *Review of Psychiatry,* **3**, 95–103.

Mandelbrote, B.M. & Folkard, S. (1961). Some problems and needs of schizophrenics in relation to a developing psychiatric community service. *Comprehensive Psychiatry,* **2**, 317–28.

Moore, E. Ball. R.A. & Kuipers, L. (1992). Expressed emotion in staff working with the long-term adult mentally ill. *British Journal of Psychiatry* (in press).

Shepherd, M., Watt, D., Falloon, I. & Smeeton, N. (1989). The natural history of schizophrenia: a five-year follow-up study of outcome and prediction in a representative sample of schizophrenics. In *Psychological Medicine, Monograph Supplement 15.*

Snyder, K.S., Wallace, C.J., Moe, K. & Liberman, R.P. (1994). Expressed emotion by residential care operators, residents' symptoms and quality of life. *Hospital and Community Psychiatry,* **45**, 1141–3.

Stevens, B. (1972). Dependence of schizophrenic patients on elderly relatives. *Psychological Medicine,* **2**, 17–32.

Tarrier, N., Barrowclough, C., Vaughn, C., Bamrah, J.S., Porceddu, K., Watts, S. & Freeman, H. (1988). The community management of schizophrenia: a controlled trial of a behavioural intervention with families to reduce relapse. *British Journal of Psychiatry,* **153**, 532–42.

Tarrier, N., Barrowclough, C., Vaughn, C., Bamrah, J.S., Porceddu, K., Watts, S. & Freeman, H. (1989). Community management of schizophrenia in a two-year follow-up of a behavioural intervention with families. *British Journal of Psychiatry,* **154**, 625–8.

Tarrier, N., Beckett, R., Harwood, S., Baker, A., Yosopoff, L. & Ugarteburn, I. (1993*a*). A trial of two cognitive behavioural methods of treating drug resistant residual psychotic symptoms in schizophrenic patients. I: outcome. *British Journal of Psychiatry,* **162**, 524–32.

Tarrier, N., Sharpe, L., Beckett, R. *et al.* (1993*b*). A trial of two cognitive behavioural methods treating drug-resistant residual psychotic symptoms in schizophrenic patients: II

Treatment specific changes in coping and problem solving skills. *Social Psychiatry and Psychiatric Epidemiology*, **28**, 5–10.

Waters, M.A. & Northover, J. (1965). Rehabilitated long-stay schizophrenics in the community. *British Journal of Psychiatry*, III, 258–67.

Wing, J.K. (1977). The management of schizophrenia in the community. In *Psychiatric Medicine*. Usdin, G., ed. New York: Brunner, Mazel.

Wing, J.K., Bennett, D.H. & Denham, J. (1964). *The Industrial Rehabilitation of Long Stay Schizophrenic Patients*. Medical Research Council Memo No. 42, London: HMSO.

Wing, J.K., Cooper, J.E. & Sartorius, N. (1974). *The Measurement and Classification of Psychiatric Symptoms*. Cambridge: Cambridge University Press.

[20] Organising continuing care of the long-term mentally ill in general practice

Tony Kendrick

Introduction

The move to community care

In the United Kingdom, as in other European countries and the United States, there has been a progressive move away from extended mental hospital inpatient care since the 1950s, so that nowadays most people with long-term mental illnesses spend nearly all their lives in the community (Chapter 14). More than 100 000 people disabled by long-term mental illnesses were estimated to be living in the community in England by 1986 (Department of Health and Social Security (DHSS), 1987) and the number is likely to have increased since then with further hospital closures.

Despite advances in treatment however, many mentally ill people still require support on a long-term basis (Chapters 16 and 18). For all their faults, the old asylums did at least provide patients with reliable food and shelter and the immediate support of trained nursing staff and psychiatrists. Outside hospitals such support is more difficult to deliver and by the 1990s there was serious concern in the UK that long-term mentally ill people might not get the continuing care they needed in the community. Researchers found that many disabled former residents of long-stay wards, with active symptoms, were living in hostels unsupported by psychiatrically trained staff (Marshall, 1989); a third of destitute men on the streets of inner London were found to be suffering from hallucinations and delusions (Weller et al., 1989); and a disproportionately high percentage of men with schizophrenia was found among those in remand prisons (Taylor & Gunn, 1984).

In the UK, community mental health teams have been asked by the government to target those with disabling long-term mental illnesses for continuing support, most recently through The Health of the Nation initiative (Department of Health, 1991). This is thought to be the best strategy to prevent suicides, most of which occur among this patient group, and to improve significantly the health and social functioning of mentally ill people. However, in practice many long-term mentally ill patients have no continuing contact with psychiatric services once they leave hospital. This represents a challenge to general practice.

General practitioners and the long-term mentally ill

The large majority of patients with chronic neurotic illnesses have always been managed in general practice, with few referrals to psychiatrists (Shepherd et al., 1966; Goldberg & Huxley, 1980). In addition to this, with the shift to community care, general practitioners have become increasingly involved in the care of patients with psychosis, not just immediately before hospital admissions (Parkes, Brown & Monck, 1962), but in the longer term too. Around a third of patients with psychosis lose contact with specialist services altogether within a year after hospital discharge and depend entirely on general practitioners for medical care (Johnstone et al., 1984; Pantelis, Taylor & Campbell, 1988; Melzer et al., 1991) (see Chapter 14). To an extent, this increase in involvement is inevitable, and there are a number of good reasons why general practitioners should play a central role in the care of people with long-term mental illnesses, including psychotic illnesses such as schizophrenia (see Chapter 18).

Even where secondary care services are involved in a person's care, there is still a role for primary care. *The Health of the National Mental Illness Key Area Handbook* (Department of Health, 1994) recommends that primary health care teams should help secondary care teams to identify and monitor the long-term mentally ill, agree protocols for referral and shared care, and join in audit, hospital discharge planning meetings and confidential reviews of suicides (Chapter 21).

However, questions have been raised about the extent to which primary health care services can contribute to the continuing care of long-term mentally ill patients, particularly those with psychoses. Goldberg and Jackson (1992) pointed out that the number of patients with chronic schizophrenia seen in a year by general practitioners in the UK Third National Morbidity Survey fell short of the known prevalence of such patients, suggesting that significant numbers were not seen by their family factors from one year to the next. In the 1970s, practice activity analysis data revealed that around half of all prescriptions for phenothiazine major tranquillisers were repeat prescriptions issued without the patient being seen, and only one-third were given in follow-up consultations (Royal College of General Practitioners' Birmingham Research Unit, 1978).

We conducted a postal survey from St George's Medical School of 507 general practitioners in the South West Thames health region, to investigate their involvement with long-term mentally ill patients (Kendrick *et al.*, 1991). Of the 369 (73%) who responded, 333 (90%) were willing to share in the care of long-term mentally ill patients with psychiatric teams and as many as 151 (41%) stated that they were willing to organise the care of such patients with psychiatric back-up as necessary. However, the large majority agreed that often the patients came to their attention only when there was a crisis in their care. Only nine doctors (2%) reported any specific practice policies for looking after the long-term mentally ill.

So how should general practitioners organise their practices to try and ensure that their long-term mentally ill patients received the continuing care they need outside hospital?

Practice organisation

The provision of care for patients with a chronic illnesses has implications for practice organisation and management. Schofield (1984) outlined the areas in which changes may have to be thought through. These include the aims of care, accessibility of the doctor, the continuity of care, the medical records and performance review.

The aims of care

Pendleton and Schofield (1983) argued that to maintain the motivation needed to provide continuing care for a chronic disease, the doctor should have a clear sense of purpose and realistic aims. The aims of tertiary prevention in long-term mental illness are to limit complications and to avoid deterioration in the patient's condition where possible, rather than to expect a cure. The aims will therefore include:

1. to identify and meet physical, psychological and social needs for treatment or care;
2. to prevent relapse;
3. to prevent suicide;
4. to enable the sufferer to live as full a life as possible;
5. to enable the relatives or other carers to support the sufferer.

A proactive approach

Many patients with long-term mental illness, particularly those with chronic psychosis, suffer from poor motivation, a lack of self-esteem, loss of concentration and social withdrawal (Wing, 1989). This explains why they may fail to attend for treatment, neglecting themselves and allowing problems to build up into crises which might have been avoided. The doctor must therefore be prepared to make an active effort to contact patients, to ensure that they do not drift out of touch. This is especially important if the patient lives alone.

To adopt this kind of proactive approach, the practice needs to set up a system for the regular review of long-term mentally ill patients. Most important is a fail-safe mechanism for dealing with non-attenders. When they begin to relapse, patients often lose insight into their illness and the significance of changes in their symptoms, and cannot be relied upon to present themselves for help just when they need it most (Birchwood *et al.*, 1989). When a patient with schizophrenia misses a follow-up appointment action by the doctor is required.

For these reasons, achieving the aims of continuing care will require a number of active steps within the practice. These include:

1. defining and identifying the vulnerable patient group;
2. operating a call-recall register, to help maintain regular contact with the patients and their carers;
3. structuring regular reviews of the patients to include a checklist of possible problem areas;
4. ensuring a high level of continuity of care, to encourage an effective doctor–patient relationship.

Just as the practice might have a disease register of patients with diabetes, for example, and a system of call and recall to ensure that their care is reviewed systemically at regular intervals, so a disease register and call/recall system for patients with long-term mental illness can be created.

Defining and identifying the long-term mentally ill
The first step is to decide how the practice wishes to define long-term mental illness, which will determine how many patients will be included and what type of problems are likely to be found.

There is no widely accepted definition of a long-term mentally ill patient. Bachrach (1988) pointed out that any definition should include consideration of the '3Ds' of diagnosis, duration, and disability. *The Mental Illness Key Area Handbook* (Department of Health, 1994) lists four different definitions, drawn up by psychiatrists, all of which include a psychotic diagnosis as one criterion for inclusion. In primary care, however, there will usually be significant numbers of patients with non-psychotic diagnoses who are nevertheless vulnerable and should therefore be included in any practice policy for the care of the long-term mentally ill. To qualify for inclusion, patients should have been ill for some time, perhaps a year or two, and be disabled by their illness. Disability is often defined by psychiatrists in terms of a previous need for hospital admission, but in primary care there will be patients who have never been admitted but are significantly disabled in terms of impaired functioning at work or in the home.

Box 20.1 shows the definition we adopted in a study of the provision of care to the long-term mentally ill conducted in 16

We define a long-term mentally ill patient as one who for two years or more has been disabled by impaired social behaviour associated with mental illness.

Duration

The patient's disability must extend for at least two years.

Disability

Disability is the most important criterion; the patients are unable to fulfil any one of four roles that might be expected of them, including:

    (i) holding down a job
    (ii) maintaining their appearance and personal hygiene
    (iii) performing necessary domestic chores
    (iv) participating in recreational activities

The abnormal social behaviour can be any one of four types:

    (i) withdrawal and inactivity
    (ii) behaviour due to hallucination or delusions
    (iii) bizarre, embarrassing behaviour
    (iv) violence towards others or self

Diagnosis

The mental illness may be any of the following:
One of the psychoses, including:

    Schizophrenia
    Paranoid psychosis
    Manic-depressive psychosis
    Psychotic depression

or it may be a non-psychotic illness which is none the less severe and chronic and disabling, including:

    Anxiety neurosis (neurasthenia, nervous debility)
    Neurotic depression
    Phobic or obsessional neurosis
    Personality disorder
    Eating disorder
    Alcohol or drug misuse

or it may be a mental illness which has not been given a specific label

Box 20.1 *Definition of a long-term mentally ill patient.*

group general practices in the South West Thames health region (Kendrick *et al.*, 1994).

In our study, we were interested in experimenting with the delivery of care to adults with functional mental illnesses, so we excluded patients under 16 or over 65, and those with dementia or learning disability. This latter group might also benefit from special practice policies (see Chapter 17), but they are outside the scope of this chapter.

Having decided on the type of patient to be included in a disease register, the next step is to identify patients for inclusion. The general practitioners will remember a proportion of patients, but more will be identified through a search of repeat prescription lists, appointment records and diagnostic data, which these days are computerised in many practices. In addition to searching practice data, local psychiatric and social service teams can be asked to examine their caseloads to identify any long-term mentally ill people known to them who are registered with the practice. The potential sources are listed in Box 20.2, together with an indication of their relative usefulness in terms of the percentage of the total identified by any one method in our study. In most practices, 90% of patients can be identified quickly through repeat prescription and diagnostic data.

Long-term mentally ill patients were identified from the following sources: (Kendrick et al., 1994)

1. *Practice data*
   (a) The repeat prescription system, if any, for patients on:
       Antipsychotic drugs (oral and depot)
       Anticholinergics
       Antidepressants
       Anxiolytics (61%)
   (b) Computer records or disease register where appropriate (23%)
   (c) Patients being seen for depot injections by the practice nurse where appropriate (5%)
   (d) Appointment lists of patients seen in surgery or on visits in the previous 3 months (to remind oneself of patients who are not on medication or seeing the nurse) (21%)

2. *Mental Health Services data*
   (a) Patients of the community psychiatric nurse (14%)
   (b) Consultant psychiatrists' case registers and outpatient records (5%)
   (c) Day Hospital patients (6%)

3. *Social Services data*
   (a) Social workers' caseloads (5%)

Box 20.2 *Identifying patients with long-term mental illness.*

The names of patients identified from all these sources should be checked, to confirm that they match the definition for inclusion, using the doctor's knowledge of the patients and information in their records The general practitioners in our 16-practice study found no difficulty in using our research definition to decide whether patients should be included.

Numbers and types and long-term mentally ill patients

Using the definition and methods of identification outlined above, we found 440 patients between the 16 practices, a mean prevalence of three per thousand patients registered, i.e. six or seven patients per doctor on average (Kendrick et al., 1994). However, the actual number of patients per individual doctor varied between zero and 20. The prevalence of patients with psychotic diagnoses was found to correlate with the practices' Jarman underprivileged area scores, which are a measure of social deprivation derived from population census data (Fig. 20.1). This means that practices in inner city and other deprived areas are likely to find themselves with more long-term mentally ill patients than those in affluent areas.

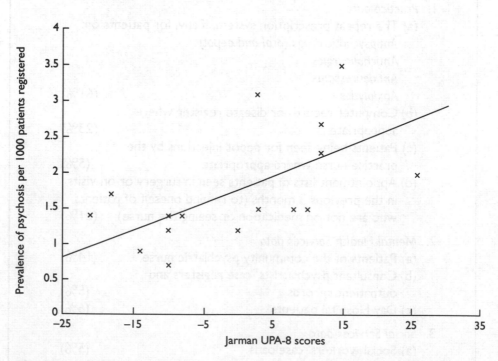

Fig. 20.1 *Relationship of prevalence of psychosis to social deprivation in 16 group general practices.* (Kendrick et al., 1994.)

The patients' diagnoses are shown in Table 20.1. Overall, 253 (57.5%) had received a psychotic diagnosis and 187 (42.5%) a non-psychotic diagnosis, confirming the impression that there are many non-psychotic patients who nevertheless are significantly disabled by their illnesses. Over one-third of the patients had had no contact with psychiatrists or community psychiatric nurses within the previous 12 months. Significantly, more of the psychotic patients were in current contact with specialist teams (73%) than the non-psychotic patients (48%), suggesting that patients in long-term contact with secondary care services cannot be taken as representative of the whole population with long-term mental illness.

Diagnosis recorded in files	Number of patients	Number (%) seen by their GPs in last 12 months	Number (%) in current contact with either psychiatrists or community psyciatric nurses
Schizophrenia/schizo-affective disorder	204	181 (89)	144 (70)
Manic-depressive psychosis	38	37 (97)	33 (87)
Psychotic depression	11	10 (91)	8 (73)
Total psychotic	253	228 (90)	185 (73)
Anxiety/depression	103	101 (98)	50 (48)
Agoraphobia	27	27(100)	11 (41)
Personality disorder	16	15 (93)	8 (50)
Alcohol abuse	15	15(100)	9 (60)
Anorexia nervosa	7	7(100)	4 (57)
Chronic psychogenic pain	6	6(100)	0 (0)
Obsessive–compulsive disorder	5	4 (80)	3 (60)
Drug abuse	4	4(100)	1 (25)
Other	4	4(100)	3 (75)
Total non-psychotic	187	183 (98)	89 (48)
Total long-term mentally ill	440	411 (93)	274 (62)

Table 20.1 *Recorded diagnosis of the long-term mentally ill and their contacts with professionals*

Call–recall systems

Table 20.1 shows that the large majority of the long-term mentally ill patients in the 16 practices we studied had been seen by their general practitioners within 12 months. Whilst virtually all the non-psychotic patients had consulted, however, 10% of the psychotic patients had not been seen in the practice for a year. The practices studied were to an extent self-selected on the basis of an interest in the long-term mentally ill, and it is quite likely that in other practices an even greater proportion of psychotic patients do not see their general practitioners from one year to the next, as suspected by Goldberg and Jackson (1992). It is therefore particularly import-ant for the practice to draw up a register of psychotic patients and to operate a call/recall system, if the primary health care team is to ensure regular contact and involvement with such patients.

Recall registers

These days, call/recall lists can be kept on computer in the majority of practices. Alternatives include a simple diary or an index of cards, one for each month, on which patients' names are entered at the required intervals. The desired interval between reviews will, of course, vary between patients, depending on the severity of their problems, their level of compliance with medication and the fre-quency of relapses in the past. What is important is that someone in the practice is given responsibility for reviewing the register of patients at intervals to check whether patients have been reviewed as required by the practice protocol. In my own practice, my partners and I adopted a policy whereby all patients with chronic schizophrenia should be seen by their general practitioners at least once every six months, although some patients would of course be seen much more frequently, as necessary. One of the senior admin-istrative staff is responsible for reviewing the list of chronic schizo-phrenia patients on the computer every quarter, and alerting the practitioners to any patient who has not consulted.

Limiting repeat prescriptions

Sometimes, too many repeat prescriptions are given without a review of the patient. Repeats are often signed at the end of morning surgery, when the doctor is in a hurry to get out on visits, and therefore may not receive the attention they deserve. The first step towards improving the regular supervision of patients is to limit the number of repeats they may have before their next review. This helps to ensure check-ups of those who seek a repeat of their prescription, but of course such a method cannot ensure that patients who give up taking medication are reviewed, since at present repeat prescription systems are not usually programmed to warn staff which patients have *not* put in for a prescription at the predicted time.

Where the practice nurse gives depot medications, it is very important that, if a patient does not turn up for their injection, the nurse alerts the doctor who can then seek out the patient, or perhaps involve a community psychiatric nurse who could attempt to trace the patient.

Structured assessments

When a health professional is seeing a long-term mentally ill patient regularly, it is remarkably easy to miss newly developed problems in the absence of a systematic search for them. To detect acute mental health problems, general practitioners are taught to use open-ended questions and allow the patient to set the agenda in consultations (Goldberg *et al.*, 1980, see Chapter 10). However, this approach may be counter-productive with the long-term mentally ill, many of whom suffer from low self-esteem, apathy, poor insight and inability to speak to a purpose (Wing, 1989) and cannot be relied upon to volunteer problems. The question 'How are you'? may be met with a bland 'Fine', from a patient who is actually seriously depressed, actively deluded or hallucinating. Wooff and Goldberg (1988) observed the interviews of community psychiatric nurses and psychiatric social workers with their long-term mentally ill patients. The interviews often took the form of a social chat, especially with the patients who were well known to the professionals concerned. Significant hallucinations and delusions were missed in these interviews and the authors stressed the need for regular systematic structured assessments of the long-term mentally ill in the community.

Such problems are even more likely to be missed by general practitioners, since there is evidence from a number of studies that they do not involve themselves in the care of chronic mental illness as frequently as they do in chronic physical illness. In our 16-practice study, a review of patients' general practice records revealed that the large majority of consultations with the long-term mentally ill were for the treatment of minor physical problems and the issuing of repeat prescriptions and certificates. Elements of the formal mental state examination (see Chapter 18) were recorded in only 20% of patients within a 12-month period, and changes in psychotropic medication in only 20% (Kendrick *et al.*, 1994). A similar pattern was found in a study of general practitioner involvement with schizophrenic patients carried out over 30 years ago (Parkes *et al.*, 1962). More recently, Nazareth and colleagues (1993) showed that general practitioners did not carry out 'disease-specific' reviews of their schizophrenia patients as frequently as they did for their diabetes patients.

The main aim of our 16-practice study was to assess the impact of teaching general practitioners to carry out structured assessments of their long-term mentally ill patients (Kendrick *et al.*, 1994). We hypothesised that this would lead to increased activity by the practitioners, particularly in changes of psychotropic drug treatment and referrals to other professionals. Having set up case registers in the 16 practices, in eight of them the practitioners were given two sessions of teaching about the problems of the long-term mentally ill and were taught to use a structured assessment designed for use in ordinary surgery appointments every six months for two years. The assessment covered psychiatric symptoms, physical symptoms, social problems and drug side-effects (see Chapter 18).

After two years, changes in psychotropic drug treatments, particularly neuroleptic prescriptions, and referrals to secondary care services, particularly to community psychiatric nurses, were more frequent in the intervention group compared to the other eight (control) practices. However, it was unclear whether the increased activity was a direct result of the structured assessments, because many of the participating general practitioners did not find them useful, thought they were time consuming, and did not repeat them on most patients. We concluded that the increased activity might be a result of heightening the practitioners' awareness of their long-term mentally ill, and of teaching them about the sorts of problems they might expect to find and the sorts of solutions available.

If structured assessments are not feasible in ordinary surgery appointments, then special sessions might be set aside, perhaps with the involvement of the practice nurse, as in primary care clinics for asthma and diabetes. Such clinics have become the rule in most practices since financial changes were introduced which facilitated the employment and training of practice nurses and provided a sessional payment for the clinics. Whether such an approach would be taken up as readily for mental illness clinics is currently being explored (Alan Cohen & Tom Burns, personal communication).

Special record cards

The general practitioner sees the patient for all sorts of problems, acute as well as chronic, which means that the important information for the continuing care of a chronic disease may get lost among all the other entries in the notes. Having a separate card in the record envelope on which to record the management of long-term mental illness allows the doctor carrying out regular review to see quickly which has been happening and prompts the next appropriate action. It also makes gathering data for audit much easier (Kendrick, 1993).

The record card used for long-term mentally ill patients in my practice has a section on baseline data, including the date of diagnosis, dates of admissions to hospital, the pattern of relapse if

Name	D.O.B.
First diagnosed	Hospital No.
Hospital admissions	
Relatives/other carers	
GP	CPN
Consultant	SW
Psychologist	OT
Pattern of relapse	
Important notes	

Fig. 20.2 *The special record card used in TK's practice (side 1).*

established, the names of the person's relatives or other carers and key professionals involved in their care (Fig. 20.2). On the other side is a checklist of problem areas to be addressed through a structured assessment at each scheduled review (Fig. 20.3).

	Date	Date	Date	Date
Medication				
Anxiety				
Depression				
Hallucinations				
Delusions				
Appearance				
Behaviour				
Preventive				
Cardiovascular				
Respiratory				
Other physical				
Housing				
Finance				
Occupation				
Social life				

Fig. 20.3 *The special record card used in TK's practice (side 2).*

Continuity of care

Patients with long-term mental illness sometimes need a lot of time and persuasion to be able to accept medical help. They may come to respond best to one particular doctor. The move to practising in groups has tended to reduce the continuity of care. Freeman and Richards (1990) showed that patients are much less likely to see the same doctor at each consultation in practices which do not operate a strict policy of personal lists, that is with a named doctor for each patient. Balint (1957) pointed out the problems which may arise from the 'dilution of responsibility' which results when no single doctor takes overall responsibility for the patient's care.

However, it is possible to agree on a policy within a group practice that a doctor seeing a patient with schizophrenia who is registered with his partner should ensure that the patient returns to his own doctor for follow-up care. To achieve this each patient must be encouraged to identify with a particular doctor. In this way Pereira-Gray (1979) managed to increase the proportion of occasions on which he personally saw his patients with chronic schizophrenia from 44% to 100% of contacts within a few years.

Appointment systems and reception

Some patients come to call at the surgery frequently enough, but fail to fit in with the system by making appointments in advance. They may be turned away, or be seen as 'fit-ins' or 'extras' by the duty partner who may have time only to deal with immediately pressing problems and not to assess the situation fully. An explicit practice policy needs to be developed to ensure continuity of care, with the involvement of the practice manager and reception staff. They can be made aware of the names of patients who may be allowed to bypass the appointment system.

Home visits

Home visiting may be essential for patients who lack the motivation, organisation or insight to attend follow-up surgery appointments. Often the general practitioner can spend longer on a home visit than a surgery appointment, which tends to be more strictly timetabled. This allows a more thorough review of the situation including obtaining the relative's viewpoint and information about the home circumstances. Pereira-Gray (1978) listed schizophrenia as one of the chronic diseases which should be managed at home as much as possible.

Performance review

Having instigated a special policy for the care of the long-term mentally ill, practices will usually wish to audit such care, to ensure they are doing what they intended to do. One approach to performance review considers the total practice population of patients with schizophrenia, whilst a different approach considers each individual case (Marinker, 1990).

The population approach

Donabedian (1980) divided the assessment of quality of care into the three areas of structure, process and outcome. Measures of structure include the number of staff available and the systems set up for continuing care. Measures of the process of care include the degree to which patients are reviewed regularly and the proportion of checks which are completed at each review. Outcome measures for the whole population include the number of admissions and the number of identified unmet needs. However, there are difficulties in defining need and determining whether a need is met or not.

It is easier to agree specific criteria for the process of care, of which the degrees of achievement are measurable. A list of criteria for the process of care of patients with chronic schizophrenia adopted in my practice is given in Box 20.3 (Kendrick, 1993).

The individual patient

Review of an individual patient may be best carried out in a case conference involving all the people involved in the person's care. Such case conferences may take place regularly, or could be

---

1. All patients with schizophrenia on the practice list should be included in the disease register

2. Each patient with schizophrenia should see the doctor with whom he is registed each time he consults. (Accept eight out of ten consultations recorded in the patient's own doctor's handwriting.)

3. All patients with schizophrenia should be seen by the general practitioner at least once every six months. (Accept that nine out of ten are seen in any six-month period, as long as all are seen every year.)

4. All patients on the register should be checked yearly for the psychiatric, physical and social problems listed on the continuation record. (Accept that nine out of ten boxes are ticked in any one calendar year.)

5. All patients on the register should have recorded in their medical record the following preventive health data:
   - *smoking habit*
   - *blood pressure within the preceding five years*
   - *estimate of weight compared to ideal weight*
   - *alcohol consumption*
   - *cervical smear result within three years for women of child-bearing age*
   - *method of contraception for women of child-bearing age*
   - *mammogram result for women aged 50–65*

Box 20.3 *Criteria for care of schizophrenia (practice example).*

organised for the review of critical events, for example when a patient relapses and is readmitted to hospital, or after a suicide (see Chapter 21).

'Section 117' multidisciplinary discharge planning meetings are mandatory for all patients admitted under the treatment sections (Sections 3 and 37) of the Mental Health Act 1983, but should also be held for any patients regarded as vulnerable and in need of long-term coordinated care. General practitioners can request such a meeting for any of their patients who are receiving specialist care, at any time. Questions to be addressed might include whether a relapse could have been predicted and prevented, whether each professional fulfilled his or her role, and whether the systems in place need changing as a result.

Liaising with the community mental health team

The practice activities described in this chapter are not designed to make community mental health teams redundant.

However, I believe that the specialist services should be reserved for those patients who really need them. If mental health teams try to take on the regular supervision of all long-term mentally ill patients, they are going to find themselves overloaded (unless there is a huge increase in the number of mental health professionals, which is unlikely due to cost). The corollary is that expert help will then be harder to access when really needed, for the most difficult and unstable patients. Many long-term mentally ill patients, once they are in remission and relatively stable, can be looked after entirely in primary care for the most part, perhaps seeing a psychiatrist for review of long-term medication every two years.

Such a policy can only work if there is good communication between primary and secondary care teams. This is facilitated where consultant psychiatrists and other mental health professions spend some of their time working on general practice premises (Strathdee & Williams, 1984). Practices which do not benefit from such an arrangement might consider taking the initiative and inviting their local mental health team into their practice.

Conclusion

Adopting the proactive approach outlined here may well involve general practitioners and their administrative staff in extra work initially, in setting up the practice recall system and making it work. However, it may *save* time in the longer run, by preventing crises which may take hours to sort out, often in out-of-hours work. In any case, there can be little doubt that patients with chronic schizophrenia are particularly disadvantaged and deserve the best efforts of a modern well-organised practice.

References

Bachrach, L.L. (1988). Defining chronic mental illness: a concept paper. *Hospital and Community Psychiatry*, **39**, 383–8.

Balint, M. (1957). *The Doctor, His Patient and the Illness*. London: Tavistock.

Birchwood M., Smith J., MacMillan, F. *et al*. (1989). Predicting relapse in schizophrenia: the development and implementation of an early signs monitoring system using patients and families as observers, a preliminary investigation. *Psychological Medicine* **19**, 649–56.

Department of Health and Social Security (1987). *On the State of the Public Health. The Annual Report of the Chief Medical Officer of the Department of Health and Social Security for the Year 1986*. London: HMSO.

Department of Health (1991). *The Health of the Nation*. London: HMSO.

Donabedian, A. (1980). *Explorations in Quality Assessment and Monitoring. Vol.1. The Definition of Quality and Approaches to its Assessment*. Ann Arbor: Health Administration Press.

Freeman, G.K. & Richards, S.C. (1990). How much personal care in four group practices? *British Medical Journal*, **301**, 1028–30.

Goldberg, D. & Huxley, P. (1980). *Mental Illness in the Community*. New York: Tavistock.

Goldberg, D. & Jackson, G. (1992). Interface between primary care and specialist mental health care. *British Journal of General Practice*, **42**, 267–9.

Goldberg, D.P., Steele, J.J., Smith, C. & Spivey, L. (1980). Training family doctors to recognise psychiatric illness with increased accuracy. *Lancet*, **ii**, 521–6.

Johnstone, E.C., Owens, D.G.C., Gold, A., Crow, T.J. & MacMillon, J.F. (1984). Schizophrenic patients discharged from hospital – a follow-up study. *British Journal of Psychiatry*, **145**, 586–90.

Kendrick, T. (1993). Care of people with schizophrenia. *British Journal of General Practice*, **43**, 259–60.

Kendrick, T., Sibbald, B., Burns, T. & Freeling, P. (1991). Role of general practitioners in care of long-term mentally ill patients. *British Medical Journal*, **302**, 508–10.

Kendrick, T., Sibbald, B., Burns, T. & Freeling, P. (1994). Provision of care to general practice patients with disabling long-term mental illness: a survey in 16 practices. *British Journal of General Practice*, **44**, 301–5.

Kendrick, T., Burns, T., Sibbald, B. & Freeling, P. (1995). Randomised controlled trial of teaching general practitioners to carry out structured assessments of their long-term mentally ill patients. *British Medical Journal*, (in press).

Marinker, M. ed. (1990). *Medical Audit and General Practice*. pp. 1–15. London: British Medical Journal Publications.

Marshall, M. (1989). Collected and neglected: are Oxford hostels for the homeless filling up with disabled psychiatric patients? *British Medical Journal*, **299**, 706–9.

Melzer, D., Hale, A.S., Malik, S.J., Hogman, G.A. & Wood, S. (1991). Community care for patients with schizophrenia one year after hospital discharge. *British Medical Journal*, **303**, 1023–6.

Nazareth, I., King, M., Haines, A., See Tai, S. & Hall, G. (1993). Care of schizophrenia in general practice. *British Medical Journal*, **307**, 910.

Pantelis, C., Taylor, J. & Campbell, P. (1988). The South Camden Schizophrenia Survey. An experience of community-based research. *Bulletin of the Royal College of Psychiatrists*, **12**, 98–101.

Parkes, C.M., Brown, G.W. & Monck, E.M. (1962). The general practitioner and the schizophrenic patient. *British Medical Journal*, **i**, 972–6.

Pendleton, D.A. & Schofield, T.P.C. (1983) Motivation and performance in general practice. In *Medical Annual*. Bristol: Wright.

Pereira-Gray, D.J. (1978) Feeling at home. *Journal of the Royal College of General Practitioners*, **28**, 6–17.

Pereira-Gray, D.J. (1979). The key to personal care. *Journal of the Royal College of General Practitioners* **29**, 666–78.

Royal College of General Practitioners. Birmingham Research Unit (178). Practice activity analysis 4. Psychotropic drugs. *Journal of the Royal College of General Practitioners*, **28**, 122–4.

Schofield, T.P.C. (1984). Implications for practice. In *Continuing Care: the Management of Chronic Disease*. Hasler, J. and Schofield T.P.C., eds. pp. 69–80. Oxford: Oxford University Press.

Shepherd, M., Cooper, B., Brown, A.C. & Kalton, G. (1966). *Psychiatric Illness in General Practice*. Oxford: Oxford University Press.

Strathdee, G. & Williams, P. (1984). A survey of psychiatrists in primary care: the silent growth of a new service. *Journal of the Royal College of General Practitioners*, **34**, 615–18.

Taylor, P.J. & Gunn, J. (1984). Violence and psychosis. I-Risk of violence among psychotic men. *British Medical Journal*, **288**, 1945–9.

Weller, M. Tobiansky, R.I., Hollander, D. & Ibrahimi, S. (1989). Psychosis and destitution at Christmas 1985–1988. *Lancet*, **ii**, 1509–11.

Wing, J.K. (1989). The concept of negative symptoms. *British Journal of Psychiatry*, **155** (suppl. 7), 10–14.

Wooff, K. & Goldberg, D. (1988). Further observations on the practice of community care in Salford. Differences between Community Psychiatric Nurses and Mental Health Social Workers. *British Journal of Psychiatry*, **153**, 30–7.

[21] The prevention of suicide

Philip Seager

Introduction

Family doctors will be familiar with people presenting with suicidal thoughts and ideas, and less commonly with acts of deliberate self-harm, parasuicide or attempted suicide. It is much rarer to hear that a patient has actually committed suicide – in the United Kingdom only one person in 6000 will do so each year (Secretary of State for Health, 1992). Thus the average British general practitioner will meet between ten and fifteen in a professional lifetime.

Is suicide preventable?

An important point to remember is that a significant proportion of people who kill themselves go to see a general practitioner in the weeks leading up to the suicidal act (Vassilas & Morgan, 1993), which allows at least the possibility of intervention. However, there is significant debate at this time about whether suicide is truly preventable (Wilkinson & Morgan, 1994). There is evidence that many primary health care professionals are dubious that they can prevent suicide among their patients. Morgan & Evans (1994) found that 31% of nurses and 27% of general practitioners evinced equivocal or negative responses to questionnaires concerning attitudes to suicide prevention.

Whatever policies primary health care teams adopt to try to prevent suicides, it will be difficult for them to tell whether they are having a worthwhile effect on their own list of patients. As suicide is a relatively rare event, any reduction in the suicide rate may not be perceived at the level of the practice – indeed, it is doubtful if it can be noticed at the level of a town, a health district or even at regional level, from one year to the next. Nevertheless, the activities described in this chapter represent good clinical practice based on the available evidence and should form part of the practice's effort to offer the best available service to patients, despite a lack of immediate feedback on how successful that effort has been.

Recognition of suicidal risk

There is no simple technique which can be applied to determine which of the many patients seen in a day's work is an immediate, a probable, or still less a possible, suicidal risk. It is not possible to distinguish absolutely those patients who feel ideas of suicidal gloom but say they would not give way to the thoughts which harass them, from those who will not keep the next appointment because they are in the mortuary. However, several factors associated with an increased risk of suicide have been identified (Box 21.1).

Demographic and personal information

An important benefit of general practice in the UK is that virtually every person is registered with a practice and there may well be medical records and reports going back to birth, or at least to the birth of the National Health Service in 1948. This means that much medical and demographic information is often available when the person makes an appointment or arrives at the surgery.

Suicide is commoner amongst men than women in all age groups in the UK. This is not necessarily true in other countries. In general, the risk of suicide increases with age, although since 1980 there has been an increase in suicides amongst younger men. There is no clear explanation for this change which has been noted in many other countries (Kingman, 1994).

It would be wrong to suggest that age or sex alone should be primary factors in alerting professionals to an increased suicidal risk. It is difficult to apply epidemiologically derived risk factors to individual patients. Nevertheless, these factors should be borne in mind in conjunction with other items of information which may be more significant and, taken together, should alert the practitioner to increased risk.

Age

Sex

Marital status

Employment status

Ethnicity

Unsupportive neighbourhood

Box 21.1 *Demographic risk factors to consider.*

Marital status and employment must also be considered. In general, suicide rates are highest in the widowed, particularly those recently bereaved. Rates are relatively increased in divorced compared to single people, and lowest in those who are married. There is evidence to suggest that having children to look after is protective against suicide as far as women are concerned. Social changes, such as the move away from marriage to cohabiting and the increase in numbers of single parent families, do not seem to have made a mark on the suicide statistics as yet.

The risk of suicide is higher amongst lower socio-economic groups, for both males and females. This may be linked to an increased risk of unemployment. Commonly cited explanations for the increasing rate of suicide in younger men include higher unemployment levels and the use of illegal drugs. It may also be that, by comparison, the relative risk of suicide is falling among women, because they are becoming more emancipated and less likely to be trapped in difficult marriages due to economic, moral and social pressures.

Suicide rates also vary between occupations. The proportional mortality ratio (PMR) is the ratio of observed deaths from suicide in a particular occupation to the expected number of suicides (Dunnell, 1994). Amongst males aged 16–64, for the years 1979–90, vets, pharmacists, dental practitioners, farmers and medical practitioners had the highest PMRs. Transport managers, glass and ceramics furnacemen, machine tool operators, education officers, school inspectors, and physiotherapists had the lowest. Some of these groups include very few people and so low suicide rates may be seen by chance. It is noteworthy that easy access to lethal methods of self-harm may well distinguish the occupations with the highest rates of suicide.

In general, members of ethnic minority groups have a higher rate of suicide in their country of immigration than that of their country of origin. Again, it may not be of much help in the assessment of an individual, but it is recognised that the incidence of suicide among those of Indian and West Indian origin in England and Wales is below average in men but above average in women, particularly young women (Raleigh & Balarajan, 1992). It is important that information about the main ethnic minority groups in a particular area is taken into account, but it should be based on reliable evidence and not on prejudice or fantasy (see Chapter 6).

Finally, the general level of social cohesion and well-being of the patient's neighbourhood can be a further item of information to consider when trying to ascertain the nature of the patient's problem and their risk of self-harm. Factors such as the strength of family ties, including the presence of an extended family, and spiritual and social support from church and other groups may be relevant. In general, suicide is commoner in urban than rural environments.

Having noted this general information about an individual, further clues can be obtained from the patient's file.

Past medical and psychiatric history

The previous medical notes are an important source of background information and should always be scanned if the doctor is not familiar with the patient. An obvious first indicator of the possibility of an emotional component to a person's illness is the thickness of the medical record envelope, which may result from frequent attendance at the practice or from a thick pack of hospital letters. The regular attender may be labelled as attention seeking, perhaps with a well-recognised family problem, an inability to cope with the demands made by life, or pressure at work from a demanding boss. It is important to recognise however that attention-seeking behaviour is often attention-needing behaviour.

Just as important to note is a new consultation with a person who has never been seen before, or rarely so. For such a person to seek advice may be significant and the question should be asked 'Why has this person come at this time?'

Mental disorders with increased suicide risk

It must be emphasised that suicide is associated with serious mental illness in at least eight out of ten cases. Traditionally suicides tended to take place in hospital environments because that is where the patients were usually to be found. This situation has changed markedly in the past decade with the move to community care and while this has brought about benefits to many people who had been deprived of their liberty for long periods, it has also brought responsibility to general practitioners and other primary care and community workers to be much more observant and conscious of the risks to people living in non-institutional settings but still suffering from serious mental illness. A history of recent or repeated episodes of deliberate self-harm is particularly relevant, since the risk of suicide is increased in the following three years, and particularly in the first six months after a previous attempt (Hawton & Fagg, 1988).

Depressive disorders

The lifetime risk of suicide in major depression is as high as 15%. The single most important predictor of a future episode of depression is a past history, especially where admission was required. Where a patient is on a prophylactic drug such as lithium or carbamazepine, it is likely the psychiatric team will wish to monitor the continuing care. It is important to ensure that this is the case, or if not that it is clear who is accepting responsibility for the review of drug dosages and carrying out regular blood checks, including drug levels and thyroid function tests.

Schizophrenia

Understandably, much is made of the dangers of people with schizophrenia in the community who have caused major public concern when they have attacked and killed innocent bystanders or therapists trying to help them. However, it is not generally appreciated by the public that the greatest danger is to themselves, since suicide is a common final outcome of their condition. Long-term follow up suggests that 8–10% of people with schizophrenia eventually kill themselves, more males than females (Roy, 1986).

Suicide appears to take place during episodes of depression, a common feature of long-term schizophrenia, perhaps arising from a perceived hopelessness and despair about the condition, as well as a recognition of the isolation and loneliness patients can expect to endure. The main features of depression such as poor appetite and weight loss and insomnia are often apparent.

However, on reviewing suicides among schizophrenia sufferers, there is often little evidence to suggest either that patients were receiving inadequate neuroleptic medication, or that the depressive element had gone unnoticed and untreated. Social isolation has been frequently noted as a major risk factor and there is now emphasis on encouraging supportive family relationships, and helping patients in bed sitters and flatlets to make social contacts, perhaps through community centres.

Personality disorder

Suicide is less common in this condition although epidemiological studies have clearly identified increased risks (Sims, 1983). Many of these individuals are people who make numerous demands on services, perhaps making spasmodic, ineffectual suicide attempts. They may raise the ire of house officers called to resuscitate them, psychiatrists who have to assess them, and general practitioners from whom they may demand medication often thought to be unwise, and usually unnecessary. Yet these contacts represent opportunities to identify impending crisis episodes and to prevent them reaching levels which precipitate repeated overdoses or other suicidal responses. Beware the situation of 'malignant alienation'. It has been shown (Flood & Seager, 1968; Watts & Morgan, 1994) that the unhappy, unco-operative, demanding individual in hospital who antagonises the staff and rejects treatment, leaving against advice, is at increased risk of suicide. There is no reason to believe a similar phenomenon does not occur outside hospital. Drug overdoses may represent manipulative action which keeps a domestic situation under control. However, it is more likely that they indicate serious personal problems, usually unresolved by the self-destructive behaviour.

In this context, we can now consider the situation of a patient presenting in primary care with symptoms which suggest that an

---

Previous suicidal thoughts or behaviour

Marked depressive symptoms

Longstanding schizophrenia, particularly with depressive symptoms

Alcohol or drug misuse

Recent psychiatric inpatient treatment

Self-discharge against medical advice

Personality disorder with impulsive behaviour and affective crises

Legal or criminal action pending

Painful or disabling physical illness

Recent social disruption
- *bereavement*
- *marital break-up*
- *job losses*

Box 21.2 *Factors indicating high risk in an individual.*

emotional condition is the main problem, and in particular the factors indicating that suicidal intent is a possibility (Box 21.2).

The medical interview

It is important that every patient be given the opportunity to set out the problems for which they require advice and help. The doctor should facilitate communication by using open-ended questions initially and allowing the patient to map out the areas of concern (see Chapter 10). At the start of the interview, patients will be inhibited by closed questions which can be answered with only a limited range of responses, driven by the doctor's need to know about particular symptoms or associated factors, rather than by the patient's need to relate what is most important to him or her (Goldberg et al., 1980; Sanson-Fisher & Maguire, 1980).

Closed diagnostic questions are often necessary later in the interview, to corroborate the opinion developing in the doctor's mind. A summary of the perceived problem should be presented by the doctor and the patient given the opportunity to ask questions and make corrections, to ensure that matters are clear to both patient and doctor.

Clear-cut depressive symptoms

Some patients will report obvious feelings of depression with lack of drive, of energy, and of interest, with sleep disturbance and weight loss (see Chapter 10). On further questioning it is likely that ideas of self-doubt, hopelessness, and pessimism about the future will be apparent. It is common to be able to elicit suicidal thoughts or ideas in such individuals and the task is to evaluate their strength and the likelihood of them being carried out.

One myth should certainly be cast out – 'People who talk about it don't do it.' This is almost entirely incorrect. It is well established that the majority of people who have committed suicide have mentioned their feelings to family and friends, and often to their doctors in recent weeks before the death. Sadly, the response too often has been that they should not be silly and that things are not as bad as all that. But they were.

It has to be recognised that the converse: 'People who talk about it always do it' – is not true either. Firstly, I believe that appropriate intervention can certainly reduce or abolish the likelihood of suicide in a given situation. Secondly, suicidal talk may be a way of manipulating the behaviour of people in one's environment. It is a well-recognised way of making lovers come to heel, children behave in desired ways, and of bringing about changes in the way a household should run. Thus, while talk of suicidal ideas or be-haviour should be taken seriously, it is important to discuss the feelings, motives, and background situation before assuming that such words will inevitably result in suicidal action.

Another concern often expressed is that asking about suicide will put the idea into someone's head and bring about the feared outcome. Anyone feeling depressed, pessimistic and hopeless has almost certainly considered ending their life in some way, or at least hoped that some accident or event will hasten death. Asking about suicidal ideas may bring about a sense of relief that the person's feelings can be expressed to someone who at least knows enough about it to be able to ask the question.

Presentation with physical symptoms

Many patients believe that the right 'ticket of admission' must be presented. To a vicar or priest, one expresses spiritual problems, to a social worker, housing or marital problems and to a doctor, physical symptoms. This naive concept may result in an initial presentation of a physical symptom, masking an underlying emo-tional problem. The situation will then be more difficult to assess and may result in an inappropriate concentration on the physical component. Symptoms such as weight loss, anorexia and constipa-tion in the elderly would understandably provoke a search for carcinoma of the colon, yet these may all be due to depression. In such a case, further enquiry should include questions about the mood, energy level and suicidal thinking. The worst that can happen is a rude comment along the lines of '*The doctor thinks I'm crazy*'.

Emotional problems, pain, and suicide

Presentation with physical symptoms may result from denial of an underlying emotional problem. Some individuals find it difficult to talk about stress and anxiety and may only express their emotional disturbance through physical symptoms such as chest pain, head-ache or abdominal pain, for example. The form of presentation of emotional distress will often depend on ethnic and cultural factors concerning attitudes towards pain and illness.

The possibility of suicide should be borne in mind in individuals with persisting disability and pain due to stroke or arthritis. There is undoubtedly an increased risk in the context of unremitting pain, particularly in terminal illness such as cancer. Yet, while there is an increase in the suicide rate in such painful conditions, it is not as great as one might expect (Allebeck & Bolund, 1991). Equally, when there is evidence of depressive illness, it is wrong to assume that such symptoms are entirely understandable in terms of the terminal condition, or to withhold antidepressants which may well allow emotional improvement if only for the short time left to the person.

Box 21.2 summarises the individual factors which may be associated with a significantly increased risk of suicide and which should prompt the health care professional to enquire after suicidal ideas. The whole range of the person's circumstances have to be considered, including demographic correlates of risk, the degree of current depression and other characteristics such as previous suicide attempts, substance misuse problems, social isolation and long-standing mental disorder.

Those who do not seek help

It is important to remember that many people do not seek help at all, either from medical services or from other appropriate sources, such as the Samaritans for example. They may discuss suicidal thoughts with relatives and friends who do not recognise the seriousness of the situation and offer casual reassurance, or they may secretly plan their death whilst avoiding giving any indication of their state of mind.

Nevertheless, in primary care the first task is to provide opportunities for people seeking help to communicate their difficulties. The next step, taking into account all the available information, is to offer appropriate action to prevent or modify any developing crisis.

Interventions

Hospital admission

When a patient indicates that they have been taking serious steps to kill themselves, with strong feelings of hopelessness, ideas that there is no future, or more specific depressive nihilistic delusions, there is little doubt that urgent admission to a psychiatric unit is indicated. If this is not accepted by the patient, compulsory admission procedures need to be implemented (see Chapter 14).

But this is not usually where the problem lies. How are lesser degrees of depression to be evaluated and what action is appropriate?

Assessing and treating depression

Several studies have concluded that significant depression is often incorrectly diagnosed or inadequately treated in primary care (see Chapter 10). Freeling (1993) has pointed out that, among those attending their general practitioners, depression goes unacknowledged in as many as half the patients who would be likely to benefit from treatment. This is partly because many patients present with somatic symptoms, but more importantly, many are perceived to have understandable causes for their depressive symptoms and are therefore not seen to merit antidepressants.

Direct help in terms of environmental manipulation may not be possible where obvious life events are involved. It should be realised however that once the depression is under control through drug treatment, people can often cope better with the life difficulties which are thought to be causing their depression (Chapter 8) (Garvey, Schaffer & Tuason, 1984).

In many cases, although psychological distress is recognised in primary care, the treatment offered is by hypnotics or tranquillisers, rather than antidepressant drugs. Symptomatic support may include hypnotics for insomnia, but these should be used only for a limited period, as they may be depressive in themselves. It may be preferable to utilise the hypnotic side-effects of an antidepressant drug.

Even where antidepressants are used, they may be used in subtherapeutic doses or for inadequate time, since they have side-effects such as dry mouth and sedation which may interfere with the patient's ability to tolerate an adequate dosage. Lack of compliance may mean that the patient has not been fully informed of potential side-effects, or that it may take two to three weeks before improvement can be expected.

Three groups of drugs should be considered, the traditional tricyclics such as amitriptyline and imipramine, newer drugs such as lofepramine and trazodone, and the selective serotonin uptake inhibitors such as fluoxetine and paroxetine. Overdosage, particularly with the earlier group of drugs, may lead to a fatal outcome, and if in doubt only a small supply should be prescribed initially. However, while the newer antidepressants have less side-effects and are less toxic in overdosage, there is still argument about their relative efficacy (Harrison, Owens & Rubin, 1994).

Relatives and friends

With the agreement of the patient, the situation should also be discussed with those near to the patient. Confirmatory information about behaviour can be obtained, and advice given about managing the situation, including necessary supervision and keeping contact and ensuring that medication is taken appropriately. The presence or absence of suitable support may well be the important factor indicating home or hospital treatment.

Other services

Support may also be available from secondary care services such as the community mental health team or day hospital where available, and social services provision including day centres. Voluntary mental health groups may also offer local support facilities which can provide activity and contact for the isolated, though these may only be suitable in less immediately serious cases.

Cognitive–behavioural therapy by a skilled therapist has been shown to be as effective as medication and should be considered for potentially suicidal patients where it is available (see Chapter 17).

Self-help groups and voluntary services

A knowledge of what is available locally may be very helpful, for example Cruse counselling for the recently bereaved (see Chapter 5). Spiritual support from local churches should be considered for people who value such help.

Special supervision

It is important to ensure that people with long-term and severe mental illness have regular and frequent visits by a key worker who will be able to seek help if there are any doubts about current status. Equally, it is important that when such a request for help is received, it is dealt with speedily, whether by the primary health care team or the community mental health care team. Disasters have occurred when no professional has taken direct responsibility and patients have fallen through the holes in the community net.

As outlined above, a history of longstanding mental disorder, whether unipolar or bipolar depression, schizophrenia, or substance misuse in particular, has significant implications for the risk of suicide and these days, under the care programme approach, all vulnerable psychiatric patients should have a written care plan devised by the community mental health team, with a named key worker with whom information can be exchanged. If there is a continuing serious risk to the patient's own life or a risk of harming others, then the individual should be placed on a supervision register, with specific arrangements made by the mental health team for monitoring the patient in collaboration with the primary health care team and the social services department. A line of contact must be clearly established, to enable emergency help to be offered at any time.

Educating primary care professionals

There may be a need to improve doctors' and other health care professionals' interviewing and treatment skills. There is evidence that where specific teaching has been offered, positive effects can be demonstrated. On the island of Gotland in Sweden an educational programme about the detection and management of depression was offered to general practitioners and in a three-year follow-up, improvements were noted in the treatment of depressive disorders, including changes in drug prescriptions and hospital admission rates (Rutz, van Knorring & Walinder, 1992). The Swedish researchers also cited a fall in the suicide rate as evidence of success of their educational programme, although the number of suicides was very small to start with and the fall may have been due to chance variation. After a further three years the initially encouraging indicators, including the suicide rate, had reverted to the original levels, which led the authors to conclude that such educational activities have to be repeated at least every two years.

More extensive training programmes are now becoming available for doctors and nurses, as well as education for the general public about the patterns and implications of depressive illness, such as the defeat depression campaign in the UK (Dillner, 1992; Priest, 1994).

The aftermath of suicide

After a practice patient commits suicide, the primary health care team should join the mental health team in a confidential inquiry aimed at reviewing the events prior to death and the roles and responsibilities of the professionals involved, to consider whether anything more could have been done to prevent the suicide. In this way, locally agreed policies and procedures can be developed to help prevent suicides in future.

Suicide obviously has an immediate effect on the family and friends and can produce feelings of guilt and responsibility, since it is rare than someone among them has not uttered glib reassurance or attempted well-meaning but unsuccessful support. The primary health care team can involve the family in a 'psychological postmortem' after a suicide, seeking information about the events leading to the death. I have noted on a number of occasions that such a meeting helps to relieve some of the tensions and anxieties of families and friends by allowing them to express their feelings.

The same is true of staff working in hospital wards, hostels, prisons and other institutions where suicides have occurred. The part played by them, their feelings of rejection, guilt and depression, and even on occasion their own suicidal thoughts, need to be considered, especially if they should report with some form of sickness themselves.

It should also be remembered that the children of someone who commits suicide may themselves be at increased risk of mental illness, including suicidal behaviour, later in life (Chapter 9).

Conclusions

In summary, the prevention of suicide in primary care depends on

(i)   a knowledge of the relevant risk factors;
(ii) careful consideration of a patient's personality difficulties, personal circumstances, and social background; and
(iii) the active treatment of depression, often with medication, or with psychological treatment where this is available.

Primary care professionals should try to develop an awareness of the issues, an optimistic and constructive attitude to those in distress, a recognition that treatment is available, and a willingness to apply it effectively and immediately to prevent what are generally avoidable fatalities among their patients.

References

Allebeck, P. & Bolund, C. (1991). Suicides and suicide attempts in cancer patients. *Psychological Medicine*, **21**, 979–84.

Dillner, L. (1992). Colleges join together to fight depression. *British Medical Journal*, **304**, 337.

Dunnell, K. (1994). Epidemiology and trends in suicide in the UK. In *The Prevention of Suicide* Jenkins, R., Griffiths, S., Wylie, I., Hawton, K., Morgan, G. and Tylee, A., eds. London: HMSO.

Flood R.A. & Seager, C.P. (1968). A retrospective examination of psychiatric case records of patients who subsequently committed suicide. *British Journal of Psychiatry* **114**, 443–50.

Freeling, P. (1993). Diagnosis of depression in general practice. *British Journal of Psychiatry*, **163**, 14–19.

Garvey, M.J., Schaffer, C. B. & Tuason, V. B. (1984). *British Journal of Psychiatry*, **145**, 363–5.

Goldberg, D.P., Steele, J.J., Smith, C. & Spivey, L. (1980). Training family doctors to recognise psychiatric illness with increased accuracy. *Lancet*, **ii**, 521–3.

Groves, T. (1990). After the asylums. The future of community care. *British Medical Journal*, **300**, 923–4.

Harrison, G., Owens, D. & Rubin, PC. (1994). Controversies in management: New or old antidepressants? *British Medical Journal*, **309**, 1280–1.

Hawton, K. & Fagg, J. (1988). Suicide and other causes of death following attempted suicide. *British Journal of Psychiatry*, **152**, 359–66.

Kingman, S. (1994). Suicide. *British Medical Journal*, **388**, 7–11.

Morgan, H.G. & Evans, M.O. (1994). How negative are we to the idea of suicide prevention? *Journal of the Royal Society of Medicine*, **87**, 622–5.

Priest, R.G. (1994). Improving the management and knowledge of depression. *British Journal of Psychiatry*, **164**, 285–7.

Raleigh, V.S. & Balarajan, R. (1992). Suicide and self-burning among Indians and West Indians in England and Wales. *British Journal of Psychiatry*, **161**, 365–8.

Roy, A. (1986). *Suicide*. Baltimore: Williams & Wilkins.

Rutz, W., van Knorring, L. & Walinder J. (1992). Long-term effects of an educational program for general practitioners given by the Swedish Committee for the Prevention and Treatment of Depression. *Acta Psychiatrica Scandinavica*, **85**, 83–8.

Sanson-Fisher, R. & Maguire P. (1980). Should skills in communication be taught in medical schools? *Lancet*, **ii**, 523–5.

Secretary of State for Health. (1992). *The Health of the Nation: A Strategy for Health in England*. London: Her Majesty's Stationery Office.

Sims, A. (1983). *Neurosis in Society*. London: Macmillan.

Vassilas, C. & Morgan H.G. (1993). General practitioners' contact with victims of suicide. *British Medical Journal*, **307**, 300–1.

Watts, D. & Morgan, G. (1994). Malignant alienation. *British Journal of Psychiatry*, **164**, 11–15.

Wilkinson, G. & Morgan G. (1994). Can suicide be prevented? *British Medical Journal*, **309**, 860–2.

Index

Page numbers in *italics* refer to boxes.

manipulative behaviour, and
    suicidal talk, 371
maprotiline, tricyclic
    antidepressant, 285
marital partner, and prevention of
    postnatal depression, 65–6
marital relationship, and postnatal
    depression, 58, 59, 61, 62,
    63–4, 69
marital status
    and anorexia nervosa, 209, 211
    and suicide risk, 366, 367
material stressors, and depression,
    43, 44
maternal loss, and adult
    depression, 47, 48, 49
Medical Council on Alcoholism,
    educational materials by,
    242
medical history
    and drug misuse 236–7
    and suicide prevention, 368
medical tertiary prevention
    interventions, 266–8
medication
    anxiolytic, 198
    in bereavement, 84, 86
    causing behavioural problems,
    123
    and cognitive therapy, 303
    for depression, 373–4; in
        adolescents and children, 164;
        long-term therapy, 283–9
    for depressive disorders, review
        of, 368
    and ethnic minority patients,
    100–1
    for long-term mental illness,
        review of, 355–6
    for mental illness and learning
        disability, 121–2, 123–4
    for psychoses: emergency
        treatment, 260; management
        of, 251–2
    repeat prescriptions, and
        long-term mental illness, 351,
        354–5
    for schizophrenia: advice for
        carers, 333, 334; dislike of,
        337; long-term, problems of,
        329

for withdrawal symptoms: in
    alcohol misuse, 235; in opiate
    drug misuse, 237–8; in
    sedative drug misuse, 239–41
medicines, prescription, and
    organic psychoses, 248
Meet-a-Mum Association
    (MAMA), and postnatal
    depression, 60
mental exercises, in management
    of anxiety disorders, 200, 201
Mental Health Act
    and detention in hospital,
    258–9, 260
    sections, and ethnic minority
        patients, 101
mental health problems
    childhood: assessment of,
        154–9; detection of, 149–55;
        management of, 160–5;
        treatment of, 157–65
    development of, 4–5
    differential diagnosis of, 8–9
    preventive approach to, 4–10
mental health services
    changes in, 13–14
    for children and adolescents,
    158–60
mental health teams, and
    schizophrenia, 339–40
mental illness
    diagnosis of, 6–7; and culture,
        91, 93–5, 99–100
    in ethnic minorities, 95–7,
        99–100
    expressed emotion of carers,
        and outcome, 330–1
    and learning disability,
        detection of, 114–16, 122,
        124–5
    long-term, identification of,
        349–53
    parental, and parenting, 29, 30,
        31
    prevention of: counselling in
        130–2; principles of, xi–xii,
        xiii
mental state, assessment of, in
    schizophrenia, 318
methadone, in treatment of opiate
    drug misuse, 237–8